Immunology

D0474387

Donald M. Weir MD FRCPE
Emeritus Professor of Microbial Immunology,
Department of Medical Microbiology,
University of Edinburgh Medical School, Edinburgh

John Stewart BSc (Hons) PhD
Senior Lecturer
Department of Medical Microbiology,
University of Edinburgh Medical School, Edinburgh

EIGHTH EDITION

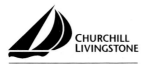
CHURCHILL
LIVINGSTONE

NEW YORK EDINBURGH LONDON MADRID MELBOURNE SAN FRANCISCO
AND TOKYO 1997

CHURCHILL LIVINGSTONE
Medical Division of Longman Group Limited

Distributed in the United States of America by Churchill
Livingstone Inc., 650 Avenue of the Americas, New York,
N.Y. 10011, and by associated companies, branches and
representatives throughout the world.

First edition 1970
Second edition 1971
Third edition 1973
Fourth edition 1977
Fifth edition 1983
Sixth edition 1988
Seventh edition 1993
Eighth edition 1997

ISBN 0 443 05452 5
International edition 0443 05563 7

British Library Cataloguing in Publication Data
A catalogue record for this book is available from the British
Library.

Library of Congress Cataloging in Publication Data
A catalog record for this book is available from the Library of
Congress.

Medical knowledge is constantly changing. As new
information becomes available, changes in treatment,
procedures, equipment and the use of drugs become
necessary. The authors and the publishers have, as far as
it is possible, taken care to ensure that the information given
in this text is accurate and up to date. However, readers are
strongly advised to confirm that the information, especially
with regard to drug usage, complies with current legislation
and standards of practice.

Produced by Longman Singapore Publishers (Pte.) Ltd
Printed in Singapore

Preface

There have been many important breakthroughs in the field of immunology over the last five years. Developments in the field of molecular biology have enabled investigators to employ sophisticated and sensitive techniques in the quest for a better understanding of the immune system. Many of the discoveries made have helped to explain puzzles that have intrigued immunologists for decades and at times have made understanding the immune system difficult. The chapters in the 'Basic Immunology' section have been updated in light of these recent findings. As before the aim is to explain the workings of the immune system in a clear and understandable way rather than to rely on complex illustrations. Figures and tables, many changed for this edition, are included to aid understanding not as a replacement for descriptive narrative.

The book is designed for medical and science students taking their first course in immunology and for those wanting to revise their immunological knowledge. It is not possible in a short text to cover the application of immunology to the enormous range of topics encompassed by clinical immunology. The material covered in the 'Immunology in Action' chapters aims to give an insight into the ways immunological knowledge has helped not only in the understanding of the pathogenesis of infectious disease but in many other medical disciplines.

The authors are indebted to the publishers for their help and encouragement during the production of this book.

For Churchill Livingstone

Publisher: Timothy Horne
Project Manager: Ninette Premdas
Project Controller: Nancy Arnott
Designer: Erik Bigland

Contents

Basic immunology

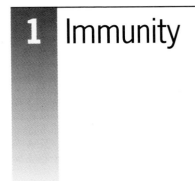

1 Immunity

The tissues and cells capable of exhibiting what is now recognized as an acquired immune response have an evolutionary history of some 400 million years and the forms taken by the response during this period have retained a remarkable constancy at both the molecular and functional levels. The basic pattern of the protein molecules involved has been retained, with the diversification that has occurred through evolutionary selective pressures being superimposed on this basic pattern.

Recognition

Immune phenomena as expressed in the higher animals have evolved from **recognition mechanisms** that enable a multicellular primitive animal to distinguish between itself and other (foreign) species. This idea of **self/non-self discrimination** lies at the foundation of immunological theory. Self recognition mechanisms appear very early in evolution and can be seen in marine organisms, such as sponges. Reaggregation of dispersed colonies is regulated by species-specific surface glycoproteins. The failure of unrelated species to adhere to each other amounts to a primitive form of graft rejection. The cells lining the cavity of sponges are able to capture and engulf (phagocytose) organisms, present in the water, drawn into this cavity. Similar mechanisms play a role in the metamorphosis of insects by removing dead and disintegrated tissue. An important recognition phenomenon occurs in the interaction between pollen grains and plant stigma that appears to depend on the nature of surface proteins. Pollination and germination only occur if the pollen and stigma are genetically compatible, and self-fertilization is prevented.

Primitive marine species, such as starfish and corals, appear to be able to reject grafts of unrelated forms. Self/non-self discrimination enables the maintenance of **specific partnerships** between cells of a multicellular organism and provides an organism with the additional benefits of recognizing and excluding changed self-constituents and potentially harmful parasitic organisms, such as fungi and bacteria. The particular cell surface molecules that are recognized and determine foreignness are often carbohydrates or glycoproteins. The recognition structures, referred to as **receptors**, are themselves proteins or glycoproteins. It is interesting to note that the production of immunoglobulin M (IgM), one of the recognition proteins in higher vertebrates, is often stimulated by carbohydrate molecules. IgM is believed to most resemble the precursor of all forms of immunoglobulin and has its origin in the most primitive vertebrate fish.

The cells of the immune system are probably derived from the primitive cellular defence mechanisms that arose with the evolution of the invertebrates. This is manifested by the engulfment and walling off of foreign particles. The phagocytic cells responsible for this do not respond by proliferation so that the animal does not become better adapted to deal more effectively with the foreign material.

Immunity

There are many different defence mechanisms that protect an individual from microorganisms and potentially harmful material. Some of these, including physical barriers like the skin, phagocytic cells and certain chemical substances and enzymes, are active before exposure to foreign material. These **innate** or **natural** immune mechanisms are not enhanced by previous exposure to, nor do they discriminate between, most foreign substances. Other defence mechanisms, collectively known as **acquired** or **adaptive** immunity, have components that are able to recognize variation in structures present on foreign material. The defence mechanism that is generated is therefore able to eliminate specifically the offending material and, in addition, subsequent exposure leads to a more efficient and effective immune response. The characteristics and constituents of innate and acquired immunity are shown in Table 1.1.

The meaning of the term immunity (from the Latin *immunitas* — exemption from civic duties afforded to senators) as it is used today derives from its earlier usage referring to exemption from military service or paying taxes. It has long been recognized that those who recovered from epidemic diseases such as smallpox and plague were exempt from further attacks and such immune individuals were often used in an epidemic to nurse those suffering from active disease. Immunization against smallpox, by the process of variolation using material from mild cases of smallpox (variola), was recorded as being practised in China in about AD 590 and was also practised in India in ancient times. Dried crusts from the pustules of sufferers from the dis-

Table 1.1 Characteristics and determinants of innate and acquired immunity

Innate immunity	Acquired immunity
Non-specific No change with repeat exposure Mechanical barriers Bactericidal substances Natural flora	Specific Memory
Humoral Acute phase proteins Lysozyme Complement	Antibody
Cell-mediated Natural killer cells Phagocytes	T-lymphocytes

ease were either inhaled into the nose, or cotton pledgets that had been stored for a year after infection with smallpox matter were placed over scratches on the skin. The procedure was introduced into England from Turkey in the reign of George I by Lady Mary Wortley Montagu, the wife of the British Ambassador to Constantinople. The matter from smallpox lesions was introduced on the point of a large needle into the vein of a recipient. The procedure was not without hazard and if the recipient did not develop the disease itself there was the danger of transmission of other infections such as leprosy or syphilis. George I was persuaded to allow the inoculation of two of his grandchildren and variolation became widespread throughout the country. The practice had been used on a small scale even at the end of the previous century in the Scottish Highlands and Wales and was introduced into America by immigrant slaves at the beginning of the eighteenth century.

Despite the hazards associated with variolation, smallpox was so widespread and feared that the small percentage of persons who developed the disease after inoculation was accepted as a worthwhile risk. In England at the time of George I, 60 of every 100 persons were likely to develop the disease and of these more than half would die. The efficacy of variolation in preventing the death of young children and women at childbirth is believed to have been largely responsible for the great increase in population in the early part of the eighteenth century. The Edinburgh physician Francis Home, who was familiar with the procedure of variolation, in 1758 applied the same principle to inoculate against measles. Home carried in his pocket-book pieces of cotton soaked in the tears, blood or tissue fluid taken from an incision into the rash of a patient. The pieces of cotton were placed over an incision in a recipient and in 7 of 15 persons immunized in this way mild measles developed after an incubation period of about 9 days.

Edward Jenner, towards the end of the eighteenth century, was the first to initiate the scientific approach to immunization. He took up observations, made 20 years earlier by a Dorchester farmer named Benjamin Jesty, that persons exposed or deliberately inoculated with cowpox were protected against smallpox. Jenner not only established the value of immunization with cowpox but was able to transmit the cowpox infection from one person to another.

The difficulties Jenner faced in gaining acceptance of vaccination (from the Latin *vaccinus* — pertaining to cows) are fully and fascinatingly described in *Victory with vaccines* (Parish 1968). Jenner's paper of 1798, giving the results and conclusions of his investigation, was refused by the Royal Society and he was subjected to crude criticisms and caricatures including a cartoonist's representation of vaccinated individuals being transformed into cows. In 1802 and 1807 he was given a parliamentary grant (less deductions for taxes and fees). Surprisingly, variolation was not made illegal until 1840. Two years after Jenner's paper was finally published, Dr Benjamin Waterhouse of Harvard obtained supplies of the vaccine and its use became widespread in America. Napoleon had his troops vaccinated and the first child to be vaccinated in Russia was named Vaccinof.

The foundations for an understanding of immunity were laid by the invention of the microscope by Leeuwenhoek, the recognition of microorganisms and the advent of Pasteur's **germ theory of disease**. Pasteur's chance observation that aged cultures of chicken cholera bacillus would not cause the expected disease in chickens led to the development of methods for reducing the virulence of pathogenic microorganisms called **attenuation**. The protection given to animals by inoculation of such attenuated organisms led to the widespread use of the method for immunization purposes.

At the end of the nineteenth century Robert Koch developed staining techniques and, later, the fixation of organisms on slides. His work on anthrax showed that the disease could be transferred from animal to animal by pure cultures. He went on to describe tubercle bacilli and the phenomenon of delayed hypersensitivity or **cell-mediated immunity** as it is known today. Immunology as a science began with the demonstration by von Behring and Kitasato at the Koch Institute in Berlin in 1890 of an antibacterial substance, called antitoxin, in the blood of animals immunized against tetanus and diphtheria organisms. Protection from the harmful effect of the bacterium could be transferred to naive (unimmunized) animals by injection of serum from animals that had recovered from infection. The active component, now known as **antibody**, is present in the cell-free portion of blood, i.e. plasma or serum, and is the basis of **humoral immunity** (humors meaning body fluids).

In the early part of this century Pfeiffer and Bordet demonstrated the activity of a serum factor called **complement**, which participates with antibody in the destruction of bacteria and has now been shown to have a wide variety of important biological activities. Paul Ehrlich proposed the first theory of antibody formation — **the side chain theory**. This proposed the existence of receptors on the surface of cells that could be released into the blood and neutralize bacterial toxins. It soon became clear that non-microbial substances could induce humoral immunity and the more general term antibody replaced antitoxin.

The specificity of antibody for the agent (i.e. the antigen) which induced its formation led to the use of antibodies as analytical tools. Thus the antigenic characters of bacterial and non-bacterial substances could be worked out and systems of classification of microorganisms were developed on this basis. Landsteiner used antibody–antigen interactions to define the **ABO blood group system** on the basis of antigenic differences in red cell membranes and was also responsible for performing the groundwork on the chemical basis of antigenic specificity.

The part played by **phagocytic cells** in clearing away and destroying bacteria was recognized by Metchnikoff, a Russian biologist working in France. Later the helpful effect of antibody (called **opsonins** by Almroth Wright) in encouraging phagocytosis became apparent, thus reconciling two opposing schools of thought on immune mechanisms — one believing the process to be brought about completely by blood factors and the other upholding an entirely cellular viewpoint.

It was not until the 1950s that reactivity to certain types of antigens was shown to be mediated by cells. George Mackaness demonstrated that resistance to the intracellular bacterium *Listeria monocytogenes* could be transferred to non-immune animals by cells and not with serum. Cell-mediated reactions are controlled and mediated either directly by lymphocytes or through molecules produced by these cells acting on other cells.

The two arms of acquired immunity, i.e. humoral and cell-mediated, are effected by two distinct types of lymphocyte. B-lymphocytes respond to antigens by differentiating into antibody-producing plasma cells while T-lymphocytes are responsible for cell-mediated immunity. Humoral immunity is effective against extracellular pathogens and their products because antibody can bind to these structures and cause their destruction. Microorganisms, such as viruses, certain bacteria and some parasites, that survive within cells are inaccessible to antibody. Cell-mediated immunity plays a major role in the elimination of these intracellular pathogens by causing the lysis of the infected cells or the intracellular destruction of the microorganism.

THE IMMUNE SYSTEM

The immune system consists of a number of organs and several different cell types. All the cells of the immune system, tissue cells and white blood cells or **leucocytes**, develop from pluripotent stem cells in the bone marrow. These haemopoietic stem cells also give rise to the red blood cells or **erythrocytes**. The production of leucocytes is through two main pathways of differentiation (Fig. 1.1). The **lymphoid** lineage produces T-lymphocytes and B-lymphocytes while the **myeloid**

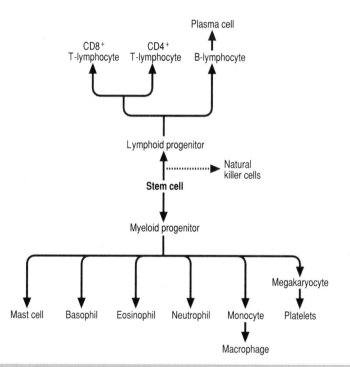

Fig. 1.1 Cells of the immune system.
The two main lineages, lymphoid and myeloid, are derived from pluripotent stem cells present in the bone marrow. A common lymphoid progenitor has the ability to give rise to both T- and B-lymphocytes. B-cells develop in the bone marrow and when terminally differentiated become antibody-producing plasma cells. Lymphoid progenitors that mature in the thymus become members of one of the T-cell subsets. Myeloid progenitors are capable of producing the granulocytes (basophils, eosinophils and neutrophils), mast cells, megakaryocytes that give rise to platelets, and monocytes that differentiate into macrophages when they enter the tissues. The precise pathway of development of natural killer cells is unknown although they do originally develop from stem cells. Stem cells also give rise to the red blood cells via the erythroid lineage (not shown).

pathway gives rise to mononuclear and polymorphonuclear leucocytes as well as platelets and mast cells. Platelets are involved in blood clotting and inflammation while mast cells are similar to basophils but are found in tissues. Natural killer (NK) cells, sometimes referred to as large granular lymphocytes, are thought to differentiate from lymphoid progenitor although the exact pathway is unknown.

Lymphoid cells

Lymphocytes make up about 20% of the white blood cells present in the adult circulation. Mature lymphoid cells are long-lived and may survive for many years as memory cells. These mononuclear cells are heterogeneous in terms of size and morphology. The typical small lymphocytes are agranular and comprise the T- and B-cell populations. The larger cells are referred to as large granular lymphocytes because they contain cytoplasmic granules. Cells within this population are able to kill certain tumour and virally infected cells (natural killing) and destroy cells coated with immunoglobulin (antibody-dependent cell-mediated cytotoxicity).

Morphologically it is quite difficult to distinguish between the different lymphoid cells and impossible to differentiate the subclasses of T-cell. Since these cells carry out different processes they possess molecules on their surfaces unique to that functional requirement. These molecules, referred to as markers, can be used to distinguish between different cell types and also identify cells at different stages of differentiation. The different cell surface molecules have been systematically named by the CD (cluster of differentiation) system and some of those expressed by different T-cell populations are shown in Table 1.2. These CD markers are identified using specific monoclonal antibodies. The presence of these specific antibodies on the cell surface is then visualized using fluorescent- or enzyme-antibody conjugates that recognize the first antibody (Fig. 1.2).

Table 1.2 **Major T-lymphocyte markers**

Marker	Distribution	Proposed function
CD2	All T-cells	Adherence to target cell
CD3	All T-cells	Signal transduction as a result of antigen recognition
CD4	MHC class II restricted T-cells	Binding to MHC class II molecules
CD7	All T-cells	Unknown
CD8	MHC class I restricted T-cells	Binding to MHC class I molecules

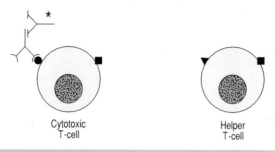

Cytotoxic
T-cell

Helper
T-cell

Fig. 1.2 Identification of T-cell subsets.
An antibody specific for a molecule present only on a cytotoxic T-cell will bind specifically to this cell type. The structure recognized by the antibody is not present on the helper T-cell, therefore no antibody is bound. The bound antibody can be detected by treating the cells with an antibody that recognizes a determinant present on the first antibody. If this second antibody is labelled with a substance that can be detected (radioisotope, enzyme or fluorescent molecule) then the cells that possess the specific antigen can be enumerated or visualized. In this example, the specific antigens could be CD8 (●) and CD4 (▲) and the common antigen CD3 (■). Label on the second antibody is depicted by an asterisk.

Myeloid cells

The second pathway of development gives rise to a variety of cell types of different morphology and function.

Mononuclear phagocytes

The common myeloid progenitor in the bone marrow gives rise to **monocytes** that circulate in the blood and migrate into organs and tissues to become **macrophages**. These two cell types are collectively known as mononuclear phagocytes. The human blood monocyte is larger than the lymphocyte and usually has a kidney-shaped nucleus. This actively phagocytic cell has a ruffled membrane and many cytoplasmic granules. These lysosomes contain enzymes and molecules that are involved in the killing of microorganisms. Mononuclear phagocytes adhere strongly to surfaces and have various cell membrane receptors to aid the binding and ingestion of foreign material. Their activities can be enhanced by molecules produced by T-lymphocytes, called **lymphokines**. Macrophages and monocytes are capable of producing various complement components and **monokines** such as interleukin-1, prostaglandins, interferons and tumour necrosis factor.

Polymorphonuclear leucocytes

These cells are sometimes referred to as **granulocytes** and are short-lived cells (2–3 days) compared to macrophages which may survive for months or years. They comprise 60–70% of the leucocytes but also migrate into tissues in response to injury or infection. The mature forms have a multilobed nucleus and many granules. They are classified as neutrophils, eosinophils and basophils on the basis of their histochemical staining.

Neutrophils are the most abundant circulating granulocytes. Their granules contain numerous microbicidal molecules and when a chemotactic factor is produced, as the result of infection or injury, in an extravascular site these cells enter the tissues.

Eosinophils are also phagocytic cells although they appear to be less efficient than neutrophils. They are present in low numbers in a healthy, normal individual (1–2% of leucocytes) but their numbers rise in certain allergic conditions. The granule contents can be released by the appropriate signal and the cytotoxic molecules can then kill parasites that are too large to be phagocytosed.

Basophils are found in extremely small numbers in the circulation (<0.2%) and have certain characteristics in common with tissue **mast cells**. Both cell types have receptors on their surface for the Fc portion of IgE and crosslinking of this immunoglobulin by antigen leads to the release of various pharmacological mediators. These molecules stimulate an inflammatory response. There are two types of mast cell; one is found in connective tissue and the other is mucosa-associated. Mast cells and basophils are both bone marrow derived but their developmental relationship is not clear.

Platelets

Platelets are also derived from myeloid progenitors. In addition to their role in clotting they are involved in inflammation.

Cytokines

In addition to cells many secreted molecules, known as **cytokines**, play a role in the induction and effector phases of immune responses. Many of these cytokines are produced by mononuclear phagocytes and are referred to as **monokines** while those produced by lymphocytes are termed **lymphokines**.

Cytokines are usually glycoproteins and share certain characteristics.

1. Cytokines are usually synthesized by a cell in response to a stimulus and once produced are secreted. They are not stored preformed within cells.

2. The same cytokine is produced by various cell types.

3. Individual cytokines act on many different cell types, i.e. they are **pleiotropic**, and may affect various cells in different ways.

4. Many similar functions are shared by different cytokines, i.e. their actions are redundant.

5. Cytokines often influence the synthesis of and affect the actions of other cytokines. They may enhance or inhibit both these criteria.

6. Cytokine action is mediated by binding to specific receptors on target cells. They tend to be very potent.

Cytokines are produced that act as mediators of innate immunity, e.g. interferon, tumour necrosis factor and interleukin-1, while others are involved mainly in acquired immunity. In the latter case they act to control the activation, growth and differentiation of cells. The production of cells of the immune system is controlled by cytokines that regulate haematopoiesis and are collectively known as **colony stimulating factors** (CSF). The role of a number of important cytokines is discussed in Chapter 4.

Characteristics of acquired immunity

In recent years, with increased knowledge of the molecular processes underlying the functioning of cells, it has become possible to explain at a cellular and molecular level the features that are the hallmark of acquired immune responses.

Specificity and diversity. Immune responses are directed against selected parts of antigens known as **antigenic determinants** or **epitopes**. As B- and T-lymphocytes develop they express on their cell membranes unique receptors that can interact with a complementary shape on an antigen. Therefore, before exposure to antigen, there exists in an individual many B- and T-lymphocytes each with a different specificity governed by the shape of its receptor. There is the capacity to generate at least 10^{11} different B-cell receptors and more than 10^{18} different T-cell receptors. The molecular mechanisms that give rise to this immense lymphocyte repertoire have recently been elucidated and are described in Chapter 3. Those lymphocytes that interact via their receptors with the antigen are therefore selected by the antigen and form the cells that mount a response against that particular foreign material. A different antigen will cause the activation of a different set of cells. This concept forms the basis of the **clonal selection theory** and explains the specificity of acquired immune responses.

Memory. The acquired immune response to a particular antigen is more effective on re-exposure than on the primary encounter. This immunological memory is characterized by a more rapid response of greater magnitude with higher affinity receptors involved.

Regulation. All normal immune responses decline with time as the stimulus, i.e. antigen, is removed. The effector cells produced have a short half-life and unless more are generated the response will wane.

Some of the cells will develop into memory cells that will be stimulated on re-exposure to antigen. A number of feedback regulatory pathways are also stimulated that dampen down the response once the antigen is eliminated.

One of the most exciting recent findings is the discovery of peptide neurotransmitter and hormone receptors on cells of the immune system indicating that the peptides that regulate the brain and endocrine system play an important role in regulating the activity of the immune system. Furthermore lymphocytes produce peptides identical to those in the brain and pituitary gland resulting in feedback inhibition of the pituitary and hypothalmic peptides. Thus the immune system can no longer be viewed in isolation and must be seen as part of an integrated system involving neural, endocrine and immune components. It is now clear that more than 20 separate neuroendocrine peptides, or their mRNAs, have been demonstrated in cells of the immune system so that at local level the immune system can act as an effective endocrine organ.

Self/non-self discrimination. The immune system is able to respond to and destroy foreign materials but yet remain unresponsive to self molecules. Immunological unresponsiveness is referred to as tolerance. Self-tolerance is an active process and occurs through a number of mechanisms that are still the subject of much research. As lymphocytes develop they pass a number of selection steps where useless or potentially dangerous cells are eliminated. A breakdown of the process responsible for self-tolerance can lead to the generation of self-destroying cells and autoimmune disease.

The acquired immune processes that lead to the elimination of foreign material involve the concerted efforts of a number of different cells and molecules and can be divided into three stages.

Recognition stage. During lymphocyte development cell surface molecules are synthesized that act as antigen receptors. B-lymphocytes express immunoglobulin molecules on their surface that can bind to foreign antigen in its native free form. The T-cell receptor recognizes fragments of antigen on the surface of host cells that are associated with self molecules coded for within the **major histocompatibility complex** (MHC).

Activation stage. Those lymphocytes that have bound antigen via their surface receptors are triggered into action. There is a phase of proliferation, i.e. cell division, leading to an expansion in the number of antigen specific cells which then differentiate and mature into cells that can aid in the elimination of the offending material. B-lymphocytes develop into plasma cells which secrete immunoglobulin of the same specificity as the surface immunoglobulin that acted as the antigen receptor. The antibody produced can therefore interact with the antigen that was responsible for initiating its production. T-lymphocytes undergo similar processes. Antigen-activated T-cells mature into cells that can directly kill infected cells or produce biologically active molecules, lymphokines, that activate other defence mechanisms. Because T-lymphocytes are stimulated by cell-associated antigen fragments their effector functions are directed against intracellular pathogens and the lymphokines are produced directly on to the cell that stimulated their release.

As the immune system develops, lymphocytes will be produced each with a different receptor. These cells circulate around the body and when the individual is exposed to a particular antigen the few cells that can bind to the foreign material will be stimulated as just described. There has to be expansion of the responsive cell so that an effective immune response can be generated. On the first, or primary, exposure to an antigen there will be very few cells that will recognize the foreign material. The immune response takes some time to get going since antigen reactive cells will have to proliferate before differentiating into effector cells. During this primary immune response, memory cells are generated and on subsequent exposures it will be these cells that are stimulated. There will be a considerable number of memory cells produced and they are at a higher state of readiness, so a secondary immune response is quicker and more effective. This fact is made use of in vaccination where the aim is to have the body primed ready to eliminate the infectious agent before disease is produced.

Effector stage. The final phase of an immune response is when the activated lymphocytes produce the molecules that eliminate the antigen. Plasma cells produce antibody and activated T-cells destroy target cells or secrete lymphokines. Many of the molecules produced by activated lymphocytes act on or in conjunction with components of innate immunity to aid the elimination of antigen. The various defence mechanisms therefore work in concert to protect the host from damaging insults from infectious and other agents.

The scope of immunology

Over the past 20 years tremendous advances have been made in the understanding of the immune system. Our knowledge of the immunological processes underlying the reactions of the body to infectious agents, to tumours and to transplanted tissues and organs has gained much ground as the result of advances in immunological techniques. Immunologists have used many of the techniques developed by biochemists and molecular biologists to study the immune system. Advances in nucleic acid technology have been used to identify the genes coding for molecules such as the T-cell receptor and MHC molecules. The genes for immunologically important molecules have been cloned and recombinant DNA technology has allowed the production of relatively large amounts of pure proteins.

It is now possible to culture many different cell types in vitro and to clone these cells so that a population with an identical genetic make-up is obtained. Many different strains of inbred mice have been developed and allow the investigation of cellular interactions to be performed with cells of identical genetic backgrounds or with known differences. The role of a number of gene products has been elucidated by producing transgenic animals and studying the effect of the introduced genes.

Immunologists have developed many new techniques including novel ways of producing a homogeneous immunoglobulin preparation, monoclonal antibody, from impure antigens. The development of these defined reagents that can be produced in large amounts has revolutionized immunoassays and detection systems that employ antibodies. Their potential in the treatment of infectious diseases and cancer patients is being actively investigated and a number of clinical trials have been performed. In addition to antibodies, other immunologically important molecules have been produced and are being developed as therapeutic agents. The introduction of flow cytometry has revolutionized the analysis of cell populations and the use of the polymerase chain reaction has increased the sensitivity of the detection of microorganisms.

The interplay between cell and molecules of the immune system is extremely complex. Some molecules appear to have many different functions depending on their location or the presence of other molecules. The possibility of harnessing these powerful reagents to aid in the elimination of not only pathogenic microorganisms but also cancer cells is being actively pursued. We are only now beginning to understand the intricacies of immune recognition. The ability to predict the minimum structures that can induce protective immunity will allow the development of better vaccines. With this knowledge it might be possible to develop novel ways of treating autoimmune diseases, allergic conditions and tumours and to develop new strategies to reduce transplant rejection.

Thus it can be seen that immunity in its original meaning, referring to resistance to infection by means of a specific immune response, is only one activity of a complex system in animals. The total activity of the cellular system is concerned with mechanisms for preserving the integrity of the individual with far-reaching implications in embryology, genetics, cell biology, tumour biology and many non-infectious disease processes.

FURTHER READING

Parish H J 1968 Victory with vaccines: The story of immunization. E & S Livingstone, Edinburgh

Paul W E 1993 A history of immunology. In: Paul W E (ed) Fundamental immunology, 3rd edn. Raven Press, New York

2 Innate immunity

The healthy individual is protected from potentially harmful microorganisms in the environment by a number of very effective mechanisms, present from birth, that do not depend upon prior exposure to any particular microorganism. The innate defence mechanisms are non-specific in the sense that they are effective against a wide range of potentially infectious agents.

DETERMINANTS OF INNATE IMMUNITY

Species and strains

Marked differences exist in the susceptibility of different species to infectious agents. The rat is strikingly resistant to diphtheria whilst the guinea-pig and humans are highly susceptible. The rabbit is particularly susceptible to myxomatosis and humans to syphilis, leprosy and meningococcal meningitis. Susceptibility to an infection does not always imply a lack of resistance to disease caused by the microorganism. For example, although humans are highly susceptible to the common cold they overcome the infection within a few days. Dogs, in contrast, are not susceptible to the virus responsible for the common cold in humans. In some diseases, it may be difficult to initiate the infection but once established the disease can progress rapidly implying a lack of resistance. For example, rabies occurs in both humans and dogs but is not readily established as the virus does not ordinarily penetrate healthy skin. Once infected, however, both species are unable to overcome the disease. Marked variations in resistance to infection have been noted between different strains of mice and it is possible to breed, by selection, rabbits of low, intermediate and high resistance to experimental tuberculosis.

In humans the habits and environment of a community affect the ability to resist particular infections by acquired immune mechanisms developing early in life. This environmentally determined type of resistance is easily confused with the genetically controlled innate immunity and makes it difficult to ascertain differences in innate immunity in different communities. There is clear evidence that Caucasians are more resistant to tuberculosis than certain other racial groups. It seems reasonable to assume that certain interspecies and interstrain differences have arisen by a process of natural selection.

Individual differences and influence of age

The role of heredity in determining resistance to infection is well illustrated by studies on tuberculosis in twins. If one homozygous twin develops tuberculosis, the other twin has a three to one chance of developing the disease compared with a one in three chance if the twins are heterozygous. Sometimes genetically controlled abnormalities are an advantage to the individual in resisting infection as, for example, in a hereditary abnormality of the red blood cells (sickling). These red blood cells cannot be parasitized by *Plasmodium falciparum*, thus conferring a degree of resistance to malaria in the affected individuals.

Infectious diseases are often more severe in early childhood and in young animals; this higher susceptibility of the young appears to be associated with immaturity of the immunological mechanisms affecting the ability of the lymphoid system to deal with and react to foreign antigens. In certain viral infections, e.g. polio and chickenpox, the clinical illness is more severe in adults than in children. This may be due to an active immune response producing greater tissue damage. In the elderly, besides a general waning of the activities of the immune system, physical abnormalities (e.g. prostatic enlargement leading to stasis of urine) or long-term exposure to environmental factors (e.g. smoking) are common causes of increased susceptibility to infection.

Hormonal influences: sex

There is decreased resistance to infection in diseases such as diabetes mellitus, hypothyroidism and adrenal dysfunction. The reasons for this decrease have not yet been clarified but may be related to enzyme or hormone activities. It is known that glucocorticoids are anti-inflammatory agents, decreasing the ability of phagocytes to ingest material. They also have beneficial effects by interfering in some way with the toxic effects of bacterial products such as endotoxin.

There are no marked differences in susceptibility to infections between the sexes. Although the overall incidence and death rate from infectious disease is greater in the male than in the female, both infectious hepatitis and whooping cough have a higher morbidity and mortality in females.

Nutritional factors

The adverse effects of poor nutrition on susceptibility to certain infectious agents is not now seriously questioned. Experimental evidence in animals has shown repeatedly that inadequate diet may be correlated with increased susceptibility to a variety of bacterial diseases, associated with decreased phagocytic activity and leucopenia (levels of leucocytes below normal levels). Studies in Scotland, for example, have shown that sheep (particularly those grazing on hill farms) can have a deficiency in the trace element copper. This results in a decrease in their leucocyte microbicidal activity and an increased susceptibility to bacterial challenge.

In the case of infectious agents such as viruses which depend on normal metabolic function of the host cells, malnutrition, if it interferes with such activities, would be expected to hinder proliferation of the potentially infectious agent. There is experimental evidence in support of this view in a number of animal species which when undernourished are less susceptible than normal animals to a variety of viruses including vaccinia virus and certain neurotropic viruses, e.g. poliovirus. The same may be true of malaria infections in humans. The parasite requires para-aminobenzoic acid for multiplication and this may be deficient in the malnourished. The exact role of nutritional factors in resistance to infectious agents in humans is difficult to determine by epidemiological data. Poor diet is often associated with poor environmental conditions and increased incidence of infection can correlate with poor sanitary conditions and overcrowding.

MECHANISMS OF INNATE IMMUNITY

Mechanical barriers and surface secretions

The intact skin and mucous membranes of the body afford a high degree of protection against pathogens. In conditions where the skin is damaged, such as in burns patients and after traumatic injury or surgery, infections can be a serious problem. The skin is a resistant barrier because of its outer horny layer consisting mainly of keratin, which is indigestible by most microorganisms, and thus shields the living cells of the epidermis from microorganisms and their toxins. The relatively dry condition of the skin and the high concentration of salt in drying sweat are inhibitory or lethal to many microorganisms.

The sebaceous secretions and sweat of the skin contain bactericidal and fungicidal fatty acids and these constitute an effective protective mechanism against many potential pathogens. The antimicrobial substances include the sweat gland secretions: lactic acid, amino acids, uric acid and ammonia (the acidity of sweat, pH 5.5, has a microbicidal effect); the sebaceous secretions: triglycerides, free fatty acids and wax alcohols; substances derived from the cornification process: steroids, amino acids, pentoses, phospholipids and complex polypeptides. Certain areas of the body such as the soles of the feet are deficient in sebaceous glands and this explains in part why such areas are susceptible to fungal infections. The protective ability of these secretions varies at different stages of life and some fungal 'ringworm' infections of children disappear at puberty with the marked increase of sebaceous secretions.

The sticky mucus covering the respiratory tract acts as a trapping mechanism for inhaled particles. The action of cilia sweeps the secretions, containing the foreign material, towards the oropharynx so that it is swallowed; in the stomach the acidic secretions destroy most of the microorganisms present. There are no cilia in the gastrointestinal tract but the layer of mucus can trap organisms and the effect of peristalsis prevents bacterial overgrowth. Slowing of normal intestinal mobility is likely to lead to increased numbers of gut bacteria and, if the mucosal barrier is damaged, leakage of microorganisms can occur with potentially serious effects. Nasal secretions and saliva contain mucopolysaccharides capable of blocking some viruses, and the tears and the mucous secretions of the respiratory, alimentary and genitourinary tracts contain lysozyme that is particularly active against some Gram-positive bacteria.

The washing action of tears and flushing of urine are effective in stopping invasion by microorganisms. Areas where there is a high flow rate of secretions such as the urinary tract and biliary tract are generally sterile in contrast to areas where the flow rate is slower, such as the oropharynx and the large bowel. Interference with flow rate in the urinary tract or biliary tract will lead to infection.

Normal bacterial flora

The normal bacterial flora of the skin may produce various antimicrobial substances such as bacteriocines and acids. At the same time the normal flora competes with potential pathogens for essential nutrients.

There are a very large number of microorganisms that live in close association with humans — around 10^{12} bacteria on the skin and about 10^{14} in the gut. Probably the most valuable function of these 'commensal' organisms is the exclusion of other microorganisms. If the commensal organisms of the gut are removed by antibiotics, pathogenic microbes can readily gain a foothold. Experiments with mice have shown that after sterilization of the gut with streptomycin the animals can be killed with 1/10 000th of the dose of *Salmonella typhimuri-*

um required to kill the untreated animals. Guinea-pigs given penicillin undergo a profound change in the microbial content of the bowel. Such organisms may get into the bloodstream and kill the animal. The lactobacilli of the vagina produce acid, during normal metabolic processes, which reduces the pH to about 4. If this flora is disturbed by antibiotics other bacteria, yeasts and parasites can become established.

Commensal organisms from the gut or bacteria normally present on the skin can cause problems if they gain access to an area that they do not normally populate. An example of this is urinary tract infections resulting from the introduction of *Escherichia coli*, a gut commensal, by means of a urinary catheter. Commensal organisms that are provided with the circumstances by which to cause infections are called **opportunistic pathogens**. Infections with these opportunists are quite widespread, often appearing as a result of medical or surgical treatment which breaches the innate defences or reduces the host's ability to respond.

Humoral defence mechanisms

A number of microbicidal substances are present in the tissue and body fluids. Some of these molecules are produced constitutively, e.g. lysozyme, and others are produced in response to infection, e.g. acute phase proteins and interferon. These molecules all show the characteristics of innate immunity — there is no specific recognition of the microorganism and the response is not enhanced on re-exposure to the same antigen.

Lysozyme

This enzyme is a basic protein of low molecular weight found in relatively high concentrations in phagocytic cells as well as in most tissue fluids, except cerebrospinal fluid, sweat and urine. It is a muramidase, splitting sugars off the peptidoglycan of the cell wall of many Gram-positive bacteria causing their lysis. It seems likely that lysozyme may also play a role in the destruction of some Gram-negative bacteria. In many pathogenic bacteria the peptidoglycan appears to be protected from the access of lysozyme by other wall components, e.g. lipopolysaccharide. The action of other enzymes from phagocytes or of complement may be needed to remove this protection and expose the peptidoglycan to the action of lysozyme.

Basic polypeptides

A variety of basic proteins, derived from tissues and blood cells, have some antibacterial properties. This group includes the basic proteins called spermine and spermidine which can kill tubercle bacilli and some staphylococci. Other toxic compounds are the arginine- and lysine-containing proteins protamine and histone. Defensins, antimicrobial peptides, containing 29–35 amino acid residues, are present in human neutrophils. The bactericidal activity of basic polypeptides probably depends on their ability to react non-specifically with acid polysaccharides at the bacterial cell surface.

Acute phase proteins

A number of molecules, known as acute phase proteins, are present at very low levels in normal serum but their concentration rises dramatically during an infection. Microbial products such as endotoxin (lipopolysaccharide) can stimulate macrophages to release endogenous pyrogen — more correctly known as interleukin-1 (IL-1). This molecule is responsible for the rise in temperature seen during infections. Interleukin-1 and other cytokines, notably interleukin-6, stimulate the liver to produce increased amounts of various acute phase proteins the concentrations of which can rise over 1000-fold. One of the best characterized acute phase proteins is C-reactive protein which binds to phosphorylcholine residues in the cell wall of certain microorganisms. This complex is very effective at activating the classical complement pathway. Also included in this group of molecules are α_1-antitrypsin, α_2-macroglobulin, fibrinogen and serum amyloid A protein, all of which act to limit the spread of the infectious agent or stimulate the host response.

Interferon

The observation that cell cultures infected with one virus resist infection by a second virus, i.e. viral interference, led to the identification of the family of antiviral agents known as **interferons**. A number of molecules have been identified and these can be divided into two types. Type 1 interferons (α and β) are part of innate immunity and type 2 interferon (γ) is produced by T-cells as part of the acquired immune response. The 15 known alpha-interferons are produced mainly by lymphocytes, and most cell types are capable of producing the one beta-interferon that has been identified. When a cell is infected with a virus it secretes interferon which then binds to receptors on uninfected neighbouring cells to induce an antiviral state. This state results from the production of enzymes that inhibit translation and destroy mRNA, therefore progeny virus cannot be produced. The virally infected cell is, in effect, isolated from healthy cells that could permit viral replication (described more fully in Ch. 5). Since interferons affect the replicative machinery of a cell they will inhibit host cell functions as well as virus production. Due to this fact they have been postulated as possible anti-cancer agents but so far they have not lived up to the expectations, mainly because of their many side-effects.

Interferons, mainly gamma-interferon, act on cells of the immune system in both a stimulatory and inhibitory fashion, depending on the cell types involved and their state of activation. Antibody responses can be affected as can the activities of natural killer cells and macrophages (see below and Ch. 4).

Complement

The existence of a heat-labile serum component with the ability to lyse red blood cells and destroy Gram-negative bacteria has been known for over 70 years. The chemical complexity of the phenomenon was not appreciated by early workers who ascribed the activity to a single component, called complement. Complement is in fact a group of serum proteins present in low concentration in normal serum. These molecules are present in an inactive form but can be activated to form an enzyme cascade, i.e. the product of the first reaction is the catalyst of the next and so on.

There are about 20 proteins involved in the complement system some of which are enzymes, some are control molecules and some are structural proteins with no enzymatic activity. A number of the molecules involved are split into two components by the product of the previous step. The smaller of the products is termed the 'a' fragment and

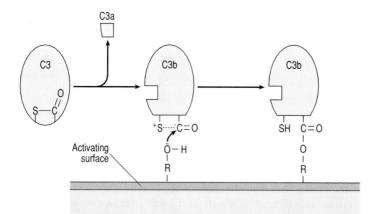

Fig. 2.1 Attachment of C3 to cell surface.
The cleavage of C3 into C3a and C3b exposes an unstable thioester bond in the C3b moiety. This exposed chemical grouping is susceptible to nucleophilic attack by oxygen or nitrogen atoms. The result is the formation of a covalent linkage to proteins and carbohydrates on a cell surface or if H_2O donates the electrons (not shown) then fluid phase C3b is produced and the process is terminated.

the larger the 'b' fragment. Complement can be regarded as an innate defence system but antibody can also be involved in its activation. There are two pathways of complement activation, the alternative and the classical, that lead to the same, physiological consequences — opsonization, cellular activation and lysis — but use different initiation processes. C3, a molecule of 195 kD, forms the connection between the two pathways and the binding of this molecule to a surface is the key process in complement activation. Host cell surfaces contain molecules that stop C3 deposition whereas non-self structures allow the rapid deposition of many molecules of activated C3. When C3a is split from C3 a reactive binding site is generated in the C3b moiety (Fig. 2.1). The majority of this reactive C3b interacts with water thus losing any biological activity. A small fraction, however, binds to hydroxyl and amino groups in adjacent proteins and carbohydrates to continue the activation process. A similar reactive binding site is generated when C4 is converted to C4b.

Classical pathway. The classical pathway of activation leading to the cleavage of C3 is initiated by the binding of two or more of the globular domains of the C1q component of C1 to its ligand–immune complexes containing IgG or IgM and certain microorganisms and their products. This causes a conformational change in the C1 com-

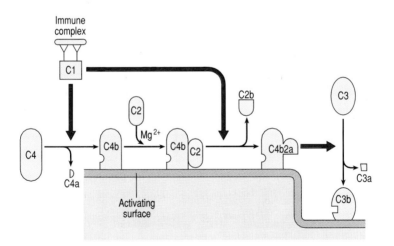

Fig. 2.2 Activation of complement cascade by classical pathway.
The binding of C1 to an immune complex changes its conformation to generate an active serine esterase. This enzyme can now cleave C4a from C4. The resulting C4b binds to a surface and joins with C2 in an Mg^{2+} ion-dependent process. The same enzyme is then able to cleave C2b from C2 to generate the C3-cleaving enzyme C4b2a. This C3 convertase removes C3a from C3 to give C3b that can bind to the activating surface. Enzymatic reactions are indicated by thick arrows.

plex that leads to the autoactivation of the C1r component. The enzyme C1r then converts C1s into an active serine esterase that acts on the thioester-containing molecule C4 to produce C4a and a reactive C4b (Fig. 2.2). C4a is released and less than 1% of the C4b becomes attached to a surface. The rest is inactivated by reacting with water. C2 binds to the surface-bound C4b, becomes a substrate for the activated C1 complex and is split into C2a and C2b. The C2b is released leaving C4b2a — the classical pathway C3 convertase. This active enzyme then generates C3a and the unstable C3b from C3. A small amount of the C3b generated will bind to the activating surface and act as a focus for further complement activation. The activation of the classical pathway is regulated by C1 inhibitor and by a number of molecules that limit the production of the 'C3 convertase'.

Alternative pathway. Intrinsically C3 undergoes a low level of hydrolysis of the internal thioester bond to generate C3i (Fig. 2.3). This molecule binds, in the presence of Mg^{2+}, with Factor B. This complex is then acted on by Factor D to produce C3iBb. This is a 'C3 convertase' capable of splitting more C3 to C3b, some of which will become membrane bound. This 'tickover' must be controlled or the process could get out of hand. There are molecules on host cell surfaces that prevent the formation of stable C3 convertase enzymes. The surface bound C3b can then act as a binding site for more Factor B and can in turn give rise to a C3 convertase, C3bBb (see below).

Amplification loop. The initial binding of C3b generated by either the classical or alternative pathways leads to an amplification loop that results in the binding of many more C3b molecules to the same sur-

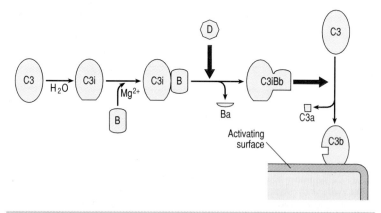

Fig. 2.3 C3 tickover.
C3 is slowly hydrolysed by water to give C3i which in the presence of Mg^{2+} ion binds Factor B (B). Factor D (D) cleaves Factor B to release Ba and generate C3iBb. This C3 convertase can directly cleave C3 into C3a and C3b. Enzymatic reactions are indicated by thick arrows.

face. Factor B binds to the surface-bound C3b to form C3bB, the substrate for Factor D — a serine esterase — that is present in very low concentrations in an already active form (Fig. 2.4). The cleavage of Factor B results in the formation of the C3 convertase, C3bBb, which dissociates rapidly unless it is stabilized by the binding of properdin (P), forming the complex C3bBbP. This convertase can cleave many more C3 molecules, some of which become surface-bound. This amplification loop is a positive feedback system that will cycle until all the C3 is used up unless it is regulated carefully.

Regulation. In solution C3bBb is unstable and Factor B is replaced by Factor H to form a complex that is the substrate for Factor I. The product iC3b has no enzymatic activity and can be further degraded by proteases in body fluids. The fate of surface-bound C3b is the critical step in the induction of further activation of C3 and the terminal components. The nature of the surface to which the C3b is bound regulates the outcome. Self cell membranes contain a number of regulatory molecules that promote the binding of Factor H rather than Factor B to C3b. This results in the inhibition of the activation process since C3bH is the substrate of the inactivating Factor I and the iC3b formed cannot lead to further activation. On non-self structures the C3b is protected since regulatory proteins are not pre-

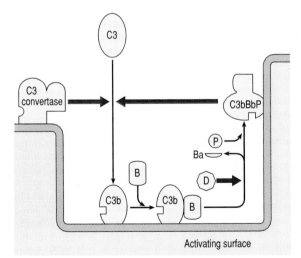

Activating surface

Fig. 2.4 Amplification loop.
C3b produced by activation through either the classical or alternative pathway binds to Factor B (B) in an Mg^{2+} ion-dependent fashion. This is acted on by Factor D (D) releasing Ba and generating the C3 convertase C3bBb. Properdin (P) binds to C3bBb stabilizing the convertase. This can in turn convert more C3 to C3b and amplify the initial complement activation. Enzymatic reactions are indicated by thick arrows.

sent and Factor B has a higher affinity for C3b than Factor H at these sites.

Thus the surface of many microorganisms can stabilize the C3bBb by protecting it from Factor H. In addition another molecule, properdin, stabilizes the complex. The deposition of a few molecules of C3b on to these surfaces is followed by the formation of the relatively stable C3bBbP complex. This C3 convertase will lead to more C3b deposition. Immune complexes composed of certain immunoglobulins, e.g. IgA and IgE, also function as protected sites for C3b and activate complement by the alternative pathway. Poor activation surfaces will be made more susceptible to deposition by the presence of antibody that generates C3b by the classical pathway.

Membrane attack complex. The next step after the formation of C3b is the cleavage of C5. The 'C5 convertases' are generated from C4b2a of the classical pathway and C3bBb of the alternative pathway by the addition of another C3b molecule (Fig. 2.5). These membrane-bound trimolecular complexes selectively bind C5 and cleave it to give fluid phase C5a and membrane-bound C5b. The formation of the rest of the membrane attack complex (MAC) is non-enzymatic. C6 binds to C5b and this joint complex is released from the C5 convertase. The formation of C5b67 generates a hydrophobic complex that inserts into the lipid bilayer in the vicinity of the initial activation site. Usually this will be on the same cell surface as the initial trigger but occasionally other cells may be involved. Therefore bystander lysis can take place giving rise to damage to surrounding tissue. There are a number of proteins present in body fluids to limit this potentially dangerous

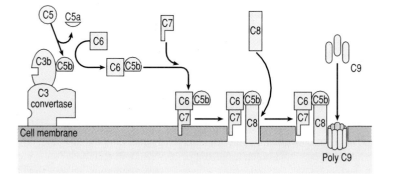

Fig. 2.5 **Membrane attack complex.**
The C5 convertase of the classical and alternative pathways binds C5 and cleaves it with the release of C5a (an anaphylatoxin) and production of C5b. C6 binds and C5b6 is released from the convertase. Subsequently the binding of C7 forms the hydrophobic C5b67 complex that can insert into the membrane in the vicinity of the initial activation site. C8 binds to a site on C5b, becomes membrane associated and directs the polymerization and membrane insertion of up to 20 C9 molecules.

process by binding to fluid phase C5b67. C8 and C9 bind to the membrane-inserted complex in sequence, resulting in the formation of a lytic polymeric complex containing up to 20 C9 monomers. A small amount of lysis can occur when C8 binds to C5b67 but it is the polymerized C9 that causes the most damage. The complete complement cascade is depicted in Figure 2.6.

Functions. The activation of complement by either pathway gives rise to C3b and the generation of a number of factors that can aid in the elimination of foreign material.

The complete insertion of the membrane attack complex into a cell will lead to membrane damage and lysis, probably by osmotic swelling. Some thin-walled pathogens, such as trypanosomes and the malaria parasite, are killed by complement-mediated lysis. Some Gram-negative bacteria can be killed by complement in conjunction with lysozyme. However, complement-mediated lysis is of limited importance as a bactericidal mechanism when compared to phagocyte destruction of bacteria. Inherited deficiencies of the terminal components are associated with infection by gonococci and meningococci which can survive inside neutrophils and for which complement-mediated killing is important.

Phagocytic cells have receptors for C3b and iC3b that facilitate the adherence of complement-coated particles. Therefore, complement is an **opsonin** and in certain circumstances this attachment may lead to phagocytosis.

Two of the molecules released during the complement cascade, C3a and C5a, have potent biological activities. These molecules, known as **anaphylatoxins**, trigger mast cells and basophils to release mediators of inflammation (see below). They also stimulate neutrophils to produce reactive oxygen intermediates while C5a on its own is a chemoattractant and acts directly on vascular endothelium to cause vasodilation and increased vascular permeability.

Complement also plays a role in the destruction and elimination of potentially harmful antigen/antibody complexes (immune complexes). Immune complexes are potentially harmful as they can be deposited in blood vessels and stimulate an inflammatory response (see below) that could damage surrounding tissues. Complement is able to interfere with this process by sterically blocking the interactions between antigen and antibodies that are involved in immune complex formation. In addition, the binding of C3b to immune complexes aids in their elimination by cells in the liver and spleen that have receptors for activated C3.

Cells

Phagocytes

Microorganisms or inert particles, such as colloidal carbon, entering

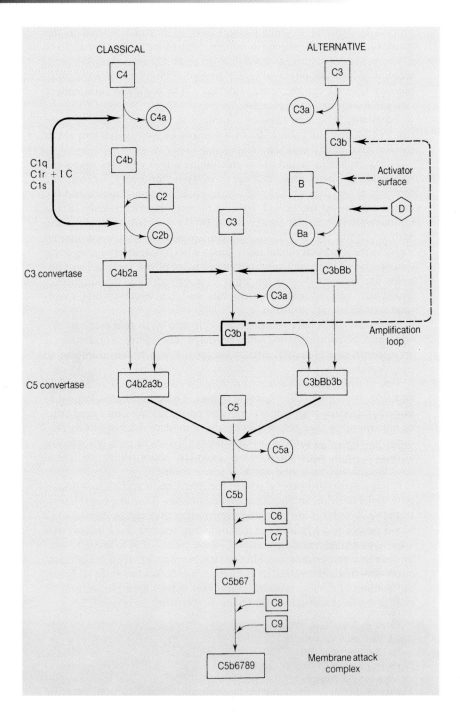

the tissue fluids or blood stream are very rapidly engulfed by various circulating and tissue phagocytic cells. These cells are of two main types, the **polymorphonuclear leucocytes** (especially **neutrophils**) and the **mononuclear phagocytes**. Neutrophils are short-lived cells that circulate in the blood and only enter the tissues when required. Mononuclear phagocytes are found in the blood and in tissues. In the blood they are known as **monocytes** while in the tissues they differentiate into **macrophages**. In connective tissue they are known as histiocytes, in kidney as mesangial cells, in bone as osteoclasts, in brain as microglia and in the spleen, lymph node and thymus as the sinus-lining macrophages. Kupffer cells of the liver, alveolar macrophages of the lungs and peritoneal macrophages are also derived from peripheral blood monocytes.

The three essential features of these cells are (1) that they are actively phagocytic, (2) that they contain digestive enzymes to degrade ingested material and (3) that they are an important link between the innate and acquired immune mechanisms. Part of their role in regard to acquired immunity is that mononuclear phagocytes can process and present antigens as well as producing molecules that stimulate lymphocyte differentiation into effector cells.

The process of phagocytosis is undoubtedly one of the earliest accomplishments of living cells. At the beginning of this century Metchnikoff first appreciated the continuity of this scavenging function through evolution and the important role of this activity in resistance to infectious agents. The role of the phagocyte in innate immunity is to engulf particles (phagocytosis) or soluble material (pinocytosis), and digest them intracellularly within specialized vacuoles. If the material is indigestible then the phagocytes store the offending agent away so that it no longer serves as a local irritant, e.g. carbon particles from a polluted atmosphere.

Fig. 2.6 Overview of complement activation.
Both pathways generate a C3-cleaving enzyme (C3 convertase): C4b2a in the classical pathway and C3bBb in the alternative pathway. The initial enzyme cascade leading to the production of these enzymes differs between the two pathways. In the classical pathway C1, composed of C1q, C1r and C1s, activation by immune complexes (IC) is the initial trigger. Activated C1 splits C4 and C2 to give C4b2a with the loss of the C4a and C2b fragments. In the alternative pathway, C3b produced by C3 tickover binds to Factor B (B) and if this complex binds to an activator surface, such as a microorganism, then the C3 convertase, C3bBb, will be formed by Factor D (D). Both C3 convertases produce C3b and C3a from C3. The C3b can combine with the C3 convertases to form the last enzyme in the pathway, the C5 convertases — C4b2a3b (classical) and C3bBb3b (alternative). The C5 convertase cleaves C5 to give C5a and C5b which goes on to direct the assembly of the membrane attack complex. During the activation process the anaphylatoxins, C3a and C5a, are produced. Enzymatic reactions are indicated by thick arrows.

The macrophages present in the walls of capillaries and vascular sinuses in spleen, liver, lungs and bone marrow serve a very important role in clearing the bloodstream of foreign particulate material such as bacteria. This process can be dramatically illustrated by injecting colloidal carbon into the circulation of a mouse. Samples of blood taken at short intervals thereafter show that there is a very rapid removal of most of the particles within a few minutes after injection and the blood is cleared within 15 to 20 minutes. Dissection of the animal will show massive localization of the carbon particles, particularly in the liver (Kupffer cells), spleen (sinus-lining macrophages) and in the macrophages of the lungs. So efficient is this process that the finding of a few microorganisms in the bloodstream usually indicates that there is a continuing release of microorganisms from an active focus such as an abscess or the valve vegetations found in bacterial endocarditis.

The ability of macrophages to ingest and destroy microorganisms can be impaired or enhanced by depression or stimulation of the phagocyte system. The destruction of phagocytic cells by chemical agents makes experimental animals temporarily susceptible to a normally non-virulent strain of pneumococcus. Some microorganisms such as mycobacteria and brucellae can resist intracellular digestion by normal macrophages, though they may be digested by 'activated' ones. The enhanced ability of macrophages from animals infected with tubercle bacilli and other intracellular bacteria to resist these and other infectious agents is discussed later.

Chemotaxis. For phagocytic cells to be effective they must be attracted to the site of infection. Once they have passed through the capillary walls they move through the tissues in response to a concentration gradient of molecules that has been produced at the site of damage. These chemotactic factors include products of injured tissue, factors from the blood (C5a), substances produced by neutrophils and mast cells (leukotrienes and histamine) and bacterial products (formyl-methionine peptides).

Chemotaxis is vital in bringing neutrophils and monocytes to sites of tissue damage. Neutrophils respond first and move in faster than monocytes. At the site of infection the neutrophils ingest the foreign material and destroy it using their battery of toxic molecules. Inevitably some of the neutrophils die and release their contents. This leads to tissue damage and the production of more chemotactic factors. Monocytes arrive on the scene, kill any remaining microorganisms, remove debris and initiate the repair process.

Phagocytosis. Phagocytosis involves (1) recognition and binding, (2) ingestion and (3) digestion. It may occur in the absence of antibody, especially on surfaces such as those of the lung alveoli and when inert particles are involved. Cell membranes carry a net negative charge that keeps them apart and stops autophagocytosis. The fact that they are composed of a lipid bilayer that must be kept intact necessitates special mechanisms to allow particles to enter. The hydrophilic nature of certain bacterial cell wall components stops them passing through the hydrophobic membrane. To overcome these difficulties the phagocytes have receptors on their surface that mediate the attachment of particles that have been coated with the correct ligand. Phagocytes have receptors for the Fc portion of certain immunoglobulin isotypes (see Ch. 4) and for some components of the complement cascade (discussed above). The presence of these molecules or **opsonins** on the particle surface markedly enhances the ingestion process and in some cases digestion (Fig. 2.7). Whether mediated by specific receptors or not, the foreign particle is surrounded by the cell membrane which then invaginates and produces an **endosome** or **phagosome** within the cell (Fig. 2.8).

The microbicidal machinery of the phagocyte is contained within organelles known as **lysosomes**. This compartmentalization of potentially toxic molecules is necessary to protect the cell from self-destruction and produce an environment where the molecules can function efficiently. The phagosome and lysosome fuse to form a **phagolysosome** in which the ingested material is killed and digested by various enzyme systems.

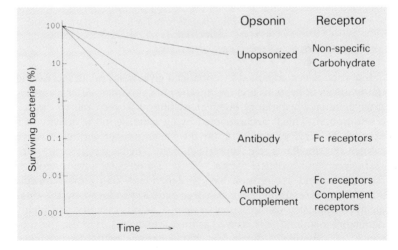

Fig. 2.7 Opsonizing activity of antibody and complement.
Unopsonized bacteria are phagocytosed slowly, possibly by non-specific mechanisms or via carbohydrate recognition molecules present on the phagocyte. Specific antibody on the surface of the foreign material can be recognized by Fc receptors on the phagocyte. This will increase adherence of the foreign particle and its subsequent ingestion and destruction. The presence of both antibody and complement components on the particle greatly increases its removal by phagocytes and can also stimulate greater intracellular killing.

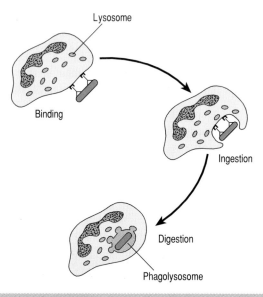

Fig. 2.8 Stages in phagocytosis.
Once attracted to the site of infection by chemoattractants the phagocyte, in this case a neutrophil, binds the foreign particle and ingestion is initiated. The binding will be mediated by receptors on the phagocyte surface. The offending material is internalized into a membrane-bound vacuole, the phagosome, that has budded off from the plasma membrane. The phagosome fuses with lysosomes and microbicidal chemicals are released into the newly formed phagolysosome where digestion takes place.

Ingestion is accompanied by enhanced glycolysis and an increase in the synthesis of proteins and membrane phospholipids. After phagocytosis there is a respiratory burst consisting of a steep rise in oxygen consumption. This is accompanied by an increase in the activity of a number of enzymes and leads to the generation of various reactive oxygen intermediates, e.g. superoxide anion, hydrogen peroxide, singlet oxygen and hydroxyl radical. All these molecules have microbicidal activity and are termed oxygen-dependent killing mechanisms. The superoxide anion, O_2^-, is a free radical produced by the one-electron reduction of molecular oxygen. It is very reactive and highly damaging to animal cells, as well as microorganisms. It is also the substrate for superoxide dismutase that generates hydrogen peroxide, H_2O_2, for subsequent use in microbial killing. Myeloperoxidase uses hydrogen peroxide and halide ions, such as iodide or chloride, to produce at least two bactericidal systems. In one, halogenation (incorporation of iodine or chlorine) of the bacterial cell wall leads to death of the organism. In the second mechanism, myeloperoxidase and H_2O_2 damage the cell wall by converting amino acids into aldehydes that have antimicrobial activity.

Recently a new antimicrobial mechanism has been described in rodent macrophages — the production of reactive nitrogen intermediates. Macrophages are able to use L-arginine as a source of nitrogen with molecular oxygen and NADPH to generate various nitrogen oxides that are toxic to microorganisms, protozoan parasites and tumour cells.

A number of oxygen independent mechanisms are also present within phagocytes that are capable of destroying ingested material. Some of these are enzymes that can damage membranes. For example, lysozyme and elastase attack peptidoglycan of the bacterial cell wall and then hydrolases are responsible for the complete digestion of the killed organism. The cationic proteins, defensins, in lysosomes bind to and damage bacterial cell walls and enveloped viruses, such as herpes simplex virus. The iron-binding protein, lactoferrin, has antimicrobial properties. It complexes with iron rendering it unavailable to bacteria that require iron for growth. The high acidity within phagolysosomes (pH 3.5–4.0) may have bactericidal effects; it probably results from lactic acid production in glycolysis. In addition, many lysosomal enzymes, such as acid hydrolases, have acid pH optima. There are significant differences between macrophages and neutrophils in the killing of microorganisms. Although macrophage lysosomes contain a variety of enzymes, including lysozyme, they lack cationic proteins and lactoferrin. Tissue macrophages do not have myeloperoxidase but probably use catalase to generate the hydrogen peroxide system. Normal macrophages are less efficient killers of certain pathogens, such as fungi, than neutrophils. The microbicidal activity of macrophages can, however, be greatly improved after contact with products of lymphocytes, known as lymphokines (see later).

Once killed, most microorganisms are digested and solubilized by lysosomal enzymes. The degradation products are then released to the exterior.

Natural killer cells

Viruses can only replicate within host cells; therefore it is advantageous to eliminate infected cells before progeny virus is released. Natural killer cells (NK cells) recognize changes on virus-infected cells and destroy them by an extracellular killing mechanism. After binding to the target cell, by an as yet undefined mechanism, the NK cell produces molecules that damage the infected cell's membrane, leading to its destruction.

Natural killing can be performed by a number of different cell types. This activity has been shown to be carried out by cells described as large granular lymphocytes and also by cells with T-cell markers, macrophage markers and others that do not have the characteristics of any of the main cells of the immune system. Natural killing is present without prior exposure to the infectious agent and shows all the characteristics of an innate defence mechanism. NK cells have also been implicated in host defence against cancers. They are thought to recognize changes in the cell membranes of transformed cells in a mechanism similar to that used to combat virus infection. Recent observations suggest that NK cells might selectively kill cells that express low levels of MHC class I molecules. Natural killing is enhanced by interferons α and β which appear to stimulate the production of NK cells and also increase the rate at which they kill the target cells. Interleukin-12, a monokine produced early in many infections, acts in synergy with tumour necrosis factor α (TNFα), also a monokine, to stimulate NK cells to release large amounts of interferon-γ. This production of interferon-γ by NK cells probably plays a critical role in controlling many infections before T-lymphocytes have been activated to produce this important cytokine.

A number of cell types that usually destroy target cells in a specific fashion can be induced to kill non-specifically if exposed to high levels of lymphokines that usually control their differentiation and maturation. The cells are usually referred to as lymphokine activated killer (LAK) cells.

Eosinophils

Eosinophils are polymorphonuclear leucocytes with a characteristic bilobed nucleus and cytoplasmic granules. They are present in the blood of normal individuals at very low levels (< 1%) but their numbers increase in patients with parasitic infections and allergies. They are not efficient phagocytic cells but their granules contain molecules that are toxic to parasites, e.g. major basic protein and eosinophil cationic protein. Large parasites such as helminths cannot be internalized by phagocytes and therefore must be killed extracellularly. Eosinophil granules contain an array of enzymes and toxic molecules that are active against parasitic worms. The release of these molecules must be controlled so that tissue damage can be avoided. The eosinophils have specific receptors, including Fc and complement receptors, that bind the labelled target, i.e. antibody- or complement-coated parasites. The granule contents are then released into the space between the cell and the parasite thus targeting the toxic molecules onto the parasite membrane.

Temperature

The temperature dependence of many microorganisms is well known and tubercle bacilli, pathogenic for mammalian species, will not infect cold-blooded animals. Conversely, the mycobacteria parasitic on cold-blooded animals, e.g. *Mycobacterium marinum*, cannot cause deep or systemic infections in humans. Fowl which are naturally immune to anthrax can be infected if their temperature is lowered. Gonococci and treponemes are readily killed at temperatures over 40°C and fever therapy was used in chronic gonococcal infections and cerebral syphilis before the advent of antibiotics. The neisseriae and treponemes are also susceptible to temperatures around freezing. The smallpox virus, which has a temperature ceiling of around 38.5°C grows mainly in the cooler skin, causing a rash, during the febrile phase of the infection. However, it grows internally, probably in the respiratory tract, during the afebrile incubation period.

It is therefore apparent that temperature is an important factor in determining the innate immunity of an animal to some infectious agents. It seems likely that the pyrexia (increased temperature) that follows so many different types of infection can function as a protective response against the infecting microorganism. The febrile response in many cases is controlled by a molecule that is produced as part of the immune response. Endogenous pyrogen, now known to be the macrophage product interleukin-1, is responsible for the increase in temperature. It is produced following infection and acts either directly or through the stimulation of prostaglandin synthesis on the temperature regulatory centre of the hypothalamus.

Inflammation

A number of the above factors are responsible for the process of inflammation. This is the body's reaction to injury such as the invasion by an infectious agent, exposure to a noxious chemical or physical trauma. The signs of inflammation are redness, heat, swelling, pain and loss of function. The molecular/cellular events that occur during an inflammatory reaction are (1) vasodilation, (2) increased vascular permeability and (3) cellular infiltration. These changes are brought about mainly by chemical mediators (Table 2.1) that are widely distributed in a sequestered or inactive form throughout the body and are released or activated locally at the site of inflammation. After release they tend to be rapidly inactivated to ensure control of the inflammatory process.

There is increased blood supply to the affected area due to the action of vasoactive amines, such as histamine and 5-hydroxytryptamine, and other mediators stored within mast cells. These molecules are released (a) as a consequence of the production of the anaphylatoxins (C3a and C5a) that trigger specific receptors on mast cells and (b) following interaction of antigen with IgE on the surface of mast cells or (c) by direct physical damage to the cells. Other mediators, such as bradykinins and prostaglandins, are produced locally or released by platelets. The vasodilation causes increased blood supply to the area giving rise to **redness** and **heat**. There is therefore an increase in the supply of the molecules and cells that can combat the agent responsible for the initial trigger.

The same molecules, vasoactive amines, prostaglandins and kinins, increase vascular permeability allowing plasma and plasma proteins to traverse the endothelial lining. The plasma proteins will include immunoglobulins and molecules of the clotting and complement cascades. This leaking of fluid will cause **swelling** (oedema) that will in turn lead to increased tissue tension and **pain**. Some of the molecules themselves, e.g. prostaglandins and histamine, stimulate the pain responses directly. The inflammatory exudate has several important functions. Bacteria often produce tissue-damaging toxins that will be diluted by the exudate. Clotting factors present result in the deposition of fibrin creating a physical obstruction to the spread of bacteria. The exudate is continuously drained off by the lymphatic vessels, and antigens, such as bacteria and their toxins, are carried

Table 2.1 **Mediators of inflammation**

Mediator	Main source	Function
Histamine[*]	Mast cells, basophils	Vasodilation, increased vascular permeability, contraction of smooth muscle
Kinins (e.g. bradykinin)	Plasma	Vasodilation, increased vascular permeability, contraction of smooth muscle, pain
Prostaglandins	Neutrophils, eosinophils, monocytes, platelets	Vasodilation, increased vascular permeability, pain
Leukotrienes	Neutrophils, mast cells, basophils	Vasodilation, increased vascular permeability, contraction of smooth muscle, induce cell adherence and chemotaxis
Complement component (e.g. C3a, C5a)	Plasma	Cause mast cells to release mediators C5a is chemotactic factor
Plasmin	Plasma	Break down fibrin, kinin formation
Cytokines	Lymphocytes, macrophages	Chemotactic factors, colony stimulation factors, macrophage activation

[*] In rodents 5-hydroxytryptamine (serotonin) is present in mast cells and basophils.

to the draining lymph node where immune responses can be generated.

Chemotactic factors produced at the site of tissue injury, including C5a, histamine, leukotrienes and molecules specific for certain cell types, will attract phagocytic cells. The increased vascular permeability will allow easier access for neutrophils and monocytes and the vasodilation means that more cells are in the vicinity. The neutrophils will arrive first and begin to destroy/remove the offending agent. Most will be successful but a few will die, releasing their tissue-damaging contents to increase the inflammatory process. Mononuclear phagocytes will arrive on the scene to finish off the removal of the residual debris and stimulate tissue repair.

When the swelling is severe there may be loss of function to the affected area. If the offending agent is quickly removed then the tissue will soon be repaired and back to its original state. The inflammatory process continues until the conditions responsible for its initiation are resolved. In most circumstances this occurs fairly rapidly with an acute inflammatory reaction lasting a matter of hours or days. If, however, the causative agent is not easily removed or is reintroduced continuously then chronic inflammation will ensue, with the possibility of tissue destruction and complete loss of function.

FURTHER READING

Brown E J 1994 Phagocytosis. Bioessays 17: 109–117

Colonna M 1996 Natural killer cell receptors specific for MHC class I molecules. Current Opinion in Immunology 8: 101–107

Gallagher R B (ed) 1991 A special issue: The biology of complement. Immunology Today 12: 291–342

Lyons C R 1995 The role of nitric oxide in inflammation. Advances in Immunology 60: 323–371

Morhenn V B 1988 Keratinocyte proliferation in wound healing and skin disease. Immunology Today 9: 104–107

Müller-Eberhard H J 1988 Molecular organisation and function of the complement system. Annual Review of Biochemistry 57: 321–347

Rotrosen D, Gallin J I 1987 Disorders of phagocyte function. Annual Review of Immunology 5: 127–150

Scott P, Trinchieri G 1995 The role of natural killer cells in host–parasite interactions. Current Opinion in Immunology 7: 34–40

Wardlaw A J, Moqbel R, Kay A B 1995. Eosinophils: Biology and role in disease. Advances in Immunology 60: 151–266

3 Antigens and antigen recognition

Historically an antigen is any material capable of provoking the lymphoid tissues of an animal to respond by generating an immune reaction specifically directed at the inducing agent and not at other unrelated substances. Complex structures, like bacteria and viruses, as well as single molecules can act as antigens but the response is not to the entire structure but to individual chemical groups that have a specific three-dimensional shape. The specificity of the response for these **antigenic determinants** or **epitopes** is an important characteristic of immune responses. With some antigens the host might respond to only a few epitopes present on a small fraction of the molecules that make up the foreign material. As long as this reaction generates molecules and cells that can protect the host then the immune response will have been effective. The reaction of an animal to contact with antigen, called the **acquired immune response,** takes two forms: (1) the **humoral** or **circulating antibody response** and (2) the **cell-mediated response.** Most of the information available on the specificity of the immune response comes from studies of the interaction of circulating antibody with antigen. An antibody directed against an epitope of a particular molecule will react only with this determinant or other very similar structures. Even minor chemical changes in the conformation of the epitope will markedly reduce the ability of the original antibody to react with the altered material.

Antibody binds directly to structures on the surface of an antigen that have a three-dimensional shape complementary to the binding site of the antibody. Cell-mediated reactions are also directed against sites within antigens. The main effector cells in this type of response, T-lymphocytes, possess a receptor (known as the T-cell receptor) that will bind to a complementary shape generated from an antigen. T-cells are stimulated by fragments of foreign material presented to them by molecules present on the surface of host cells. The T-cell receptor recognizes both the antigen fragment and the self-structure to which it is bound. Therefore, T-lymphocytes recognize small pieces of foreign material attached to host cell surface molecules.

The term antigen, referring either to substances acting as stimulants of the immune response or to substances reacting with preformed antibody, is used rather loosely by immunologists. Use is made of the functional classification of antigens into: (1) substances which are able to generate an immune response by themselves and are termed **immunogens** and (2) molecules which are able to react with antibodies but are unable to stimulate their production directly. The latter substances are often low molecular weight chemicals, termed **haptens,** that will react with preformed antibodies but only become immunogenic when attached to large molecules, called **carriers** (Fig. 3.1). The hapten forms an epitope on the carrier molecule that is recognized by the immune system and stimulates the production of antibody. In other words, the ability of a chemical grouping to interact with an antibody is not enough to stimulate an immune response. As we will see later, when discussing the sites on molecules recognized by antibody, all antigens can be considered to be composed of haptens, i.e. the parts that actually interact with immunoglobulin, on larger carrier structures.

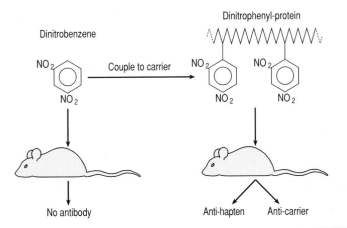

Fig. 3.1 Hapten and carrier.
Dinitrobenzene on its own is a hapten, i.e. it will not induce antibody production. When this chemical group is linked to a larger molecule, the carrier, antibodies will be produced that react with the hapten. In addition, antibodies will be produced to carrier determinants since the larger protein is immunogenic on its own.

General properties of antigens

A substance that acts as an antigen in one species of animal may not do so in another because it is represented in the tissues or fluids of the second species. This underlines the requirement that the antigen must be a foreign substance to elicit an immune response. For example, egg albumin, whilst an excellent antigen in rabbits, fails to induce an antibody response in fowls. The more foreign, evolutionarily distant, a substance is to a particular species the more likely it is to be a powerful antigen.

A widely recognized requirement for a substance to be antigenic in its own right, without having to be attached to a carrier molecule, is that it should have a molecular weight in excess of 5000. It is, however, possible to induce an immune response to substances of lower molecular weight. For example, glucagon (mol. wt. 3800) can stimulate antibody production but only if special measures are taken such as the use of an adjuvant (Ch. 4) which gives an additional stimulus to the immune system. Very large proteins, such as the crustacean respiratory pigment haemocyanin, are very powerful antigens and have been widely used in experimental immunology. Polysaccharides vary in antigenicity, for example dextran of mol. wt. 600 000 is a good antigen, whereas dextran of mol. wt. 100 000 is not. Yet these two materials are made up of identical building blocks and do not differ as far as the type of antigenic determinant is concerned.

Some low molecular weight chemical substances appear to contradict the requirement that an antigen be large. Among these are included picryl chloride, formaldehyde and drugs such as aspirin, penicillin and sulphonamides. These substances are highly antigenic, particularly if applied to the skin. The reason for this appears to be that such materials form complexes by means of covalent bonds with tissue proteins. The complex of these substances, acting as haptens, with a tissue protein, acting as a carrier, forms a complete antigen. This phenomenon has important implications in the development of certain types of hypersensitivity (Ch. 9).

Antigenic determinants

The immune system does not recognize an infectious agent or foreign molecule as a whole but reacts to structurally distinct areas — the antigenic determinants or epitopes. Thus exposure to a microorganism will generate an immune response to many different epitopes (Fig. 3.2A). The antiserum produced will contain different antibodies reactive with each determinant. This will ensure that an individual will be protected from the microorganism by producing a response to at least a few of the possible determinants. If the host only reacted to the organism as a whole then failure to react to this one site would have

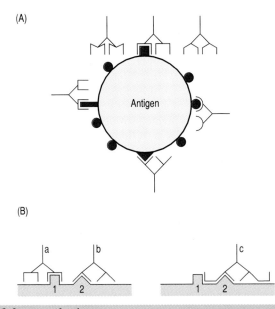

Fig. 3.2 Structure of antigens.
(A) Foreign material, antigen, will contain a mosaic of structures formed from its chemical constituents that can induce an immune response. Antibodies, with a complementary shape, will be formed that combine specifically with these epitopes on the antigen. Some of the epitopes may be unique but others (●) will be present as multiple copies. Certain epitopes (■) will stimulate the production of various antibodies, the three shown at the top, that combine with different strengths depending on the ease of fit. (B) Two epitopes (1 and 2) on an antigen induce the formation of three antibodies (a, b and c). Antibody a combines specifically with epitope 1 and antibody b with epitope 2. Antibody c recognizes an epitope composed of residues from epitopes 1 and 2. Since antibody c interacts with these overlapping residues it will compete with antibodies a and b for binding.

dire consequences, i.e. it would not be able to eliminate the pathogen. Certain antibodies may react with an epitope composed of residues that can also be part of two other epitopes recognized by different antibodies (Fig. 3.2B).

A response to antigen involves the specific interaction of components of the immune system, antibodies and lymphocytes, with epitopes on the antigen. The lymphocytes have receptors on their surface that function as the recognition units — on B-lymphocytes surface-bound antibody acts as receptors and on T-lymphocytes the recognition unit is the T-cell receptor. The interaction between an antibody (or cell-bound receptor) and antigen is governed by the complementarity of the electron cloud surrounding the determinants. The overall configuration of the outer electrons, not the chemical nature of the constituent residues, determines the shape of the epitope and its complementary **paratope** (part of the antibody or T-cell receptor that interacts with the epitope). The better the fit between the epitope and the paratope the stronger the non-covalent bonds formed and consequently the higher the affinity of the interaction.

Antigenic determinants have to be topographical, i.e. composed of structures on the surface of molecules or cells, and can be constructed in two ways. They may be contained within a single segment of primary sequence or assembled from residues far apart in the primary sequence but brought together on the surface by the folding of the molecule into its native conformation. The former are known as **sequential** epitopes and those formed from distant residues are **conformational** epitopes.

Gell and Benacerraf studied the immune response to protein antigens. The antibodies produced were specific for the form of antigen used for immunization (native vs. denatured). Antibodies formed against a native antigen react only with native antigen while antibodies produced by immunizing with denatured antigen only bind to the denatured form. However cell-mediated, i.e. T-cell, responses with identical specificities can be elicited equally well with either form of antigen. Thus the antigenic structures seen by antibody depend on the tertiary configuration of the immunogen (conformational), while epitopes seen by T-cells are defined by primary structure (sequential).

Antigenic specificity

Foreignness of a substance to an animal can depend on the presence of chemical groupings that are not normally found in the animal's body. Arsenic acid, for example, can be chemically introduced into a protein molecule and, as a hapten, acts as a determinant of antigenic specificity of the molecule. This type of chemically defined determinant enabled Karl Landsteiner early in this century to study antigenic specificity in fine detail. By a slight chemical modification of the antigenic determinant he was able to demonstrate how critical and precise was the fit between antibody and an antigenic determinant (Fig. 3.3). Thus, changes as minor as the replacement in the benzene ring of an SO_3H group by a COOH or an AsO_3H_2 group were sufficient to affect substantially the ability of the determinant to react with antibody to the original hapten.

There are many other examples which have validated Landsteiner's classical studies including experiments with simple sugars coupled to proteins. The antisera, produced by immunizing animals, were found to be able to distinguish between glucose and galactose which differ only by the interchange of H and OH on one carbon atom.

The ability of antibody (or T-cell receptors) to form a high affinity

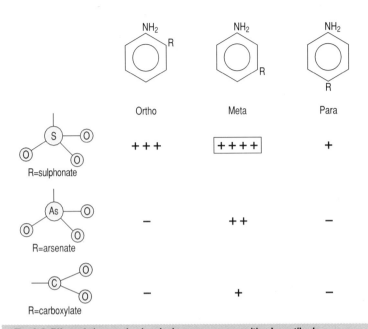

Fig. 3.3 Effect of changes in chemical groups on recognition by antibody.
Variations in the position and nature of chemical substituents of a hapten affect the strength
of binding to an antiserum raised against m-aminobenzene sulphonate. Antibodies react
most strongly with the immunizing antigen (shown by box), i.e. the sulphonate group in the
meta position, but will give a weaker cross-reaction with sulphonate in the ortho position.
Still weaker reactions occur with substitutions of arsenate and carboxylate groups.
Therefore, the overall shape of the epitopes is as important as the individual chemical
groupings. Strength of binding: more +s stronger binding; − no binding.

interaction with an antigen depends on intermolecular forces which
act strongly only when the two molecules come together in a very precise manner. The better the fit, the stronger the bond. An antibody
molecule directed against a particularly shaped antigenic determinant
might be able to react with another similar but not quite identical
determinant as shown in Figure 3.4A. This type of cross-reaction does
occur but the strength of the bond between the two molecules will be
diminished in the case of the less well fitting determinant.

A common source of confusion with respect to the specificity of
antibodies arises when an antibody to a particular antigen is found to
be capable of combining with an apparently unrelated antigen. For
example, an antibody that binds to a glucose determinant in antigen
X-glucose would be likely to react with the glucose group in antigen
Y-glucose provided the two determinants are equally accessible. The
antibody directed against the glucose determinant is not a non-specific

(A)

(B)

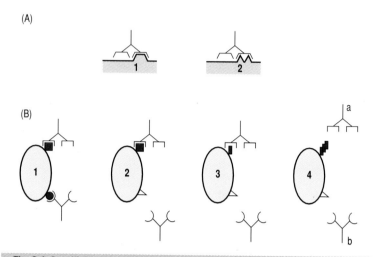

Fig. 3.4 Specificity and cross-reactions.
(A) The same antibody is able to combine with two distinct epitopes (1 and 2). The antibody was produced in response to an antigen that contained epitope 1 but the antibody will also combine with epitope 2 (and hence the antigen on which it is found). The strength of the binding will depend on how well the epitope fits the paratope and on the summation of the attractive forces and degree of repulsion. Best fit and most attraction for 1, therefore strongest interaction, i.e. higher affinity. (B) The original antigen, 1, induced the production of an antiserum containing antibodies a and b. This antiserum will cross-react with antigen 2 because it shares an epitope (■) with antigen 1. Antigen 3 has an epitope that is similar but not identical to the same epitope on antigen 1, therefore there is also cross-reaction between the antiserum and antigen 3. There is no structural similarity between antigen 4 and antigen 1 so antigen 4 does not react with the antiserum. The antiserum will react most strongly with 1 > 2 > 3 and not with 4.

type of antibody but is simply reacting with an identical chemical determinant, epitope, in another antigen molecule (cf. Fig. 3.4B).

In laboratory practice cross-reactivity is often found between antisera to certain bacterial antigens and antigens present on cells such as erythrocytes. Antigens shared in this way are known as **heterophile antigens.** Antibodies to such antigens will cross-react with cells or fluids of different species of animal and with various microorganisms. The chemical determinants responsible for this cross-reactivity are not known but are presumed to be similar or identical groupings, possibly mucopolysaccharide or lipid in nature, present in molecules which are part of the structure of the cells. The best known of the heterophile antigens is the Forssman antigen which is present on the red cells of many species as well as in bacteria such as pneumococci and salmonellae. Another heterophile antigen is found in *Escherichia coli* and human red cells of blood group B individuals. These cross-reactivities are probably responsible for the generation of antibodies found in individuals of a certain blood group that bind to the red blood cells of individuals of a different blood group. These antibodies are known as **isohaemagglutinins** because they are able to bind the red blood cells and clump them together, i.e. cause agglutination (Ch. 6).

IMMUNOGLOBULINS

Towards the end of the nineteenth century Von Behring and Kitasato in Berlin found that the blood serum of an appropriately immunized animal contained specific neutralizing substances or antitoxins. This was the first demonstration of the activity of what are now known as **antibodies** or **immunoglobulins**. Antibodies are glycoproteins that bind specifically to the antigen that induced their formation. They are produced when immunogenic molecules enter the host's lymphoid system and are present in the blood plasma, body fluids and attached to the surface of certain cell types. The terms antibody and immunoglobulin are interchangeable.

The liquid collected from blood that has been allowed to clot is known as **serum**. It contains a number of molecules but no cells or clotting factors. If serum is prepared from an animal that has been exposed to an antigen then it is known as an **antiserum** since it will contain antibodies reactive with the inducing antigen. When the components of serum are separated electrophoretically due to differences in their charge then the heterogeneity of immunoglobulins can be seen, i.e. they appear as broad bands (Fig. 3.5). This technique separates serum components into various fractions; most of the antibody molecules are present within the gamma-globulin fraction and have sometimes been referred to as gamma-globulins.

There are five distinct **classes** or **isotypes** of immunoglobulins, namely IgG, IgA, IgM, IgD and IgE. They differ from each other in size, charge, carbohydrate content and, of course, amino acid composition (Table 3.1). Within certain classes there are subclasses that show slight differences in structure and function from other members of the class. These classes and subclasses can be separated from each other serologically, i.e. using antibody. If injected into the correct species they will induce the formation of antibodies that can be used to differentiate between the different isotypes.

Antibody structure

All antibody molecules have the same basic four chain structure composed of two light chains and two heavy chains (Fig. 3.6). The light chains (mol. wt. 25 000) are one of two types designated kappa (κ) and lambda (λ) and only one type is found in one antibody. The heavy chains vary in molecular weight from 50 to 75 kD and it is these chains

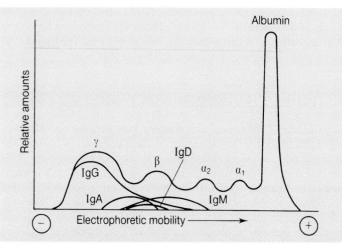

Fig. 3.5 Separation of serum proteins by electrophoresis.
Serum proteins applied to a solid support are separated according to their charge in an electric field. They are classified on the basis of their mobility as α_1, α_2, β and γ. IgG shows most charge heterogeneity. IgE has a similar mobility to IgD but it cannot be distinguished because of its low level in normal serum.

Table 3.1 Physicochemical properties of human immunoglobulins. The immunoglobulin isotype is determined by the type of heavy chain present. The different characteristics observed are also controlled by the heavy chain. Variation within a class gives rise to subclasses.

	Immunoglobulin isotype				
Characteristic	IgA	IgD	IgE	IgG	IgM*
Mean serum concentration (mg/dl)†	300	5	0.005	1400	150
Molecular weight (kD)	160	184	188	160	970
Carbohydrate (%)	7–11	9–14	12	2–3	12
Half-life (days)	6	3	2	21	5
Heavy chain	α	δ	ϵ	γ	μ

* Data for IgM as a pentamer
† dl = 100 ml

IgA is also found as a dimer and in secretions IgA is present in dimeric form associated with a protein known as secretory component.

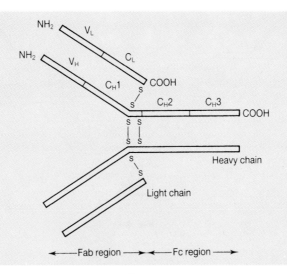

Fig. 3.6 Basic structure of an immunoglobulin molecule.
The basic structure is common to all classes of immunoglobulin and consists of two identical light polypeptide chains and two identical heavy chains linked together by disulfide bonds (S–S). The orientation of the carboxyl- (COOH) and amino- (NH$_2$) terminal ends of the chains are shown. The heavy and light chains are divided into variable (V) and constant (C) regions or domains of about 110 amino acids. These are known as V$_L$, and C$_L$, for the light chain and V$_H$, C$_H$1, C$_H$2, etc. for the heavy chain.`

that determine the isotype. The chains are held together by disulfide bridges and non-covalent interactions.

When individual light chains were studied it was found that they were composed of two distinct areas or **domains** of approximately 110 amino acids (Fig. 3.7). One end of the chain was found to be identical in all members of the same isotype and is termed the constant domain of the light chain, C$_L$. The other end shows considerable sequence variation and is known as the variable domain, V$_L$. The heavy chains are also split into domains of approximately the same size, the number varying between the five types of heavy chain. One of these domains will show considerable sequence variation (V$_H$) while the others (C$_H$) are similar for the same isotype. The tertiary structure generated by the combination of the V$_L$ and V$_H$ domains determines the shape of the antigen-combining site or paratope. Since the two light and two heavy chains are identical, each antibody unit will have two identical paratopes, situated at the amino-terminal end of the molecule, that recognize the antigen. The carboxyl end of the antibody will be the same for all members of the same class or subclass and is involved in the biological activities of the molecule.

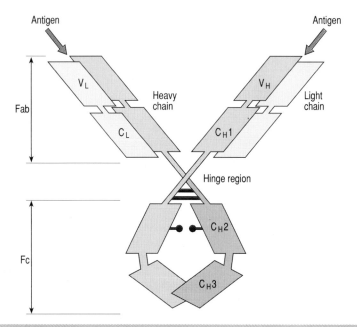

Fig. 3.7 Immunoglobulin domains.
The basic immunoglobulin chains fold into globular domains. All domains are stabilized by intrachain disulfide bonds. There are also interchain disulfide bonds between the light and heavy and between the two heavy chains (latter shown as black bars). The number of disulfide bonds varies with different classes and subclasses. For example, IgG$_3$ has at least 14 disulfide bonds linking the heavy chains and therefore has an extremely long hinge region. Various other non-covalent interactions hold the equivalent domains of the light and heavy chains together. The close apposition of the C$_H$3 domains and separation of the C$_H$2 domains are thought to be important in allowing the chains to interact with each other. The carbohydrate (━●) found in the C$_H$2 domain is necessary for the proper functioning of the antibody. It appears to act by keeping the C$_H$2 domains apart thus allowing the others to interact correctly. The arrow indicates where antigen is bound.

The area of the heavy chains between the C$_H$1 and C$_H$2 domains contains a varying number of interchain disulphide bonds and is known as the **hinge region**. A number of enzymes cleave immunoglobulins at distinct points to generate different peptide fragments (Fig. 3.8). These have been used to study the structure and function of immunoglobulins and generate useful reagents. The sites of cleavage of pepsin are to the carboxyl side of the hinge. This enzyme generates a single F(ab')$_2$ fragment, containing two paratopes joined at the hinge, and a number of small peptides from the Fc portion. Papain cleaves the molecule in the hinge region to generate two identical Fab fragments, each containing a paratope, and a single Fc fragment.

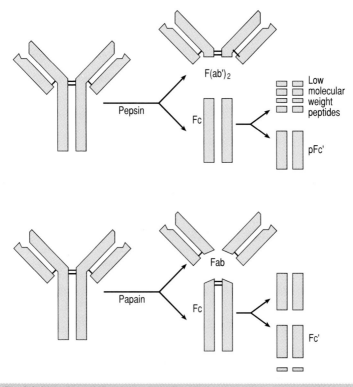

Fig. 3.8 Digestion of IgG with pepsin and papain.
Pepsin cleaves the heavy chain at the carboxyl-terminal side of the hinge region disulphide bonds. This generates a large fragment, F(ab')₂, containing two paratopes and a number of small peptides including the pFc' fragment. Treatment with papain splits the heavy chain on the amino-terminal side of the interchain disulphide bonds of the hinge region. This yields two identical Fab (antigen binding) fragments and the Fc (crystallizable) fragment. Secondary action on the Fc gives rise to Fc'.

IgG

This is the major immunoglobulin of serum making up 75% of the total and having a molecular weight of 150 000 D in humans. The molecule is composed of a single basic unit with γ heavy chains (Fig. 3.9). Four subclasses are found in humans — IgG_1, IgG_2, IgG_3 and IgG_4 — that differ in their relative concentrations, amino acid composition, number and position of interchain disulfide bonds and biological function. IgG is the major antibody of the secondary response (see Ch. 4) and is found in both the serum and tissue fluids.

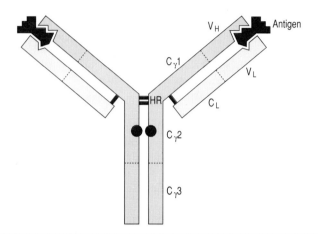

Fig. 3.9 Structure of IgG.
A simple model of IgG$_1$ showing the various domains of the light and heavy chains. The association of the V$_H$ and V$_L$ domains forms the antigen binding site into which the complementary epitope will fit. The position of the carbohydrate is shown by the black circles and disulphide bonds that join the chains are depicted by black bars. In all IgG molecules there is a hinge region (HR) between the C$_\gamma$I and C$_\gamma$2 domains.

IgA

In humans most of the serum IgA occurs as a monomer but in many other mammals it is mostly found as a dimer. The dimer is held together by a J chain which is produced by the antibody-producing plasma cells. IgA is the predominant antibody class in seromucous secretions such as saliva, tears, colostrum and respiratory, gastrointestinal and genitourinary secretions. This secretory IgA (sIgA) is always in the dimeric form and is composed of two basic four-chain units (two light chains and two α heavy chains), a J chain and the secretory component (Fig. 3.10). The secretory component is the part of the molecule that transports the dimer produced by a submucosal plasma cell to the mucosal surface (Fig. 3.11). It not only facilitates passage through the epithelial cells but protects the secreted molecule from proteolytic digestion. There are two subclasses of IgA — IgA$_1$ and IgA$_2$.

IgM

IgM is a pentamer of the basic unit with μ heavy chains that are composed of five domains (Fig. 3.12). The five basic units are held together by disulphide bonds between their C$_\mu$3 domains, and the complete pentamer also contains a single J chain. Because of its large size this isotype is mainly confined to the intravascular pool and is the first antibody type to be produced during an immune response.

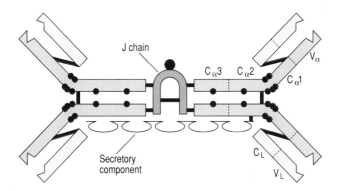

Fig. 3.10 Structure of secretory IgA.
In the dimeric form two IgA molecules are joined together by a J chain. The secretory component is held in place by non-covalent interactions and by a disulphide bond (black bar) to the $C_\alpha 2$ domain. Disulphide bonds also join the light chain to the heavy chain, hold the two heavy chains together and link the J chain to the two IgA monomers. The positions of carbohydrate residues are shown by black circles.

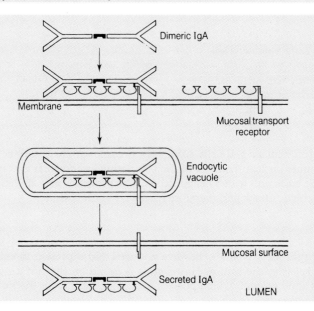

Fig. 3.11 Transport of secretory IgA.
Mucosal cells produce a receptor (also known as poly Ig receptor) that is inserted into the membrane at the basal surface. Dimeric IgA, with attached J chain, produced by sub-mucosal plasma cells becomes covalently attached to the receptor and is transported via an endocytic process to the mucosal surface. A membrane protease cleaves the complex leading to the release of IgA with a portion of the receptor, the secretory component, still attached.

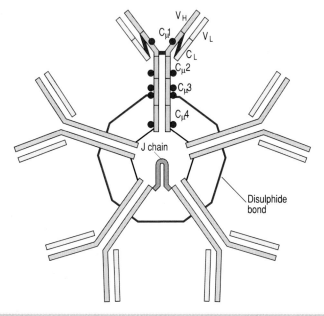

Fig. 3.12 Structure of IgM.
The polymeric form of IgM consists of five monomer subunits joined by disulphide bridges linking adjacent $C_\mu 3$ and $C_\mu 4$ domains. A J chain is also present. There is no hinge region in the subunits. The position of the carbohydrate is shown by black circles.

IgD

Many circulating B-cells have IgD present on their surface but it accounts for less than 1% of the circulating antibody. It is composed of the basic unit with δ heavy chains. The protein is very susceptible to proteolytic attack and therefore has a very short half-life.

IgE

The IgE heavy chain, ε, has five domains and is present in extremely low levels in the serum. However, it is found on the surface of mast cells and basophils which possess a receptor specific for the Fc part of this molecule.

Antigen binding

Despite the different characteristics of the various isotypes, as shown in Table 3.1, all antibody molecules are composed of the same basic unit structure with the Fab portion containing the antigen-recognizing paratope and the Fc region carrying out the activities that protect the host, i.e. effector functions. The diversity seen in the Fc region between the various heavy chains is responsible for the different biological activities of the antibody isotypes. However, the amino acid sequences found within the variable domains, i.e. parts responsible for binding antigen, of different antibody molecules exhibit considerable diversity.

The variability in amino acid sequence in the V domains of light and heavy chains is not spread evenly over their entire length but is restricted to short segments. These segments show considerable variation and are termed **hypervariable regions** (Fig. 3.13). Hypervariable regions are now known to contain the residues that make direct contact with the antigen and are referred to as **comple-**

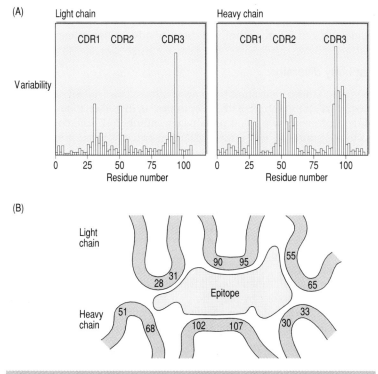

Fig. 3.13 Positions of complementarity determining regions.
(A) The degree of variability found at each residue in the variable domain in a number of different antibodies is plotted against the amino acid residue number from the N-terminus. The analysis of both light and heavy chain variable domains is shown. Three hypervariable regions are found on each chain and are referred to as complementarity determining regions (CDR). (B) The tertiary structure of the variable domains forms the CDRs in the paratope which forms the contact points with the epitope of the antigen.

mentarity determining regions (CDR). Although the remaining **framework** residues do not come into direct contact with the antigen, they are essential for the formation of the correct tertiary structure of the V domain and maintenance of the integrity of the binding site. In both light and heavy chains there are three CDRs which, in combination, form the paratope.

The antigen and antibody are held together by various individually weak non-covalent interactions. However, the formation of a large number of hydrogen bonds and electrostatic, van der Waals and hydrophobic interactions leads to a considerable binding energy. These attractive forces are only active over extremely short distances and therefore the epitope and paratope must have complementary structures to enable them to combine. If the electron clouds overlap or residues of similar charge are brought together then repulsive forces will come into play. The balance of attraction against repulsion will dictate the strength of the interaction between an antibody and a particular antigen, i.e. the affinity of the antibody for the antigen.

Antibody diversity

It is now known that an antigen selects from the available antibodies those that can combine with its epitopes. It therefore follows that an individual must have an extremely large number of different antibodies to cope with the vast array of different antigens present in the environment. It has been estimated that more than 10^{11} different combining sites can be produced. There are not enough genes in a cell for each antibody molecule to have its own unique set of genes. In addition, it must be remembered that half of each light and a quarter of each heavy chain are variable but the rest is constant for a particular isotype. The solutions to these problems have been worked out over the last two decades. The genes for the light and heavy chains are composed of coding exons separated by non-coding (silent) introns. A relatively small number of different germ line genes are present with the variable domain coded for by separate gene segments. The diversity is increased by somatic mutation and by introducing variable recombinations when the complete antibody variable exon is being assembled. Each constant domain is coded for by a different exon.

Immunoglobulin variability

The paratope is produced by the CDRs of the light and heavy chains generating a specific three-dimensional shape. Any light chain can join with any heavy chain to produce a different paratope. Thus theoretically with 10^5 different light chains and 10^5 different heavy chains 10^{10} different specificities could be generated. To understand how a small number of variable genes can give rise to the observed diversity the structure of the genetic material must be studied.

The germ line DNA is the structure of the gene as it is inherited, i.e. in the sperm or ovum. All cells in the body contain all the inherited genes but various genes become active in different cells at different times — some genes only become active in certain cells, i.e. immunoglobulin genes in B-lymphocytes. Antibodies are produced by B-lymphocytes and therefore the structure of the immunoglobulin genes within these cells as they develop reveals how antibody diversity is generated.

Light chain genes. Light chains are composed of two domains, C_L and V_L. The structure of the constant region will determine if the light chain will be κ or λ and the primary amino acid sequence of the variable domain dictates its antigen specificity.

The genes for the κ chain are on chromosome 2 in humans. In cells not producing antibodies the gene segments that form the complete light chain are separate (Fig. 3.14). Even in a fully differentiated B-lymphocyte the V_κ and C_κ gene segments are not joined together. Between the V and C gene segments and joined to the V gene segment is a small section of DNA known as the J gene segment.

In humans, there are about 100 V_κ and 5 J_κ gene segments associated with a single C_κ gene segment. As the B-cell develops a DNA rearrangement takes place to bring a V_κ and J_κ gene segment together. If this V–J joining is successful in producing a variable exon that can give rise to a functional product then this is the structure present in the mature B-cell. If no product could be formed, e.g. due to the generation of a stop codon, then the V_κ and J_κ gene segments on the other chromosome can be used. The intervening DNA has been deleted in this process. The rearranged DNA will then be transcribed into a large primary transcript known as heterogeneous nuclear mRNA. Mature mRNA will be formed after splicing out the non-coding regions, i.e. introns, and any extra gene segments between the variable and constant exons. Translation of this mRNA will generate a κ light chain where the V domain is formed from the V and J gene segments. Two CDRs will have come from the V gene segment and the third generated at the site of V–J joining. Therefore, the combination of different V_κ and J_κ segments will generate different antigen-combining sites. Thus the number of possible κ light chains is at least 500 (100 × 5). The same V gene segment associating with different J gene segments will also give two different paratopes but might recognize similar epitopes since they share two CDRs.

A similar mechanism for generating diversity applies to the λ light chains (Fig. 3.15). In the germ line configuration there are more than 100 V_λ gene segments and there are 6 functional J_λ gene segments each associated with its own C gene segment. As with κ the first event is V–J joining to give a functional variable exon. After transcription

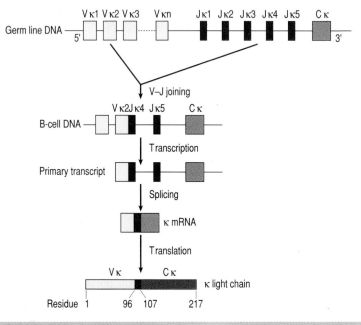

Fig. 3.14 Production of kappa chains.
The exon coding for the variable domain of a κ light chain is generated during B-cell differentiation by the joining together of a V$_\kappa$ and a J$_\kappa$ gene segment. This V–J joining is brought about by complementary base sequences 3' to V pairing with sequences 5' to J. In the mature B-cell the rearranged V exon is still separate from the C region gene segment. All that has been deleted is the part between the selected V and J segments. The final joining occurs when the intervening intron is spliced out of the primary mRNA transcript. Two CDRs are coded for in the V gene segment and the third is generated at the junction of V and J gene segments. Residues 1–95, 96–106 and 107–217 are coded for by V, J and C gene segments respectively. The κ genes are present on chromosome 2 in humans and 6 in mice. Dashed lines show parts that contain other gene segments.

and splicing this gives rise to mRNA that can be translated into a functional γ light chain.

Heavy chain genes. The heavy chain V domain is generated by the same mechanisms as outlined for the light chain. In addition to the V and J gene segments there are D gene segments (Fig. 3.16). In humans there are 12 germ line D gene segments together with 100–200 V$_H$ gene segments and 6 functional J$_H$ gene segments. The rearrangements take place in a defined order: a D gene segment joins with a J gene segment and then a V gene segment is joined. Again two CDRs are coded for in the V$_H$ segment and the site of the third is generated by the combination of V, D and J.

Once a functional V$_H$ exon has been constructed from the V, D and

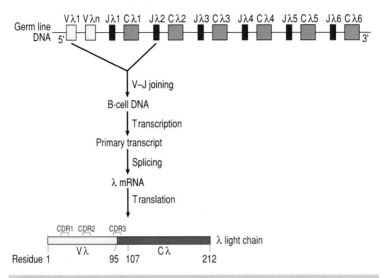

Fig. 3.15 Production of lambda chains.
The λ genes are present on chromosome 22. During B-cell development the exon coding for the variable domain is formed by the joining of a V_λ and a J_λ gene segment. A primary transcript is produced that contains the VJ gene segment separated from the associated C_λ gene segment by an intron. The primary transcript is then spliced to bring the exons together and the mRNA is translated into the final product. In the λ light chain, residues 1–95 are coded for by the V segment, the J gene segment codes for residues 96–106 and residues 107–212 come from the C gene segment. The positions of the three CDR are also indicated.

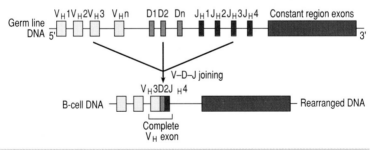

Fig. 3.16 Generation of functional heavy chain variable exons in the mouse.
The genes for the heavy chain are on chromosome 12. The exon coding for the V_H domain is produced by the recombination of a V_H, D and J_H gene segment. In humans, the heavy chain locus is on chromosome 14. Dashed lines show parts that contain other gene segments.

J gene segments on one chromosome then rearrangements of the gene segments on the other chromosome are inhibited. This is known as **allelic exclusion.** Allelic exclusion also acts on light chain genes which are also restricted to the production of only one isotype per cell, i.e. **light chain isotype exclusion.** This ensures that one particular cell, and its progeny, will produce antibody with a single specificity.

Thus the mature B-cell has a rearranged heavy chain with a complete V_H exon, composed of V_H, D and J_H gene segments, upstream of the C_H gene segments. The light chain will be produced from either a successfully rearranged κ or γ gene.

Additional diversity. The random joining together of any V with any D and any J gene segments gives a vast number of possible combinations (Table 3.2). However, in addition to this, the exact place where these recombinations occur can vary. In certain cases **imprecise joining** will result in the formation of a modified codon and the subsequent insertion of a different amino acid (Fig. 3.17). This has increased importance when it is remembered that V–J and V–D–J joining produce one of the CDRs. There is also evidence that additional random nucleotides can be inserted between D and J_H, and between V_H and D. These non-template insertions are known as **N region additions** and are catalysed by the enzyme terminal deoxyribonucleotidyl transferase. Again the amino acid changes that occur will be to residues forming the third CDR and could therefore affect the antibody specificity.

Table 3.2 Diversity in immunoglobulin (Ig) and T-cell receptor (TCR) genes. TCR has fewer germ line V gene segments but a much greater junctional diversity.

Mechanism	Ig		TCR		TCR	
	H	κ	α	β	γ	δ
V gene segments	100–250	100	75	75	8	4
Diversity in V gene segments	H × κ 10 000–25 000		α × β 5625		γ × δ 32	
D gene segments	10	0	0	2	0	2*
D read in cell frames	rarely	—	—	often	—	often
J gene segments	6	5	75	12	5	3
N-region additions	V–D D–J	—	V–J	V–D D–J	V–J	V–D D–D D–J
Potential using all mechanisms†	10^{11}		10^{16}		10^{18}	

* In all δ chains more than one D gene segment can be included.
† Somatic mutations not included.

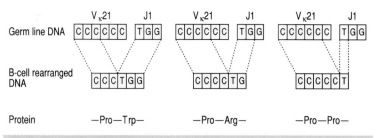

Fig. 3.17 Variable recombination.
The same V_κ and J_κ gene segment can produce three different amino acid sequences when they are joined at different nucleotides. This imprecise joining gives rise to changes in residues 95 and 96 of the κ chains produced. Since these form part of the third CDR they could alter the three-dimensional shape of the paratope and, therefore, its binding characteristics. In this example, the last complete codon from the V gene segment gives rise to a proline (Pro) residue but the next amino acid can be tryptophan (Trp), arginine (Arg) or proline (Pro) depending on where the joining takes place. Imprecise joining is also seen when D to J_H and V_H to DJ_H recombinations occur and in λ light chain rearrangements.

The substitution of one nucleotide for another can lead to a mutation, i.e. a change, in the final protein. In cells that are growing and dividing rapidly, such as antibody-producing plasma cells, this becomes more likely. There is evidence that the gene segments for the variable domains of immunoglobulins are particularly susceptible to somatic mutations. This can lead to subtle changes in specificity and/or affinity that are important as an immune response develops (see Ch. 4).

Therefore, we have a number of mechanisms to generate antibody diversity (Table 3.3). Multiple germ line variable gene segments combine with J and D gene segments. There are inaccuracies in these recombination events that generate the part of the protein that contains the third complementarity determining region. Somatic point

---

Table 3.3 Generation of antibody diversity. During the production of the V gene segment all of these mechanisms can occur.

---

1. Multiple germ line V gene segments
2. V–J and V–D–J recombinations
3. Junctional diversity a. imprecise joining
                                  b. N-region additions
4. Somatic mutation
5. Assorted heavy and light chain combinations

mutations occur introducing additional variation in specificity. Finally, since any light chain can associate with any heavy chain, diversity is increased enormously.

Heavy chain constant region genes

A particular plasma cell and its progeny will produce different classes of antibody as an immune response develops (see Ch. 4). However, the same variable exon generated by V–D–J joining will be used. All that is altered, or **switched,** is the heavy chain constant region. The gene segments that code for the different types of heavy chain are arranged downstream from the J_H gene segments (Fig. 3.18). Various switch sequences present 5′ to each gene segment control the recombination processes that mediate class switch.

The first primary transcripts to be produced as a B-cell develops, after V–D–J joining, contain the exon for V_H and the exons for the constant region domains of μ and δ (Fig. 3.19). These products are differentially spliced to give initially μ mRNAs which will be translated into μ heavy chains. These products will combine with light chains to give IgM molecules which are inserted into the plasma membrane. The next stage in the differentiation process of the B-cell involves splicing other primary transcripts to give δ mRNAs containing the same V_H exon as the μ mRNAs but with the C_H exons for a δ heavy chain. The δ heavy chains produced from this message will combine with the light chains to give membrane-bound IgD. Since the IgM and IgD molecules contain the same V_H and V_L domains they will have

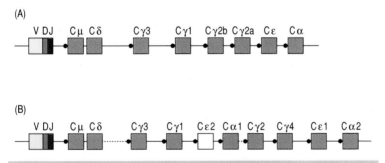

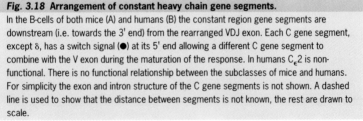

Fig. 3.18 Arrangement of constant heavy chain gene segments.
In the B-cells of both mice (A) and humans (B) the constant region gene segments are downstream (i.e. towards the 3′ end) from the rearranged VDJ exon. Each C gene segment, except δ, has a switch signal (●) at its 5′ end allowing a different C gene segment to combine with the V exon during the maturation of the response. In humans $C_\varepsilon 2$ is non-functional. There is no functional relationship between the subclasses of mice and humans. For simplicity the exon and intron structure of the C gene segments is not shown. A dashed line is used to show that the distance between segments is not known, the rest are drawn to scale.

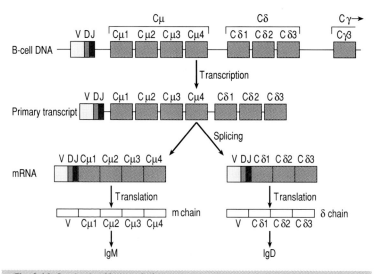

Fig. 3.19 Synthesis of heavy chains.
The V exon has been constructed from V, D and J gene segments as the B-cell develops and is now proximal to the constant region gene segments. The initial RNA produced contains the sequences coding for V_H, C_μ and C_δ still separated by introns. This primary transcript is then spliced to give two different mRNA products both with the same V_H. One has V_H joined to C_μ, and in the other V_H and C_δ are adjacent. Translation of the former will give a μ heavy chain and the latter gives δ heavy chains. The two heavy chains can then combine with the light chain produced by the cell to give IgM and IgD respectively. The differential splicing is controlled by sequences known as poly-A tails (a number of adenosine molecules joined together) but the exact mechanism is unknown.

identical paratopes and therefore bind to the same epitope. When first stimulated by antigen the B-cell will initially secrete IgM in a pentameric form. As the immune response develops the class of antibody being produced changes. There are further DNA rearrangements resulting in the bringing together of a different constant region gene segment to the original V_H exon and the elimination of intervening DNA with its μ and δ heavy chain gene segments (Fig. 3.20). Thus the progeny of a single B-cell will produce different immunoglobulin isotypes as the response to a particular antigen develops but each will have the same paratope.

Secreted and membrane immunoglobulins

At different stages in its development a B-cell will produce immunoglobulins that have to be inserted into the membrane or secreted. The membrane-bound immunoglobulin will be used as the B-cell's antigen receptor and a cell that binds antigen through this

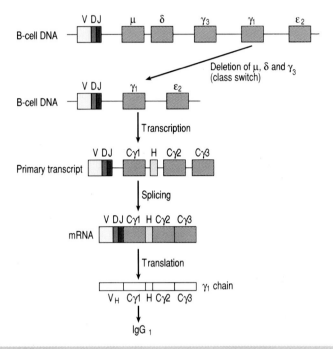

Fig. 3.20 Isotype switching.

A single B-cell can produce different isotypes as an immune response develops. During maturation different constant region gene segments can be brought close to the VDJ \ segment. This process is controlled by T-cell factors and involves recognition through switch sequences. In this example the γ_1 gene segment is positioned next to the complete V_H exon. This process results in the deletion of the intervening gene segments, i.e. μ, δ and γ_3. A primary transcript is produced from this rearranged DNA that is then spliced to give mRNA with the original V_H exon joined directly to the exon coding for the γ_1 constant domains. The mRNA is then translated into γ_1 heavy chains that can combine with light chains to give IgG_1. The exons present within the γ_1 gene segment are shown in the primary transcript.

molecule will then secrete immunoglobulin of the same specificity. The only difference between the two types of antibody is to be found at the carboxyl terminus (Fig. 3.21). The transcript that directs the production of the membrane form has an additional part to code for the transmembrane portion.

Antibody function

Knowledge gained from the structural studies discussed above has gone some way towards an understanding of the biological activities of the immunoglobulin molecule. It is now possible to pinpoint areas of the molecule responsible for different activities.

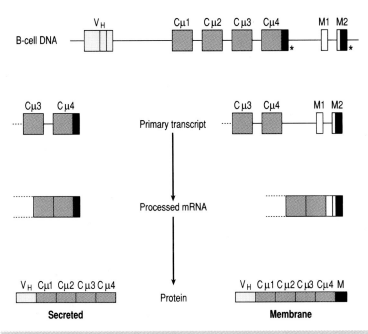

Fig. 3.21 Secreted and membrane IgM.
In the B-cell DNA two exons (M) are found 3' to the last heavy chain constant domain exon. These exons code for the transmembrane portion of membrane immunoglobulin. There are also two translation stop signals (black boxes) and two possible poly-adenylation sites (*). If the second poly-adenylation site is used (right-hand side in figure) a primary transcript is produced that includes both membrane exons. During modification of the primary transcript MI is spliced to a site within $C_\mu 4$ exon to remove the stop signal. In this example, translation of this mRNA will give rise to membrane IgM. The secreted form is produced by using the first poly-adenylation site and the stop codon adjacent to the $C_\mu 4$ exon. Similar membrane exons are found adjacent to the heavy chain gene segment for each isotype.

The primary function of an antibody is to bind the antigen that induced its formation. Apart from cases where this results in direct neutralization (e.g. inhibition of toxin activity or of microbial attachment), other effector functions must be generated. The binding of antigen is mediated by the Fab portion and the Fc region controls the biological defence mechanisms. For every antibody the paratope will be different and it will therefore recognize different epitopes. However, for every antibody of the same isotype the heavy chain constant domains will be the same and they will therefore all perform the same functions (Table 3.4).

Neutralization

The fact that antibodies are at least divalent means that they can

Table 3.4 Biological properties of human immunoglobulins. These activities are determined by the Fc portion of the molecules.

Function	IgA	IgD	IgE	IgG$_1$	IgG$_2$	IgG$_3$	IgG$_4$	IgM
Complement fixation	±*	−	−	++	+	+++	−	+++
Placental transfer	−	−	−	+	±	+	+	−
Binding to phagocytes	±†	−	−	+++	±	+++	+	−
Binding to mast cells	−	−	+++	−	−	−	+	−

* IgA will activate alternative pathway.
† Receptors for Fc portion of IgA have been found on neutrophils and alveolar macrophages.

form a complex with a multivalent antigen. Depending on the physical nature of the antigen these **immune complexes** exist in various forms (Fig. 3.22). If the antibody is directed against surface antigens of particulate material, such as microorganisms or erythrocytes, then **agglutination** will occur. This is a clump or aggregate that will isolate the potential pathogen, stop its dissemination and stimulate its removal by other mechanisms. If the antigen is soluble then the size of the complex will determine its physical state. Small complexes will remain soluble while large complexes will form **precipitates.**

As might be expected from knowledge of the structure of IgM, its 10 combining sites make it a very efficient agglutinating antibody molecule. Rabbit IgM has been shown to be more than 20 times as active as IgG (mole for mole) in bringing about bacterial agglutination. Because of its large size IgM is largely confined to the bloodstream and probably plays an important role in protecting against blood invasion by microorganisms. Agglutination of microorganisms will reduce the number of separate infectious units and limit their spread. For small microbes, clumping the particles into a larger mass may help in recognition and therefore elimination. Certain sites on microorganisms are critical to the establishment of an infection. Antibody bound to these sites will interfere with attachment processes and could, therefore, stop infection by the microbe. The binding of an antibody to functionally important residues in a toxin or other virulence factor will neutralize their harmful effects. Antibodies attached to structures that have a role in nutrient transport or motility will help kill and eradicate the foreign material.

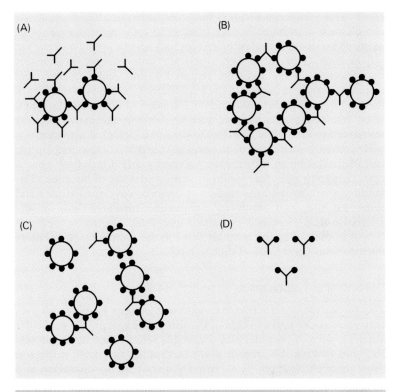

Fig. 3.22 **Immune complex formation.**
The composition of an immune complex is dictated by the valency of the antigen and the antibody. (A) In antibody excess, the epitopes are saturated and small complexes are formed. (B) At equivalence, a large lattice is formed that will clump or agglutinate a particulate antigen. A soluble antigen will be precipitated, i.e. come out of solution, due to changes in size and alterations in solute interactions. (C) In antigen excess, the paratopes of the antibody become saturated and small complexes form. (D) With a monovalent antigen crosslinking by antibody is not possible.

Complement activation

The activation of the complement system is one of the most important antibody effector mechanisms. The complement cascade is a complex group of serum proteins that mediate inflammatory reactions and cell lysis. It is discussed more fully in Chapter 2. The Fc portion of certain isotypes (Table 3.4), once antigen has been bound, will activate complement. Activation requires that C1q, a subunit of the first complement component, crosslinks two antibody Fc portions. For this to happen the two Fc regions must be in close proximity. It has been calculated that a single IgM molecule attached to a red cell can bring about lysis whereas 1000 IgG molecules are required for the same effect. This is because two IgG molecules must be close together for complement activation. A large number of IgG molecules would be required for this to occur as the epitopes are spread evenly over the red cell surface. Not all isotypes activate complement, presumably because they do not have the required amino acid sequence, and therefore tertiary structure, in the Fc portion. C1q binds to residues in the C_H3 domain of IgM and the C_H2 domain of IgG. Some isotypes, when interacting with antigen, can activate the alternative pathway that does not use C1 but gives rise to the same biological activities.

By combining with microbes, antibody can activate the complement cascade, inducing an inflammatory response that brings fresh phagocytes, antibody and other serum proteins to the site of infection. The binding of antibody to the surface of bacteria, enveloped viruses and some parasites can result in complement-mediated lysis of the microorganism. Host cells expressing microbial antigens on their surface as a result of an infection are lysed in the same way, often before the infectious agent has had time to replicate.

Cell binding and opsonization

The Fc portion of certain immunoglobulin isotypes is able to interact with various cell types (Table 3.4). Antibodies specific for particular antigens, such as bacteria, play a valuable role by binding to the surface and making the antigen more susceptible to phagocytosis and subsequent elimination. This process is known as **opsonization** and is again mediated by the Fc portion of the antibody. A specific conformation on the Fc region of certain isotypes is recognized by **Fc receptors** on the surface of the phagocyte. The important residues are in the C_H2 domain near the hinge region. Individually the interactions are not strong enough to signal the uptake of the antibody molecule, therefore free immunoglobulin is not internalized. However, when an antigen is coated by many antibody molecules then the summation of all the interactions stimulates phagocytosis or other effector mechanisms.

Certain phagocytic cells have receptors for activated complement components, **complement receptors.** If the binding of antibody to the antigen can activate the complement cascade then various complement components will be deposited on the antigen/antibody complex. Phagocytic cells that have receptors for these complement components will then ingest the complexes.

Certain cells are able to kill microorganisms, parasites and infected cells by a process known as antibody-dependent cell-mediated cytotoxicity (ADCC). The so-called killer cells have a Fc receptor that recognizes antibody bound to the foreign material or infected host cell. The target cell is too large to be engulfed and the effector cell releases toxic molecules into the space between itself and the bound target.

The above-mentioned processes require that the antibody is first complexed with antigen before they can occur. However, certain cell types will bind free antibody. Mast cells and basophils have Fc receptors that are specific for IgE. These cells perform a protective function by inducing an inflammatory response but are also involved in hypersensitivity reactions, described in Chapter 9. In human beings, IgG has the ability to cross the placenta and reach the fetal circulation. This is a passive mediated process involving specific Fc receptors. This route is limited to primates whereas in ruminants immunoglobulin from colostrum is absorbed through the intestinal epithelium. Another Fc-mediated mechanism, already described, is found for IgA, which is selectively transported into mucosal secretions by the poly Ig receptor of mucosal epithelial cells (Fig. 3.11).

Genetic markers on antibodies

Immunoglobulins are glycoproteins and can behave as antigens if injected into the correct host, i.e. antibodies will be made against epitopes on the immunoglobulin. The parts of the immunoglobulin that the immune system reacts against will depend on the species used to generate the antibody. The type of epitope that these anti-immunoglobulins recognize is given a specific name depending on its position on the molecule (Fig. 3.23).

Antibodies that detect variations between the different classes of immunoglobulin define the **isotype.** The residues that are recognized will be on the constant portions of the heavy and light chains. These anti-isotypic antibodies will be produced by injecting the immunoglobulin of one species into another. Antibodies can also be generated that differentiate between the various subclasses of IgG and IgA.

Allotypes are differences that exist between members of the same species. Allotypic markers are also found on the constant regions of heavy and light chains. The sequences recognized do not appear to influence the activity of the immunoglobulin as marked differences in

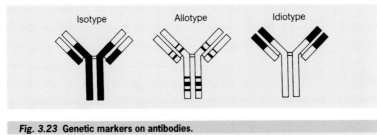

Isotype   Allotype   Idiotype

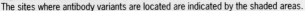

Fig. 3.23 **Genetic markers on antibodies.**
The sites where antibody variants are located are indicated by the shaded areas.

function between allotypes have not been found. These markers can be used to identify the products, present in the offspring of hybrids or chimeras, that were coded for by the different parents or donors.

The variable regions of immunoglobulin molecules exhibit, as described above, immense structural variation. The immune system of the host or a different individual or species can recognize these variations and the antibodies generated are known as anti-idiotypic antibodies. Each immunoglobulin variable domain contains a number of epitopes that stimulate the production of anti-idiotypic antibodies (Fig. 3.24). Each epitope is known as an **idiotope** and the collection of idiotopes on an immunoglobulin determines its **idiotype**.

Thus each immunoglobulin produced by an individual is capable of stimulating the production of other immunoglobulins, anti-idiotypic antibodies, and a network of interaction is generated within the individual. This process was first described by Neils Jerne and may have a role in the regulation of immune responses (see Ch. 4). Included in the network hypothesis is an important premise that has applications in other areas such as vaccine development. When an antigen is introduced the host will respond by producing specific immunoglobulin. This immunoglobulin will then stimulate the production of anti-idiotypic antibodies and so on. In Figure 3.25 it can be seen that some of these anti-idiotypic antibodies have a paratope that is similar in shape

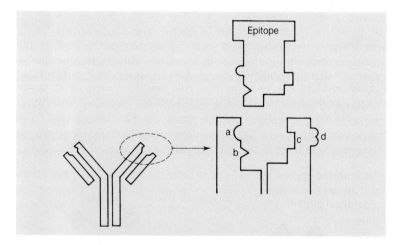

Fig. 3.24 **Antibody variable domains.**
Within the antibody variable region, shown by ellipse and in enlarged form, there are structures that can be recognized by other antibody variable regions. These determinants are known as idiotopes. In this figure some idiotopes (a, b and c) are located within the paratope (paratope associated) and d is outwith the antigen-combining site (paratope non-associated). The collection of idiotopes is referred to as the idiotype of the antibody.

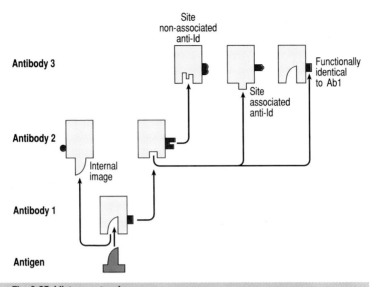

Fig. 3.25 Idiotype network.
Antigen induces an antibody (antibody 1) expressing a number of paratope associated and paratope non-associated idiotopes. These idiotopes are recognized by a set of anti-idiotypes (antibody 2) that in turn stimulate anti-anti-idiotypic antibodies (antibody 3). In this limited network one of the antibody 2 molecules mimics the original epitope and is, therefore, its internal image. Some of the antibody 3 population may be identical to antibody 1 (some antibody 4 will be identical to antibody 2). This interconnecting network may involve any part of the antibody variable domains and include interactions between parts outwith the paratope.

to the antigen that triggered the process. This antibody is known as the **internal image** and this molecule could be used to vaccinate against agents that are otherwise too difficult or dangerous to obtain.

ANTIGEN RECOGNITION

The immune system has evolved to protect us from potentially harmful material but it must not respond to self molecules. Two separate recognition systems are present that allow this to occur efficiently — humoral immunity and cell-mediated immunity. Antibody is the recognition molecule of humoral immunity. This glycoprotein is produced by plasma cells and circulates in the blood and other body fluids. Antibody is also present on the surface of B-lymphocytes. The interaction of this surface immunoglobulin with its specific antigen is responsible for the differentiation of these cells into plasma cells. Antibody molecules whether free or on the surface of a B-cell will recognize free native antigen. This contrasts dramatically with the situation in cell-mediated immunity. The T-lymphocyte antigen receptor will only bind to fragments of antigen that are associated with products of the major histocompatibility complex (MHC). T-cell recognition of antigen is said to be **MHC restricted.** These MHC products are present on the surface of cells, therefore T-cells only recognize cell-associated antigens. This MHC restricted recognition mechanism has evolved because of the functions carried out by T-lymphocytes. Some T-cells produce immunoregulatory molecules, **lymphokines,** some of which influence the activities of host cells and others that directly kill infected or foreign cells. Therefore, it would be inefficient or dangerous to produce these effects in response to either free antigen or antigen sitting idly on a cell membrane. The joint recognition of MHC molecules and antigen ensures that the T-cell makes contact with antigen on the surface of the appropriate target cell. Indeed it is important to remember that we have immunoglobulins that are capable of eliminating free antigens.

B-cell receptor

Antibody is found free in body fluids and as a transmembrane protein on the surface of B-lymphocytes, i.e. surface immunoglobulin, where it acts as the B-cell antigen receptor. The antibody present on the surface of the B-cell is exactly the same molecule as will be secreted when the cell develops into a plasma cell except for the extreme C-terminal end as described above (Fig. 3.21). It should be noted that the molecules present on the cell surface are present as monomers even though they are secreted in a polymeric form. The surface immunoglobulin is associated on the cell membrane with a number of other molecules that are thought to be involved in signal transduction leading to cell activation.

T-cell receptor

The complex on T-lymphocytes that is involved in antigen recognition is composed of a number of glycoproteins. Some of these molecules have been systematically named by CD (cluster of differentiation) nomenclature using antibodies. These generic names will be used in preference to the other symbols sometimes found in the literature since the molecules have various designations in different species.

The T-cell antigen receptor (TCR), also known as Ti, is a heterodimer composed of an α and a β, or a γ and a δ chain. The majority of human T-cells (~95%) use the $\alpha\beta$ heterodimer in antigen recognition. The role of cells that possess the $\gamma\delta$ molecules is unknown but they may be involved in the immune response to particular types of antigens at specific anatomical sites. The two glycoprotein chains that form the T-cell receptor are linked together by

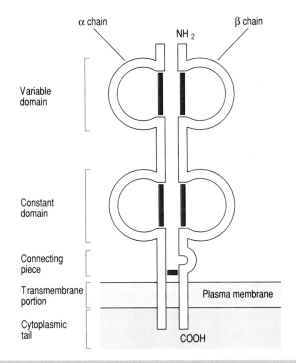

Fig. 3.26 Schematic representation of the T-cell receptor heterodimer.
The constituent glycoprotein chains, in this case α and β, fold into two immunoglobulin-like domains with intrachain disulphide bonds (black box). The N-terminal domain has a similar structure to an immunoglobulin variable (V) domain and the other is like an immunoglobulin constant (C) domain. A disulphide bond in the connecting piece joins the two chains together. The rest of the molecule is composed of a transmembrane portion and a cytoplasmic tail.

disulphide bonds (Fig. 3.26). These molecules are structurally similar to immunoglobulin, having a variable and a constant region. Within these regions, domains are present that fold into a secondary structure with many of the characteristics of immunoglobulin variable and constant domains. A number of other molecules, many involved in immune recognition, show similar structures and are members of the immunoglobulin superfamily (see p. 82).

The V region forms a domain that contains the antigen-binding site of the T-cell receptor. The C region contains four areas. The most amino-terminal portion forms an immunoglobulin constant-like domain with an intrachain disulphide bond. There is a short hinge or connecting peptide, a transmembrane portion with many hydrophobic amino acids and a short cytoplasmic tail. The transmembrane portion contains positively charged amino acid residues which appear to be involved with the interaction of the T-cell receptor with other membrane components.

The T-cell receptor is the molecule that is responsible for the recognition of specific MHC/antigen complexes and will be different for every T-cell. Therefore, as for antibody, there are mechanisms for the generation of diversity. In humans, the α genes are on chromosome 14 and are arranged in a similar way to the antibody light chain genes (Fig. 3.27). There are about 100 V_α segments, around 100 J_α segments and a single C_α gene segment. On chromosome 7 the β variable gene segments are orientated in a similar manner to that found for the antibody heavy chain gene. There are between 75 and 100 V_β, 2 D_β and about 14 J_β gene segments upstream of two C_β gene segments. The γ chain locus, on chromosome 13, is similar to the λ light chain locus with two functional C_γ segments, each associated with two to three J_γ segments, and eight known V_γ segments. The δ chain locus is found between V_α and J_α. There are four V_δ, three J_δ, two D_δ and a single C_δ gene segment.

Genetic rearrangements of these multiple germ line gene segments, similar to those seen in B-cells, is necessary before a functional T-cell receptor can be produced. The β chain locus rearranges prior to the α locus, with the joining of D_β and J_β as the first step. This is followed by the formation of a complete V exon (VDJ gene segments joined

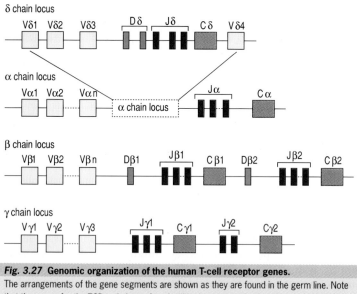

Fig. 3.27 Genomic organization of the human T-cell receptor genes.
The arrangements of the gene segments are shown as they are found in the germ line. Note that the genes for the TCR δ chain are found within the α locus. Dashed lines show parts that contain other gene segments.

together) and allelic exclusion occurs if the V exon formed is functional. Production of a β gene product stimulates rearrangements at the α locus where the V exon is formed by the joining of a V_α and a J_α gene segment. The primary nuclear transcript of the T-cell receptor genes contains the V and C exons separated by an intron. As with immunoglobulin genes this large RNA is processed to give mRNA that is then translated into the final product. In some developing T-cells the γ chain locus rearranges first and cells with a γδ T-cell receptor develop. In this case some kind of silencer molecule is produced to stop rearrangements at the α and β loci. When α gene segments are rearranged the δ locus is spliced out since it is found within this region of DNA. Imprecise joining and N-region additions (discussed above for immunoglobulins) add to the diversity of structures that can be generated. In addition, more than one D_β and D_δ gene segment can be used.

There are many fewer V gene segments for the T-cell receptor compared to those present in the immunoglobulin loci. Since the first two CDRs are present within the V gene segment this suggests that there will be less diversity in these areas of the T-cell receptor compared to immunoglobulin (Table 3.2). However, there is great potential to develop variation in the amino acid sequence of the third CDR because of the large contribution to diversity generation by imprecise joining, N-region additions and the use of multiple D gene segments in T-cells. This imbalance in diversity between CDR1/CDR2 and CDR3 may be important in T-cell recognition. The T-cell binds antigen fragments associated with MHC molecules, its receptor interacting with both the antigen fragment and MHC molecule. It is thought that the CDR1/CDR2 portion, which exhibits less diversity, might interact with the MHC molecule, and the CDR3 with the antigen fragment.

A number of processes associated with the production of immunoglobulins do not operate in T-cells.

As an immune response develops, the class of antibody produced by the plasma cell changes, i.e. class switch. This allows for the production of different isotypes that have different effector functions or tissue distribution. The effector function performed by a particular T-cell is governed by the specificity of its cell surface molecules for different ligands, e.g. CD4 or CD8 binding to MHC molecules, and these do not change. In a number of species γδ T-cells show specific tissue distribution but there is no mechanism to change T-cell receptor types as an immune response develops.

During an immune response genes for the variable portion of immunoglobulin undergo somatic hypermutations. These give rise to antibody molecules with an altered primary sequence. The B-cells that now produce an antibody with greater affinity for the antigen will be preferentially selected and are partly responsible for what is known as affinity maturation (see Ch. 4). The recognition of antigen by T-cells involves joint recognition of antigen and MHC molecules. As T-cells develop in the thymus a selection process occurs (see Ch. 4) to ensure that the cells that are produced have specificity for self MHC molecules and also do not destroy self components. If T-cells were allowed to mutate their T-cell receptor genes after they left the thymus they might lose their MHC binding capacity or become self-reactive.

By differential splicing of the primary nuclear transcript of the immunoglobulin heavy chain gene, secretory or membrane immunoglobulin can be produced. This is because antibody has two functions: (1) to activate the B-cell when membrane-bound and (2) in secreted form to carry out effector activities. In T-cells the receptor acts as the recognition molecule and the cell is responsible for the effector functions. Production of a secreted T-cell receptor would produce a molecule with no protective role.

The T-cell receptor heterodimer gives specificity for antigen recognition to the T-cell but other cell membrane molecules are needed for T-cells to function. The CD3 complex (T3 in humans) is present on all T-cells and has a constant structure. It is composed of four non-covalently associated polypeptide chains (γ, δ, ϵ and ζ) and may also transiently associate with another peptide termed eta (η) (Fig. 3.28). The constituent molecules have a negative charge in their transmembrane portion. These are thought to be important in the association of the complex with the T-cells receptor which has positively charged residues in the corresponding region. The CD3 complex is thought to be involved in signal transduction. Residues present in the cytoplasmic domain are susceptible to phosphorylation which is a commonly used activation signal.

CD4 and CD8 are mutually exclusive molecules. They are present on T-cells that are restricted in their recognition of antigen by MHC class II and class I molecules, respectively. CD4 is a monomeric transmembrane glycoprotein that folds into four extracellular immunoglobulin-like domains. CD8 is a disulphide-linked dimer. Each chain has a N-terminal immunoglobulin-like domain, a non-immunoglobulin-like domain, a transmembrane portion and a cytoplasmic tail. Due to their almost exclusive correlation with a specific MHC class it is thought that these molecules bind to non-polymorphic determinants on the MHC molecules. This interaction could stabilize the binding of the T-cell receptor to the MHC/antigen complex or it may in fact have a co-receptor function. In the former case the CD4 or CD8 molecule could interact with the same MHC molecule as the TCR or with a different one, and this interaction does not generate a stimulatory signal, i.e. it solely stabilizes the specific interaction (TCR with antigen/MHC). In the latter case the T-cell receptor and CD4 or CD8 bind to the same MHC molecule but at different sites and the joint signal that is generated leads to the stimulation of the T-cell. T-cells that have an

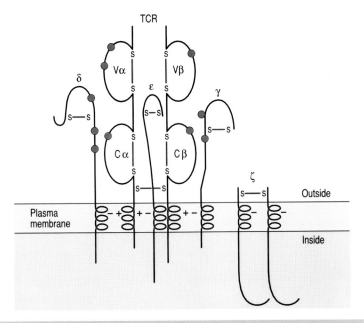

Fig. 3.28 T-cell receptor/CD3 complex.
The CD3 complex is closely associated with the T-cell receptor (TCR). A signal generated by the binding of ligand to the TCR is thought to be transmitted across the plasma membrane. The TCR heterodimer may relay this signal through the invariant CD3 proteins. CD3 is composed of at least 4 transmembrane proteins, gamma (γ), delta (δ), epsilon (ϵ) and zeta (ζ). In this schematic representation the TCR/CD3 complex is shown using the TCR α and β peptides and the non-covalently associated CD3 molecules. Disulphide bonds (S–S) and glycosylation sites (●) are shown. In immature T-cells in the thymus an eta chain (η) may replace one of the zeta chains.

$\alpha\beta$ receptor possess CD4 or CD8 while only a few $\gamma\delta$ T-cells have been shown to be CD8$^+$ and none appear to have the CD4 molecule.

A number of other adhesion molecules also appear to be involved in the interaction between the T-cell and its target. These molecules, including CD2 (leucocyte function-associated antigen-2: LFA-2) and CD 11b/CD18 (LFA-1), are responsible for mediating the initial interaction between the T-cell and other cells but will contribute nothing to the specificity of the interaction. CD2 interacts with CD58 (LFA-3) and the CD11b/CD18 molecule binds to intercellular adhesion molecule-1 (ICAM-1).

MAJOR HISTOCOMPATIBILITY COMPLEX

The major histocompatibility complex (MHC) is part of the genome that codes for molecules that are important in immune recognition including interactions between lymphoid cells and other cell types. The major histocompatibility complex of a number of species has been studied but most is known about mice and humans.

The gene complex contains a large number of individual genes that can be grouped into three classes on the basis of the structure and function of their products. The products of the genes are sometimes referred to as **MHC antigens** because they were first defined by serological analysis, i.e. using antibodies.

MHC class I and class II molecules are involved in immune recognition by presenting antigen fragments to T-lymphocytes. MHC class I molecules bind peptides generated from endogenously produced proteins, e.g. viral protein, and present them to $CD8^+$ T-cells. Exogenous antigens, i.e. foreign material taken into a cell by endocytosis, are processed within cells and the resultant peptides presented by MHC class II molecules to $CD4^+$ T-cells. Other genes that play a role in generating the antigen fragments have recently been mapped to the MHC.

The MHC of humans is known as the **human leucocyte group A** (HLA) complex and in mice it is referred to as the **histocompatibility-2** (H-2) complex. The MHC was first identified through its role in controlling graft rejection. There are other histocompatibility loci (e.g. H-1, H-3, H-4, etc.) that mediate graft rejection but the reactions they stimulate are much weaker. These so-called minor histocompatibility antigens are not involved in immunological recognition of pathogenic organisms.

MHC antigen structure and distribution

The MHC class I molecule is a dimer composed of a glycosylated transmembrane peptide of molecular weight 45 000, coded for within the MHC, non-covalently linked to a 12 kD peptide, β_2-microglobulin (Fig. 3.29). The globular protein formed by these two peptides is present on the surface of virtually all nucleated cells, except neurons, in humans. β_2-microglobulin is required for the processing and expression of MHC encoded molecules on the cell membrane. The complete molecule has four extracellular domains, three formed by the MHC encoded α or heavy chain and one by β_2-microglobulin. In addition, the heavy chain has a transmembrane portion and a cytoplasmic tail of about 30 amino acids. In the late 1980s Bjorkman and colleagues published the crystal structure of a MHC class I molecule. From this and other subsequent studies the tertiary structure of the MHC class I molecule has been elucidated (Fig. 3.30). The extracellular portion has an immunoglobulin-like region composed of the α_3 domain and β_2-microglobulin and a peptide-binding region formed by the α_1 and α_2 domains. The polypeptide backbones of the α_1 and α_2 domains fold

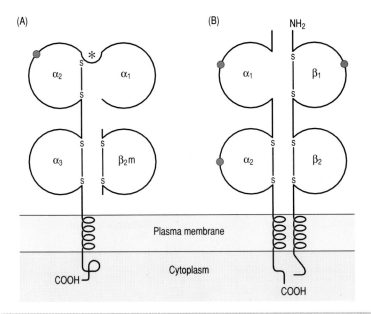

Fig. 3.29 Structure of MHC class I and class II molecules.
Schematic representations of (A) class I and (B) class II molecules as found in the plasma membrane. The MHC-encoded class I glycoprotein folds into three globular domains (α_1, α_2 and α_3) held in place by disulphide bonds and non-covalent interactions. These globular domains are found on the outer surface of the cell. There is a short cytoplasmic tail and a transmembrane portion. β_2-microglobulin (β_2m) is non-covalently associated with the α_3 domain. The MHC class II molecule consists of two non-covalently associated peptides, α and β. Each chain is composed of two extracellular domains, a transmembrane portion and a cytoplasmic tail. Both molecules contain carbohydrate moieties depicted as black circles. X-ray crystallography of class I molecules has shown that there is an antigen-binding cleft formed by the α_1 and α_2 domains (*). A similar cleft is present within the class II molecule.

in such a way that they form a platform of a β-pleated sheet supporting a peptide binding cleft. The sides of this cleft are formed by two α-helices, one from α_1 and one from α_2. It is within this cleft that antigen fragments are held and presented to T-cells.

The MHC class II molecules consist of two polypeptide chains (α 34 kD and β 28 kD) held together by non-covalent interactions (Fig. 3.29). They have a much more limited cellular distribution being limited to the surface of certain cells of the immune system. In humans, they are normally found on B-lymphocytes, macrophages, monocytes and activated T-lymphocytes. Each polypeptide chain has two extracellular domains, a transmembrane portion and a cytoplasmic tail. MHC class II molecules have now also been crystallized and shown to possess a similar overall tertiary structure to MHC class I

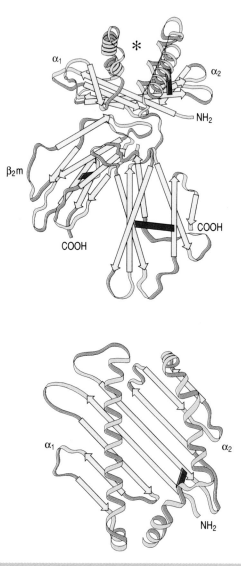

Fig. 3.30 Tertiary structure of MHC class I molecules.
The peptide folding pattern has been elucidated from X-ray crystallographic studies of an MHC class I molecule cleaved by enzymes from the cell surface. (Top) Side view with the membrane proximal part to the bottom. The peptide binding cleft (*) formed by α helices (coils) sitting on a platform of a β-pleated sheet (arrows). (Bottom) Top view looking down on to the peptide binding cleft. Disulphide bonds represented by solid lines. (Adapted with permission from Bjorkman P J et al 1987 Nature 329: 506–512. Macmillan Magazines Ltd.)

molecules. In this case the peptide binding groove is constructed from residues in the α_1 and β_1 domains.

Gene organization

The genes that code for the HLA antigens are found on the short arm of chromosome 6. They are arranged over a region of between 2000k and 4000k base pairs containing enough DNA for over 200 genes. The MHC genes are contained within regions known as A, B, C and D (Fig. 3.31). An MHC class I gene that codes for the heavy chain is

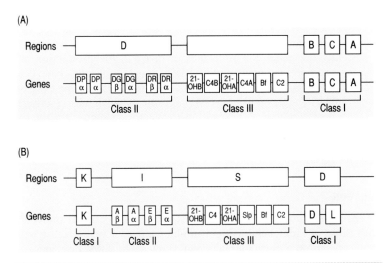

Fig. 3.31 Major histocompatibility complex gene map.
Maps of (A) the human MHC (HLA) and (B) the murine MHC (H-2). Each region contains a number of genes that produce polypeptides of a particular class. (A) The HLA genes are found on chromosome 6. The class I 'heavy chain' polypeptides are coded for by genes present in the A, B and C regions. The D region contains the genes that produce both chains of the MHC class II molecules, HLA-DP, -DQ and -DR. The HLA region coding for class III molecules does not have a particular letter designation. The class III genes include those for the complement components C4, factor B (Bf) and C2 as well as the two forms of the enzyme cytochrome P_{450} 21-hydroxylase (21-OH). (B) The H-2 complex is on chromosome 17. The two separate class I loci (K and D) contain three genes K, D and L. The I region contains the class II genes that code for both chains of the class II molecules A and E. The class III genes are found in the S region and include S1p in addition to those found in humans. S1p is a sex-linked protein, of unknown function, only found in male mice of certain strains. In both species a number of pseudogenes have been found in both the class I and class II regions. In addition the genes coding for the two tumour necrosis factors are found between the class III and class I regions. At the 3' end of the complex is a region containing class I-like genes, known as Qa in the mouse (not shown). There appear to be a number of these genes (at least 20 in mice) but only a few produce a product. The function of these molecules is unknown.

present in the A, B and C regions while β_2-microglobulin is coded for elsewhere in the genome. The genes that code for class II molecules are found within the D region. There are three class II molecules DP, DQ and DR. The class III genes that code for a number of complement components and other molecules are grouped together in a region between D and B.

The H-2 complex on chromosome 17 contains the same types of genes but they are arranged slightly differently. The class I genes are present in the K and D regions that are at either extremity of the locus. The I region contains the genes that code for the two class II molecules A and E (sometimes referred to as I-A and I-E). MHC class II molecules are sometimes known as Ia (immune associated) antigens because they are coded for by the H-2 I region. There is also a region in the mouse coding for class III molecules known as the S region.

Recently the genes for molecules involved in the production and transport of peptides presented by MHC class I molecules have been located within the MHC class II regions of humans and mice. Other genes are also present within the MHC, most of which have nothing to do with host defences. An exception to this are the genes for the two types of tumour necrosis factor and heat shock proteins. Not all the MHC has been mapped and there is a strong possibility that a number of other genes will be located in this area.

Function

There are a number of different MHC class I and class II molecules with those of each class having a similar basic structure. Each type of molecule within a particular class will show slight differences in structure, i.e. overall all HLA-A molecules will be very similar but they will exhibit differences from HLA-B and HLA-C molecules. However, fine structural differences can be detected in the α_1 and α_2 domains of all class I molecules and in α_1 and β_1 domains of all class II molecules. The variations found are due to differences in the amino acid sequence and can be detected serologically. The variable residues will give rise to different three-dimensional shapes on the MHC molecules. Since most of the residues involved form part of the peptide binding cleft this will influence the way antigen fragments can bind to the MHC molecule, i.e. different MHC molecules will bind different peptides. There are therefore many different forms of each of these molecules in a population — they are highly **polymorphic.** Thus it is highly unlikely that two individuals will have exactly the same MHC antigens. The MHC molecules of a particular individual, their haplotype, can be given a designation using tissue typing reagents. On each chromosome 6 an individual will have the genes that code for an HLA-A, -B, -C, -DP, -DQ and -DR molecule. The MHC genes are co-dominant therefore the products of both alleles are expressed on the cell surface. All the nucleated cells in the body will therefore express multiple copies of two HLA-A, two HLA-B and two HLA-C molecules. On certain cells there will also be HLA-DP, -DQ and -DR molecules that were inherited from both parents. The polymorphism maps mainly to the α_1 and α_2 domains of MHC class I molecules and to the α_1 and β_1 domains of MHC class II. The rest of the molecules are conserved. Since CD4 and CD8 are monomorphic it is likely that they bind to conserved regions. Experimental evidence suggests that CD8 binds to a site on the α_3 domain of MHC class I molecules and CD4 to a site in the α_2 or β_2 domains of MHC class II molecules.

The MHC antigens are essential for immune recognition by T-lymphocytes which are only able to bind to antigens when they are associated with these molecules. The different classes of MHC antigen are involved in the restriction of different T-cell types or subsets. T-lymphocytes that have CD4 molecules on their surface recognize antigen in association with MHC class II molecules while those that have CD8 molecules are restricted by MHC class I molecules.

The T-lymphocyte subsets perform different functions but the division is not absolute. The one thing that they have in common is that they recognize, through their T-cell receptor complex (CD3, CD4 or CD8, TCR), antigen fragments in association with MHC molecules (Fig. 3.32). In general terms CD4 positive cells produce molecules, lymphokines, that stimulate and support the production of immune system cells while the CD8 positive fraction is involved in the destruction of virally infected cells. MHC antigens are involved to make the processes more efficient. They guide the T-lymphocytes to the surface of the target cell where they function most effectively.

Viruses replicate within host cells. During this process fragments of viral proteins become associated with MHC class I molecules and these complexes are then transported to the surface of the infected cell. The CD8 T-cell recognizes this complex and destroys the infected cell before it can release progeny virus. If the T-cell could bind intact proteins not associated with MHC products then free virus would also bind, and the elimination of the infected cell and the vast number of viruses it could produce would be inhibited. Thus MHC restricted recognition of peptide fragments is responsible for directing the effector cells on to infected targets. These cytotoxic cells are also capable of destroying tissue grafts from MHC incompatible donors.

The CD4 positive cells produce molecules that stimulate growth and differentiation of other cells. These molecules are most effective over short distances since they will be more concentrated. This will happen when the two cells involved are actually joined together or in close proximity. The stimulation of CD4 T-cells by antigen fragments on the surface of a responsive cell will make sure the lymphokines are directed on to the correct cell surface.

The possession by an individual of a number of different MHC class

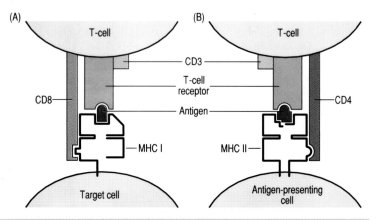

Fig. 3.32 Molecules involved in T-cell recognition.
T-cells only recognize antigen in association with products of the major histocompatibility complex, i.e. MHC restricted recognition. Antigen is usually broken down into small fragments that become associated with MHC molecules. The type of antigen and the way it enters the cell dictate whether it will associate with MHC class I or class II. (A) Antigen fragments that associate with class I molecules are recognized by T-cells that have the CD8 molecule. CD8 is thought to bind to a non-polymorphic determinant on the class I molecule. The T-cell receptor binds to the antigen that is held in the cleft formed by the α_1 and α_2 domains of the MHC class I molecule and to the MHC class I molecule itself. The interaction of the T-cell receptor with antigen/MHC class I and CD8 with the MHC class I molecule generates a signal that is probably transmitted into the cell by the associated CD3 complex. (B) Antigen fragments that associate with MHC class II molecules are recognized by T-cells that have the CD4 molecule on their surface. Again the T-cell receptor binds to both antigen and MHC molecule and CD3 is involved in signal transduction. In both cases the T-cell will only recognize antigen that is present on a cell surface since that is where the MHC molecules are found.

I and class II molecules probably ensures that at least one of the molecules will be able to bind a peptide produced from an infectious agent. An immune response will therefore be generated to eliminate the foreign material. The polymorphism will protect the species since it is likely that at least some members of the species will be able to respond to a particular pathogen.

Immunoglobulin gene superfamily

Many of the molecules mentioned above share certain structural similarities and are therefore thought to have evolved from a common ancestral gene. Other molecules involved in immune recognition, adhesion and binding, as well as several from outside the immune system, are also apparently derived from this precursor. These molecules are members of the **immunoglobulin superfamily** and their genes comprise the **immunoglobulin gene superfamily.** Members of a

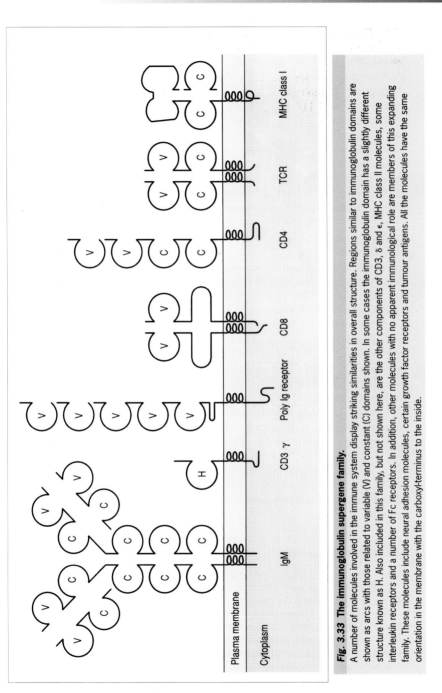

Plasma membrane

Cytoplasm

| IgM | CD3 γ | Poly Ig receptor | CD8 | CD4 | TCR | MHC class I |

Fig. 3.33 The immunoglobulin supergene family.

A number of molecules involved in the immune system display striking similarities in overall structure. Regions similar to immunoglobulin domains are shown as arcs with those related to variable (V) and constant (C) domains shown. In some cases the immunoglobulin domain has a slightly different structure known as H. Also included in this family, but not shown here, are the other components of CD3, δ and ε, MHC class II molecules, some interleukin receptors and a number of Fc receptors. In addition, other molecules with no apparent immunological role are members of this expanding family. These molecules include neural adhesion molecules, certain growth factor receptors and tumour antigens. All the molecules have the same orientation in the membrane with the carboxyl-terminus to the inside.

gene superfamily are evolutionarily related and therefore share structural similarities but they need not be on the same chromosome or necessarily perform the same functions. All members of the immunoglobulin superfamily possess at least one immunoglobulin domain or homology unit. An immunoglobulin domain contains between 70 and 110 amino acid residues that assume a globular tertiary structure containing a characteristic antibody fold comprising two antiparallel β-pleated sheets. There is also a conserved disulphide bond. These immunoglobulin domains can be either similar to immunoglobulin variable domains or constant domains that differ in the number of β-strands making up the immunoglobulin fold and also in the length of the stretches joining the β-strands together. A third type of domain, named H, present in some members is shorter and more compact than the other two types.

Most members of the immunoglobulin superfamily are integral plasma membrane glycoproteins with the immunoglobulin domain in the extracellular region. They usually also possess a transmembrane portion containing hydrophobic amino acid residues and a cytoplasmic tail. Some of the members are monomers, some are dimers and others form parts of large complexes (Fig. 3.33).

Members of the immunoglobulin superfamily are involved in functions as diverse as acting as receptor for foreign material to cartilage formation. This suggests that there is great versatility in the common structure. Immunoglobulin, T-cell receptors and MHC class I and class II molecules are members of the superfamily. Other molecules associated with the immune system, such as CD4, CD8, CD28 and CD3γδε are also members. The superfamily includes a number of receptor molecules associated with the immune system, e.g. poly Ig receptor, receptors for certain colony-stimulating factors and Fcγ receptors. Some members are involved in cell–cell interactions in the nervous system, e.g. neural cell adhesion molecule (NCAM) and myelin-associated glycoprotein (MAG), and others in cell growth and differentiation, e.g. platelet-derived growth factor receptor.

FURTHER READING

Alzari P M, Lascombe M-B, Poljak R J 1988 Three-dimensional structure of antibodies. Annual Review of Immunology 6: 555–580

Bentley G A, Mariuzza R A 1996 The structure of the T-cell antigen receptor. Annual Review of Immunology 14: 563–590

Berck C, Milstein C 1987 Mutation drift and repertoire shift in the maturation of the immune response. Immunological Review 96: 23–41

Bjorkman P J, Parham P 1990 Structure, function and diversity of class I major histocompatibility complex molecules. Annual Review of Biochemistry 59: 253–288

Bjorkman P J, Saper M A, Samraoui B, Bennett W S, Strominger J L, Wiley D C

1987 Structure of the human class I histocompatibility antigen, HLA-A2. Nature 329: 506–512

Brown J H, Jardetzky T, Gorga J C, Stern L J, Urban R G, Strominger J L, Wiley D C 1993 Three-dimensional structure of the human class II histocompatibility antigen HLA-DR1. Nature 364: 33–39

Davis M M 1990 T-cell receptor gene diversity and selection. Annual Review of Biochemistry 59: 475–496

Davis M M, Bjorkman P J 1988 T-cell antigen receptor genes and T-cell recognition. Nature 334: 395–402

French D L, Laskov R, Scharff M D 1989 The role of the somatic hypermutation in the generation of antibody diversity. Science 244: 1152–1157

Hunkapiller T, Hood L 1989 Diversity of the immunoglobulin gene superfamily. Advances in Immunology 44: 1–63

Janeway C A 1993 How the immune system recognises invaders. Scientific American September: 41–47

Lawlor D A, Zemmour J, Ennis P D, Parham P 1990 Evolution of class I MHC genes and proteins: from natural selection to thymic selection. Annual Review of Immunology 8: 23–63

Lopez de Castro J A 1989 HLA-B27 and HLA-A2 subtypes: structure, evolution and function. Immunology Today 10: 239–246

Nossal G J V 1993 Life, death and the immune system. Scientific American September: 21–30

Porcelli S, Brenner M B, Band H 1991 Biology of the human $\gamma\delta$ T-cell receptor. Immunological Reviews 120: 137–183

Raulet D H 1994 How $\gamma\delta$ T-cells make a living. Current Biology 4: 246–248

Tonegawa S 1983 Somatic generation of antibody diversity. Nature 302: 575–581

Trowsdale J, Ragoussis J, Campbell R D 1991 Map of the human MHC. Immunology Today 12: 443–446

Van Regenmortel M H V 1989 Structural and functional approaches to the study of protein antigenicity. Immunology Today 10: 266–272

4 Acquired immunity

Microorganisms that overcome or circumvent the innate non-specific defence mechanisms or are administered deliberately, i.e. active vaccination, come up against the host's second line of defence, **acquired immunity**. To give expression to this acquired form of immunity it is necessary that the antigens of the invading microorganism should come into contact with cells of the immune system (macrophages and lymphocytes) and so initiate an immune response specific for the foreign material. The cells that respond are precommitted, because of their surface receptors, to respond to a particular epitope on the antigen. This response takes two forms that usually develop in parallel. The part played by each will depend on a number of factors including the nature of the antigen, the route of entry and the individual who is infected. The existence of the two forms of acquired immunity — **humoral** and **cell-mediated** — results from the presence of the two major classes of lymphocyte, B-cells and T-cells.

Humoral immunity depends on the appearance in the blood of glycoproteins known as antibodies or immunoglobulins. These molecules are produced by plasma cells, which have developed from B-cells, and combine specifically with the antigen that stimulated their production. This union can lead to a number of consequences. For example, the antigen molecules or particles may become clumped, their toxins may be neutralized and their uptake by phagocytes and subsequent digestion facilitated whilst antigens such as cells or bacteria may also be lysed as a result of complement activation.

It is important to note that the antibody response is a physiological reaction to the introduction into the body of foreign material, irrespective of whether it is harmful or not. Further, antibodies can be generated against internal antigens that have been liberated from disintegrated microorganisms or produced during their replicative cycle. In the intact microorganism these antigens are inaccessible to the antibody which, therefore, cannot perform a protective role. Even antibodies directed against surface structures can be ineffective if they do not bind to critical sites or are of an isotype that does not stimulate an effector function that can eliminate the antigen. Therefore the presence in an individual of antibody against a microorganism does not necessarily mean that they are immune. The antibody must be shown to be able to neutralize or destroy the infectious agent.

The processes that lead to production of immunoglobulins, effector cells and cytokines by the interaction of specialised lymphocytes, require coordinated interaction between the cells in specific microenvironments and involve signals that adjust lymphocyte availability in the blood, alter lymphocyte migration in tissues, determine their retention and recirculation as well as their interaction with each other and endothelial surfaces of blood vessels. The major components of the neuroendocrine pathways controlling lymphocyte activity are the nerves of the autonomic nervous system and corticotrophin-releasing hormone from the anterior pituitary. The sharing of peptide hormones, peptide, neurotransmitters, cytokines and their receptors between the cells of the immune and neuroendocrine systems has only been established in the last 10 years with the recognition that the hypothalmic-pituitary-adrenal (HPA) axis plays a key role in the coordination of neural information into physiological responses, the details of which are described below.

The term cell-mediated immunity was originally coined to describe localized reactions to organisms mediated by T-lymphocytes and phagocytes rather than by antibody. It is now used to describe any response in which antibody plays a subordinate role. Cell-mediated immunity depends mainly on the development of T-cells that are specifically responsive to the inducing agent and is generally active against intracellular organisms. The effector cells can interact directly with the infected cell and destroy it, i.e. a cytotoxic effect, or produce molecules that stimulate other cells to destroy the intracellular parasite.

Specific immunity may be acquired in two main ways: (1) it may be induced by overt clinical infection, inapparent infection or deliberate artificial immunization. This is **active acquired immunity** and contrasts with (2) **passive acquired immunity** which is the transfer of pre-formed antibodies to a non-immune individual by means of blood, serum components or lymphoid cells.

Actively acquired immunity due to infectious agents falls into two general categories. Some infections, such as diphtheria, whooping cough and mumps, usually induce a long-lasting immunity. Others confer immunity lasting only for a short time. Failure of the second group of infections to induce long-lasting immunity is due particularly to the fact that different serotypes of the same species of organism may be involved and the immunity to one serotype may not prevent infection by another serotype of the same organism because of differences in their surface antigens.

Passively acquired immunity involves the administration of antibody often from a convalescent patient or from an immunized animal. The convalescent serum is used since this patient is recovering from the disease and has therefore produced an effective response. The extra circulating antibody, added to those that might be actively produced, may help to curtail an infection or neutralize a toxin and so moderate the illness. Passive immunization has the disadvantage that it provides only temporary protection and if an animal serum is used it is liable to provoke a response to the injected antibody.

In practice, passive immunization has been most efficiently exploited in the prophylaxis or treatment of infections caused by bacteria that produce exotoxins, such as diphtheria, botulism and tetanus. It was used in lobar pneumonia and gas gangrene until the advent of antibiotics. Tetanus antitoxin is used prophylactically in accidental wounds that may be contaminated with tetanus spores.

Passive immunity is transferred to the fetus by the passage of maternal antibodies across the placenta in some species, such as humans and rabbit. In other species, such as the rat and dog, antibodies are transferred in the colostrum via the intestine as well as across the placenta. Other animals, notably the lamb and calf, receive this form of immunity only by means of colostrum. Purified pooled human immunoglobulin is also used as a source of antibody in a number of infections including measles and infectious hepatitis, when it is given during the incubation period to modify or prevent the attack in highly susceptible individuals. Human immunoglobulin is also given to patients with a congenital inability to make their own immunoglobulin.

Tissues involved in immune reactions

For the generation of an immune response antigen must interact with and activate a number of different cells. In addition, these cells must interact with each other. The cells involved in immune responses are organized into tissues and organs in order that these complex cellular interactions can occur most effectively. These structures are collectively referred to as the **lymphoid system** and comprise lymphocytes, epithelial and stromal cells arranged into discrete capsulated organs, or accumulations of diffuse lymphoid tissue. Lymphoid organs contain lymphocytes at various stages of development and are classified into primary and secondary lymphoid organs.

Primary lymphoid organs

The primary lymphoid organs are the major sites of lymphopoiesis.

Here lymphocytes differentiate from lymphoid progenitor cells, proliferate and mature into functional effector cells. In mammals, T-lymphocytes develop in the thymus and B-lymphocytes in the bone marrow (and fetal liver). It is in the primary lymphoid organs that the lymphocytes acquire their repertoire of specific antigen receptors in order to cope with the antigenic challenges that the individual receives during its life. The ability to differentiate between self and non-self is also acquired in these tissues.

Thymus. The thymus in mammals arises from the endoderm of the third or fourth pharyngeal pouch and is the tissue in which lymphocytes can first be recognized. The thymus increases in size until puberty and then slowly atrophies although it is still readily recognizable in the adult. The cells of the thymus are of three main types — thymocytes, morphologically similar to blood lymphocytes, phagocytic reticulum and reticular epithelial cells. The thymus is organized into an outer cortex where the immature proliferating thymocytes are found and an inner medulla that contains more mature cells. Interdigitating cells of bone marrow origin are found in the connective tissue, especially in the medulla. These cells are rich in MHC class II molecules and may be involved in thymic selection that eliminates self-reactive and useless cells. It is here that the T-cell repertoire is generated. Lymphoid progenitor cells produced in the bone marrow migrate to the thymus and begin to develop into thymocytes under the influence of the thymic environment. DNA rearrangements take place leading to the formation of a T-cell antigen receptor and the expression of other T-cell markers such as CD4, CD8 and CD2. The vast majority of T-cells that develop in the thymus never leave the organ. These cells are thought to represent cells that are unable to interact correctly with MHC antigens, an activity that is essential for their correct functioning (see Development of immune system, p. 92). Mature T-cells leave the thymus via the post-capillary venules at the cortico-medullary junction. They then migrate by the blood into specific areas of the secondary lymphoid organs.

Bone marrow. Bone marrow is the source of all types of blood cells and provides the microenvironment to support the antigen-independent development of B-lymphocytes from progenitor cells. The immunoglobulin genes are rearranged as the cell differentiates and the mature B-cell leaves the bone marrow, with an antigen receptor (membrane immunoglobulin), ready to respond to antigen if necessary.

Secondary lymphoid organs

The secondary lymphoid organs create the environment in which lymphocytes can interact with each other and with antigen, and then disseminate the effector cells and molecules generated. Secondary lymphoid organs include lymph nodes, spleen and mucosal-associated lymphoid tissue (MALT), e.g. tonsils and Peyer's patches of the gut. These organs have a characteristic structure which relates to the function they carry out, with areas composed mainly of B-cells and others of T-cells.

Lymph nodes. The lymph nodes of humans are round or bean-shaped organs, 1–25 mm in diameter, that are strategically placed to filter antigens from tissues. Tissue fluids collected from limbs and organs flow in the lymphatics through the lymph nodes on their way to the main lymphatics of the neck and the union with the venous circulation.

Lymph nodes are surrounded by a collagenous capsule with trabeculae extending radially from the subcapsular marginal sinus through the cortex to the medulla (Fig. 4.1). The tissues of the gland consist of

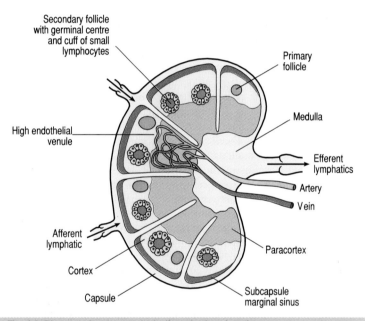

Fig. 4.1 Diagram of an immunologically active lymph node.
Cells and antigen from surrounding tissue pass into the subcapsule marginal sinuses via the afferent lymphatics. Antigen may be taken up by the phagocytes that line these sinuses. B-cells are the predominant cells of the cortex. Unstimulated B-cells are present as a primary follicle whereas antigen-stimulated, proliferating B-cells are found within the germinal centre of a secondary follicle. The paracortex contains mainly T-cells, many of which are in close association with interdigitating cells. Lymphocytes can enter the node from the circulation through specialized high endothelial venules. The medulla contains both T- and B-cells and most of the plasma cells. Cells that enter the node can only leave by the efferent lymphatics.

a meshwork of reticular cells in which large numbers of lymphocytes are embedded. B-cells are found mainly in the cortex where they are grouped in nodules or follicles. In an unstimulated node the B-cells are organized into a primary follicle that develops into a secondary follicle with a germinal centre when stimulated by antigen. The germinal centres contain actively proliferating B-cells as well as follicular dendritic cells and macrophages that are involved in antigen presentation. The paracortex is the main T-cell area which also contains many antigen-presenting cells (interdigitating cells). Although most of the lymphoid cells are found in the cortex and paracortex, some form interconnecting strands in the medulla known as medullary cords. Most of the plasma cells are present in the medullary sinuses that are formed between the medullary cords. Macrophages are present throughout the gland, many being found along the sinuses especially in the medulla.

Cells enter the lymph node in two ways: (1) via the afferent lymphatics that bring cells from the body spaces or other lymph nodes or (2) from the blood. Lymphocytes leave the blood vessels by passing through specialized cells, known as **high wall endothelium**, that are found in the post-capillary venule. These high endothelial venules (HEV) are found predominantly in the paracortex with some in the cortex. They are not present in the medulla. Cells can only leave a lymph node by the efferent lymphatics and eventually re-enter the blood at the thoracic duct.

The afferent lymph also carries antigens into the lymph node from the surrounding tissue spaces. During its passage across the node from the afferent to the efferent lymphatics, particulate antigen is removed by the various specialized antigen-presenting cells and phagocytes. Antigen can also enter a lymph node already associated with cells. Langerhans cells from the skin and dendritic cells are able to pick up antigens and transport them to the draining lymph node. Once there these cells can initiate an immune response by presenting the antigen to T-cells.

Spleen. The spleen, like the lymph nodes, is enclosed by a capsule and divided by trabeculae into communicating compartments. The tissue consists of (a) the white pulp found around the branches of the splenic artery and (b) the red pulp composed of splenic sinuses filled with blood and splenic cords. The cords make up bands of tissues — reticulum cells, erythrocytes, lymphocytes and phagocytes — lying between the sinuses, which are themselves lined by 'sinus-lining cells' held together by a network of reticular fibres. The red pulp is concerned mainly with the destruction of old erythrocytes.

The area around the splenic artery that comprises the white pulp is known as the periarteriolar lymphoid sheath (PALS). This lymphoid tissue is composed of T-cell areas around the central arteriole with B-cells being found beyond this zone. The B-cells are present as either primary 'unstimulated' follicles or secondary, 'stimulated' follicles that contain a germinal centre. There are also a number of specialized cells that are able to act as antigen-presenting cells. These cells filter antigen from the blood. Macrophages and follicular dendritic cells are found in the germinal centres. There are also macrophages in the marginal zone that separates the periarteriolar lymphoid sheath from the red pulp.

Blood enters the spleen via the branching capillaries; some of these end in the white pulp and a few in the red pulp but most empty into the marginal zone. Lymphocytes enter and leave the periarteriolar lymphoid sheath via capillary branches in the marginal zone and both T- and B-cells are found in this area. The blood is finally collected up in the venous sinuses and drains into venules and veins, leaving by the splenic vein. Some lymphocytes, especially mature plasma cells, can cross the marginal zone into the red pulp and from there back into the circulation.

Mucosal-associated lymphoid tissue. The submucosal areas of the gastrointestinal, respiratory and genitourinary tracts are protected by dispersed aggregates of non-encapsulated lymphoid tissue. This mucosal-associated lymphoid tissue (MALT) provides protection at the main portal of entry into the body for foreign microorganisms. The lymphoid cells are either present as diffuse aggregates or are organized into nodules containing germinal centres. The more organized tissues include the tonsils, appendix and Peyer's patches. In the gut, antigen enters the Peyer's patch through specialized cells (M-cells) and stimulates the antigen-specific lymphocytes. After activation these cells enter the lymphatics, pass into the circulation and back to the lamina propria of the gut where they secrete IgA that can be transported into the lumen of the gut to prevent colonization by microorganisms. Mucosal-associated lymphoid tissue is therefore important in the local immune response at mucosal surfaces.

Development of the immune system

During embryogenesis the initial site of haemopoiesis is the yolk sac. Later, haemopoiesis moves to the fetal liver and finally to the bone marrow. In the fully developed animal the bone marrow provides the haemopoietic stem cells from which all blood cells are derived. The first stage of differentiation of stem cells is controlled by various factors derived from mature leucocytes and gives rise to a cell type known as a progenitor cell. The progenitor cells differ from stem cells in that they are responsive to cytokines, hormone-like factors, that lead to development down defined pathways. The process involves progressive expansion and irreversible differentiation, therefore once committed to a particular pathway the cells are unable to mature into another cell type. Lymphoid progenitor cells seed the different lymphoid organs where the later stages of differentiation take place. These are called haemopoiesis-inducing environments. Certain epithelial cells in these microenvironments, as well as mature leucocytes, produce cytokines which are thought to act on the progenitor cells to induce a particular pathway of differentiation. These growth factors are collectively known as **colony stimulating factors** (CSFs). Different CSFs act on bone marrow cells at different stages of development and preferentially direct the maturation of specific cell types. Many of these molecules are produced by T-lymphocytes and mononuclear phagocytes during an immune response or as the result of inflammation. This leads to the production of more cells at a time when they are needed to help destroy a foreign agent.

The process of differentiation is a continuous one because of the rapid turnover of blood cells. For example, in human beings 1.6×10^9 neutrophils/kg of body weight are produced each day. There is great flexibility in the process so that even greater numbers of cells can be produced when required.

In mammals the bone marrow is the specific microenvironment where B-cells differentiate from lymphoid progenitors. Some 80% of the marrow small lymphocytes are of the B-cell lineage. In the fetal liver and bone marrow the precursor cells cluster in the vicinity of macrophages and stromal cells. These cells seem essential for B-cell development but the mechanisms are unknown. B-lymphocytes develop without contact with antigen and move from the peripheral areas of the bone marrow to the centre.

There is an ordered rearrangement of the immunoglobulin gene segments during B-cell development. The D–J gene segments of the heavy chain coding regions are joined together first followed by a V–DJ rearrangement. If this is successful in generating a functional product then a μ heavy chain can be produced and the gene of the other chromosome is silenced, i.e. allelic exclusion. Immature rapidly dividing B-cell precursors therefore first produce cytoplasmic μ heavy chains. Next, rearrangement occurs at the κ light chain gene loci followed by λ if κ rearrangements are unsuccessful. Again allelic exclusion ensures that only one light chain is produced per cell. The cell is now capable of producing an IgM molecule which can be expressed on the surface of the developing B-cell. At this stage of development these immature B-cells, which express only IgM, will be eliminated or inactivated if they bind to molecules via the surface immunoglobulin. This process eliminates autoreactive B-cells since the molecules these cells encounter in the bone marrow will be of self origin. In the surviving cells the addition of surface IgD marks the last stage in the differentiation process, which occurs in the absence of antigen. The IgM and IgD will have identical V domains and therefore the same specificity. These mature B-lymphocytes, which are now responsive to antigen, can now leave the bone marrow and enter the peripheral circulation and lymphoid tissues. These naive B-cells, i.e. they have never seen antigen, will die with a half-life of about 4 days if they do not encounter the foreign material to which they can bind. B-cell differentiation is also characterized by progressive acquisition of various cell surface molecules. These include MHC class II molecules, Fc receptors and complement receptors.

The final stage of the maturation of B-cells is the antigen-driven development into antibody-producing plasma cells and memory cells. The antigen-stimulated B-cells, i.e. activated B-cells, proliferate and differentiate into plasma cells. As this occurs there is a progressive increase in the percentage of the antibody produced being secreted rather than inserted in the membrane. Some of the activated B-cells undergo class switch and begin to produce other isotypes but again with the same V domain. Other activated B-cells do not secrete antibody but become memory cells that can survive for months without further antigen stimulation. On re-exposure to antigen some of these cells become antibody-secreting plasma cells and others become memory cells. Fully mature plasma cells lose their surface immunoglobulin and MHC class II molecules.

The thymus provides the environment for bone marrow-derived prothymocytes to develop into mature T-lymphocytes. Immature cells are found in the cortex and pass into the medulla as they mature. Maturation of T-cells during the period they spend in the thymus is associated with changes in cell surface molecules. The cells must acquire the antigen receptor, CD3 and CD4 or CD8 as well as other molecules characteristic of T-lymphocytes. The first T-cell receptor gene rearrangements are detected at about 8–9 weeks' gestation, in humans, and involve γ and δ genes. The rearranged genes are transcribed and the protein produced, i.e. T-cell receptor $\gamma\delta$ heterodimer, is expressed on the cell surface in association with CD3 polypeptides. At about 10 weeks' gestation β gene rearrangements can be detected, followed soon after by the α genes. Expression of the $\alpha\beta$ receptor rapidly increases as the fetus develops and at birth most T-cell receptor:CD3 expressing thymocytes have $\alpha\beta$ receptors. There is strong evidence that $\alpha\beta$- and $\gamma\delta$-producing thymocytes are separate lineages with a common precursor.

T-cell precursors that enter the thymus are CD4$^-$ CD8$^-$ but soon begin to express both molecules. These cells undergo rapid cell division giving rise to many cells each of which will acquire a unique T-cell receptor conferring a distinct antigen-binding specificity. The CD4$^+$CD8$^+$ cells rearrange their α and β genes and undergo a selection process before they leave the thymus. This is because the $\alpha\beta$ T-cells that leave the thymus are either CD4$^+$ or CD8$^+$ and must be able to recognize antigen fragments in association with MHC molecules but not bind to self MHC molecules on normal cells.

The CD4/CD8 double positive thymocytes that interact with MHC molecules on thymic epithelium via their T-cell receptors are positively selected to differentiate into $CD4^+CD8^-$ or $CD4^-CD8^+$. The CD4 molecule is lost from those cells with a T-cell receptor that interacts with MHC class I, and interaction with MHC class II leads to CD4 being retained with a loss of CD8. Cells that do not interact with MHC molecules will not develop further but die. This positive selection produces cells that interact with MHC molecules with varying strengths. Those that bind very strongly could cause autoreactivity when they leave the thymus since they bind MHC molecules irrespective of the peptide that is held in the peptide binding groove. Other T-cell receptors interact strongly with peptides derived from self molecules associated with MHC molecules. These cells with high affinity receptors are eliminated in the thymus if they bind to MHC molecules present on bone marrow-derived medullary cells. Hence the T-lymphocytes that leave the thymus are also being negatively selected. The only thymocytes that are left are those with a T-cell receptor that will possibly bind to foreign material associated with self MHC molecules. Therefore mature T-lymphocytes are self MHC restricted and self tolerant.

In humans, lymphoid tissue appears first in the thymus at about 8 weeks' gestation and by the tenth week some T-cell functions can be demonstrated. Peyer's patches are distinguishable by the fifth month and immunoglobulin-secreting cells appear in the spleen and lymph nodes at about 20 weeks. From this period onwards IgM and IgD are synthesized by the fetus (Fig. 4.2). At birth the infant has a blood concentration of IgG comparable to that of the maternal circulation, having received IgG but not IgM via the placenta. The rate of synthesis of IgM in the infant increases rapidly within the first few days of life but does not reach adult levels until about a year. This compares with a much slower rise in IgG and IgA, which do not reach adult levels for some considerable time. Serum IgG does not reach adult levels until after the second year and IgA takes even longer. There is an actual drop in the level of IgG from birth due to the decay of maternal antibody with lowest levels of total IgG at around 3 months of age. This corresponds to an age of marked susceptibility to a number of infections. Cell-mediated immunity can be stimulated at birth but these reactions may not be as powerful as in the adult.

It is now clear that the thymic hormones thymulin, thymosins, thymopoietin and thymic humoral factor gamma 2 are responsible as modulators of T cell differentiation. Most of these hormones induce terminal deoxynucleotidyl transferase activity in immature thymocytes, as well as expression of membrane markers such as Thy-1. Thymulin secretion is influenced by peptide hormones and neuropeptides. Thyroid hormone, for example, can be shown to upregulate thymulin production even in older individuals. Prolactin and growth hormone from the pituitary have a similar effect. In vitro experiments

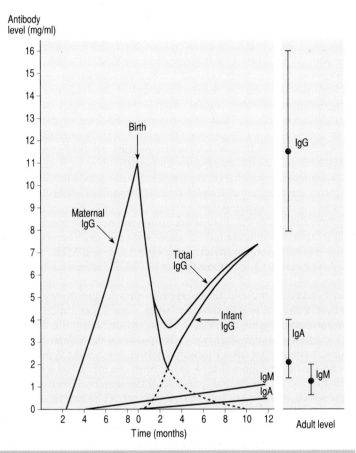

Fig. 4.2 Immunoglobulin levels in fetus and neonate.
In the fetus the serum IgG is derived solely from the maternal circulation by a passive
mediated process. This involves Fc receptors binding the maternal IgG and transporting it
down a concentration gradient into the fetus. At birth the IgG level will be the same as in the
mother but this maternal antibody disappears rapidly due to natural catabolism and has
completely disappeared by about 10 months. From birth the infant is able to synthesize its
own IgG but even at 12 months the serum level is only about 60% of that seen in adults. The
other classes of antibody cannot cross the placenta so that those present are solely of fetal
origin. The fetus can produce small amounts of IgM during gestation and the neonate
continues to do so after birth. The infant will start to produce other isotypes after birth. At
12 months IgM has reached about 75% of the adult level. IgA appears much more slowly
with only about 20% of the adult level being present at the end of the first year of life. The
adult level of the major isotypes is shown as the mean serum level (●) and the normal
range.

have shown that ACTH and Beta endorphin can be shown to modulate thymulin production from thymic fragments. Thymic hormones have also been shown to act on the neuroendocrine tissues indicating a complex bidirectional circuitry involving thymic peptides and neurohormones.

Macrophages and neutrophils develop from the same progenitor cells. Both in the monocyte/macrophage and neutrophil lineages there is a progressive acquisition and expression of functional competence with maturation. In the newborn infant the granulocyte and monocyte populations have not reached their full protective potential but this is attained during the first few weeks of life.

Lymphocyte trafficking

Lymphocytes differentiate and mature in the primary lymphoid organs and then enter the blood lymphocyte pool. B-cells are produced in the bone marrow and mature there before proceeding via the circulation to the secondary lymphoid organs. T-cell precursors leave the bone marrow and mature in the thymus before migrating to the secondary lymphoid organs. Once in the secondary lymphoid tissues the lymphocytes do not simply remain there but move from one lymphoid organ to another through the blood and lymphatics (Fig. 4.3). One of the main advantages of this **lymphocyte recirculation** is that during the course of a natural infection the continual trafficking of lymphocytes enables very many different lymphocytes to have access to the antigen. The passage of lymphocytes through an area where antigen has been localized and concentrated on the dendritic processes of macrophages or on the surface of antigen-presenting cells facilitates the induction of an immune response.

Another possible role of this recirculation process is that it can be used to replenish the lymphoid tissue of, for example, the spleen that might have been depleted by infection, X-irradiation or trauma. There is convincing evidence that lymphoid tissues can recruit lymphocytes from the recirculating pool. If rat spleen is irradiated (a procedure that stops cell division) immediately after an intravenous injection of sheep red blood cells, the antibody response is only slightly delayed. However, if whole body irradiation (all dividing cells in the body will be affected) is given after the initial splenic irradiation there is complete suppression of the anti-sheep cell response. It thus seems likely that without the whole body irradiation the irradiated spleen can recruit a fresh supply of lymphocytes from the circulating pool.

Lymphoid organs are innervated by nonadrenergic autonomic nerves and these have effects on migration and interactions between lymphocytes. Disruption of the nerve supply reduces the ability of lymphocytes to accumulate in lymphoid tissues in rats. The release of corticosteroids from the adrenal glands under the influence of corti-

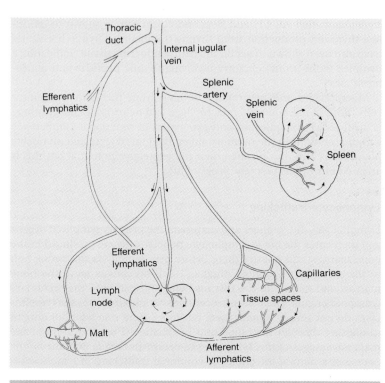

Fig. 4.3 Lymphocyte recirculation.
Lymphocytes in a mature animal continuously move between the blood and the lymphoid tissues. Lymphocytes can leave the blood and enter the secondary lymphoid organs directly or enter tissue spaces and then move via the afferent lymphatics to the draining lymph node. The lymphocytes that enter the organs become resident in particular specialized areas but eventually re-enter the blood stream to circulate again. Lymphocytes leave the vasculature through the high wall endothelial cells of the post capillary venules in the MALT and lymph nodes. In the capillaries it is thought that they also pass into tissue spaces within high endothelial venules. These tissue lymphocytes are then collected up in the lymph that will drain into a lymph node to meet up with cells that entered directly from the circulation and from other lymphoid tissues. The lymphocytes leave the node by the efferent lymphatics and ultimately rejoin the venous circulation through the thoracic duct. Lymphocytes enter the spleen from the arterial circulation mainly into the marginal zone of the periarteriolar lymphoid sheath. They leave through the marginal zone bridging channels into the red pulp sinuses and back into the venous circulation.

cotrophin from the pituitary, decreases the recruitment of lymphocytes in lymphoid tissues and those that do arrive are retained for longer periods than normal. Corticosteroids alter the adhesive properties of endothelial cells. Endothelial cell E-selectin and ICAM-1 adhesion molecules are reduced on exposure of endothelial cell cultures to corticosteroids. This would be likely to interfere with the response of endothelial cells to local inflammatory signals and the adhesion and migration of lymphocytes into the tissues.

There are three main areas where the migration or transfer of lymphocytes from the blood takes place: lymph nodes and Peyer's patches, the spleen, and the peripheral blood vessels. In lymph nodes and non-capsulated lymphoid tissue, lymphocytes actually pass through the cuboidal endothelial cells of the post-capillary venules. These post-capillary venules are unusual in that their endothelial cells are hypertrophied and cuboidal in appearance in comparison with the endothelium of the normal post-capillary venules found elsewhere. Lymphocytes have specialized adherence molecules or homing receptors which interact with molecules on the endothelial cells of high endothelial venules (HEV). The lymphocytes are transported through the high walled endothelial cells and emerge into the surrounding tissue or organ. In lymph nodes all lymphocytes return to the circulation by the efferent lymphatics and pass via the thoracic duct into the left subclavian vein. Some lymphocytes arrive by afferent lymphatics; this is the main route of entry of antigen.

Under normal conditions there is a continuous active flow of lymphoid traffic through lymph nodes but when antigen and antigen-reactive cells enter there is a temporary shutdown of the exit. Thus, antigen specific cells are preferentially retained in the node, draining the source of the antigen. This is partly responsible for the swollen glands (lymph nodes) that can sometimes be found during an infection.

Lymphocyte recirculation is also important since, as we will see later, a number of different cells and molecules must all be in close proximity so that an immune response can be generated. The chance of this happening is greatly increased if the cells are continuously being brought together in organs that are specialized to allow effective interactions to occur. This is particularly important since lymphoid cells are monospecific, i.e. they recognize one shape, and there is a finite number of lymphocytes capable of recognizing any particular epitope.

There is now evidence for non-random migration of lymphocytes to particular lymphoid compartments. For example, lymphocytes that home to the gut are selectively transported across the endothelial cells of venules in the intestine. It appears that lymphocytes have specific molecules on their surfaces that preferentially interact with high-walled endothelial cells in different anatomical sites. A lymphocyte that was initially stimulated by antigen in the Peyer's patch will be activated and some memory cells will be produced. It is important that these memory cells migrate back to the area where the same pathogen might be encountered again. Therefore, they possess receptors that direct them preferentially to the mucosal-associated lymphoid tissue.

The precise routes of lymphocyte migration in the peripheral blood circulation are not clear but the migration seems to be on a much smaller scale than in lymphoid tissues and almost certainly takes place across capillary walls. The flow of lymphocytes from the circulation will be increased if, for example, a local inflammatory response is initiated by the presence of foreign material. Then the migration from blood to lymph can be as great as in the lymph nodes themselves.

In the spleen small lymphocytes seem to enter the periarteriolar lymphoid sheath from the blood, passing between the cells rather than through them as in the post-capillary venules. The cells later re-enter the blood within the spleen rather than leaving via the lymphatics.

Clonal selection

During their development in the primary lymphoid tissues both T- and B-lymphocytes acquire specific cell surface receptors that commit them to a single antigenic specificity. For T-cells these receptors will remain the same for the life of the cells but the surface immunoglobulin on B-cells can be modified due to somatic mutations. In the B-cell this is mirrored in the modification of the antibody that the cell produces on exposure to its specific antigen. The cell is activated when it binds its specific antigen; the lymphocytes then proliferate, differentiate and mature into effector cells.

Each lymphocyte produced has a unique receptor capable of recognizing a particularly shaped epitope. Since the immune system can specifically recognize a very large number of antigens this means that the lymphocytes reactive to any particular antigen are only a small proportion of the total pool. Therefore, antigen binds to the small number of cells that can recognize it and **selects** them to proliferate (multiply) so that sufficient cells are formed to mount an adequate immune response (Fig. 4.4). A cell that responds to an antigenic trigger and proliferates will give rise to daughter cells having a genetically identical make-up, i.e. **clones**. This phenomenon is known as **clonal selection**. All the cells whose receptors did not recognize the antigen are left to wait in an unstimulated state until an epitope that they can bind to is encountered.

Lymphocyte receptors appear to be created in a random fashion so there is no reason why they should not recognize 'self' molecules. It is an important attribute of the immune system that it is able to discriminate 'self' and 'non-self' since failure to do so would lead to self-destruction. From a theoretical point of view the body can only know what is 'self' and as described earlier lymphocytes that develop self-reactive receptors are not allowed to develop. There are other mechanisms that control any cells that escape this main selection process (discussed later, see p. 142). So to the immune system anything that is not 'self' must be 'non-self' and should be destroyed. The body must both tolerate its own tissues and react effectively against all infectious agents if disease is to be avoided.

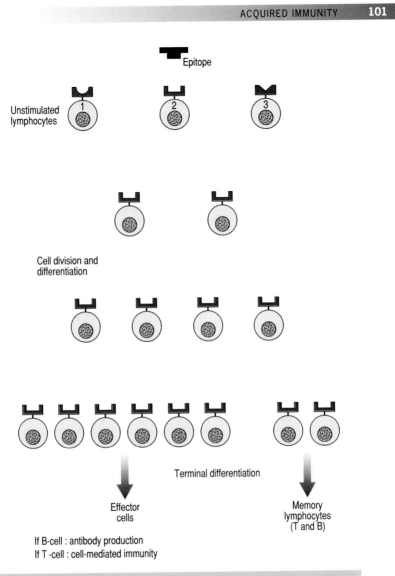

Fig. 4.4 Clonal selection.
Each lymphocyte has a receptor on its surface that is specific for a particular complementary antigenic determinant or epitope. When an antigen, containing this epitope, is introduced into the body then the antigen selects those cells (cell 2 in this illustration) that can respond to it by binding to the surface receptor. The cells selected in this way are stimulated to divide and differentiate into mature effector cells and longer-lived memory cells.

Cellular activation

When an individual is exposed to an antigen those cells with receptors that recognize parts of the foreign material are selected to respond. B-lymphocytes must proliferate and differentiate into antibody-producing plasma cells and memory cells. T-lymphocytes will be stimulated to become effector cells that can directly eliminate the foreign material or produce molecules that help other cells destroy the pathogen. The type (immunity or tolerance) and magnitude of the response, if generated, will depend on a number of factors including the nature, dose and route of entry of the antigen and the individual's genetic make-up and previous exposure to the antigen.

The first stage in the production of effector cells and molecules is the activation of the resting cells. This involves various cellular interactions with maturation of the response leading to a coordinated, efficient production of effector T-cells, immunoglobulin and memory cells.

B-cell activation

Crosslinking of the B-cell antigen receptor, surface immunoglobulin, is the initial trigger for activation. When this happens a number of biochemical changes are instigated including stimulation of phosphatidyl inositol turnover and mobilization of intracellular Ca^{2+} ions. These changes probably act through protein kinases that cause the synthesis of RNA and ultimately immunoglobulin production. In a number of cases this is all that is required to stimulate antibody production. However, for the majority of antigens this initial crosslinking is not enough and molecules produced by T-cells are also required.

Thymus-independent antigens

A number of antigens will stimulate specific immunoglobulin production directly. These T-independent antigens are of two types.

Mitogens are substances that cause cells, particularly lymphocytes, to undergo cell division, i.e. proliferation. Certain glycoproteins, called lectins, derived from plant seeds have mitogenic activity. These molecules have specificity for sugars and bind to the cell surface and will activate all responsive cells. Certain of the lectins specifically activate cells of the immune system (Table 4.1). The response to the mitogens will therefore be polyclonal since lymphocytes of many different specificities will be activated. At high concentrations a number of mitogens are able to non-specifically activate all B-cells irrespective of their antigen specificity. At low concentrations these mitogens do not cause polyclonal activation but can lead to the stimulation of specific B-cells. The surface immunoglobulin specifically binds to an

Table 4.1 Lymphocyte mitogens

Mitogen	Sugar specificity	Cell type activated*
Phytohaemagglutinin	Oligosaccharides	T-lymphocyte
Concanavalin A	α-methyl-D-mannose	T-lymphocyte
Pokeweed mitogen	N-acetylglucosamine	T- and B-lymphocyte
Lipopolysaccharide	—	B-lymphocyte

* Ability to stimulate selectively varies with species and cell source suggesting that only a subpopulation is capable of responding to mitogen.

epitope on the mitogen and this increases the local concentration of the active part of the molecule that then interacts with its receptor to cause B-cell activation (Fig. 4.5A). Such responses probably play an important role in defence against Gram-negative bacterial infections when lipopolysaccharide can act as a T-independent antigen.

Certain large molecules with regularly repeating epitopes, for example polymers of D-amino acids and simple sugars such as pneumococcal polysaccharide and dextran, tend to persist for long periods in the body. These molecules can interact directly with the B-cell surface immunoglobulin. They may also be held on the surface of specialized macrophages in secondary lymphoid tissues and the B-cells interact with them there. The multiple repeats of the epitope interact with a large number of surface immunoglobulin molecules and the signal that is generated is sufficient to stimulate antibody production (Fig. 4.5B).

The immune response generated to these antigens tends to be similar on each exposure, i.e. IgM is the main antibody and response shows little memory. This suggests that class switch and memory production require additional factors.

Thymus-dependent antigens

Most antigens do not stimulate B-cells to produce antibody without the help of T-lymphocytes. Epitopes on these antigens will bind to the surface immunoglobulin but are unable to directly stimulate antibody production, i.e. they act like haptens. It is now known that other parts of the antigen act like carriers and stimulate T-cells to provide signals that cause the B-cell with antigen bound to its surface immunoglobulin to differentiate into an antibody-producing plasma cell. Therefore the B-cell must bind antigen as a first signal and then be exposed to T-cell derived lymphokines, i.e. helper factors, before antibody can be

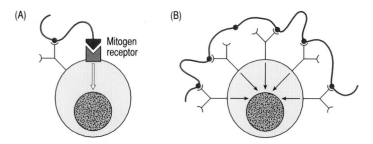

Fig. 4.5 B-lymphocyte activation by T-independent antigens.
(A) Mitogens at concentrations too low to activate B-cells polyclonally can affect specific B-cells. If the antigen receptor is specific for a separate part of the mitogen then this will focus the molecule onto the specific B-cell at a level that can give rise to a stimulatory signal via the mitogen receptor. (B) Some antigens tend to be large molecules with identical repeating epitopes. These molecules can activate B-cells directly by crosslinking a number of antigen receptors, i.e. surface immunoglobulin. The crosslinking generates a signal that causes the cell to differentiate into an IgM-producing plasma cell. In both these cases the B-cell activation has occurred without the need for T-cells and is, therefore, T-independent activation.

produced. For the second activation signal, i.e. help, to be effectively targeted at the B-cell, the T-cell epitope and the B-cell epitope must be physically linked. The experiments that lead to these conclusions are summarized in Figure 4.6. In addition, direct contact between the T-cell and the B-cell is needed for transfer of the second signal. The requirements for activation are probably slightly different between the first and subsequent exposure to a particular antigen since on first exposure to an antigen the number of cells that can respond will be low and their responsiveness to various factors is different from that seen in a secondary response (see below).

The physical need for the B- and T-cell epitopes to be on the same molecule to get an optimal response introduces problems when it comes to considering the requirements for T-cell recognition (described in Ch. 3). It will be remembered that T-cells recognize antigen that has been processed and is presented in association with products of the major histocompatibility complex (MHC). It is therefore impossible for native antigen to form a bridge between surface immunoglobulin and the T-cell receptor. The B-cell binds to its epitope on free antigen but there is no site on this molecule that the T-cell can bind to since it requires antigen associated with MHC products. The answer to this problem can be seen when the requirements for antigen presentation in T-cell recognition are considered.

T-cell activation

The development of an antibody response to a T-dependent antigen

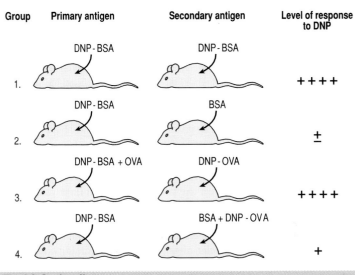

Group	Primary antigen	Secondary antigen	Level of response to DNP
1.	DNP-BSA	DNP-BSA	++++
2.	DNP-BSA	BSA	±
3.	DNP-BSA + OVA	DNP-OVA	++++
4.	DNP-BSA	BSA + DNP-OVA	+

Fig. 4.6 Carrier effect.

Four groups of mice were immunized (primary antigen) with bovine serum albumin (BSA) to which dinitrophenyl (DNP) had been chemically complexed. Group 3 also received ovalbumin (OVA). Each group was challenged (a second injection) some time later with various combinations of the primary antigens and the antibody response to DNP (hapten) measured. Optimal amounts of antibody were produced following challenge with the antigen used in the primary injection (group 1). The first injection caused B-cells specific for DNP to be activated through the binding of DNP to their surface immunoglobulin and with help from BSA specific T-cells. Antibody would have been produced and memory cell populations (B- and T-cells) would have been generated. Following a second injection of the same antigen these primed cell populations, i.e. the memory B- and T-cells, were restimulated and a high level (++++) of antibody against DNP produced. Note that antibodies against carrier epitopes, i.e. BSA, will also be produced but are not measured in the assay. Challenge of DNP-BSA primed mice with BSA gave very low levels of anti-DNP antibody (group 2). Although memory B-cells specific for DNP have been produced after the primary exposure, in the secondary challenge these cells will not be stimulated because they were not exposed to DNP. The antibody measured was residual antibody from the primary response. In group 3 the mice were primed with DNP-BSA and OVA, therefore B-cells specific for DNP would be stimulated to produce antibody and memory cells. T-cells specific for carrier determinants on BSA and OVA are also activated. On re-exposure to DNP-OVA the hapten specific B-cells can be triggered and help will be provided by activation of OVA-specific T-cells (carrier). In group 4, although DNP memory cells were produced after primary exposure to DNP BSA, no antibody is produced following challenge with DNP coupled to a different carrier (OVA) even though BSA is also present. Here memory B-cells specific for DNP have been produced. (Memory T-cells for BSA are also produced.) In the challenge these memory B-cells will be exposed to DNP but there are no primed (memory) T-cells to the carrier, OVA, to produce help. Some unprimed T-cells specific for OVA will be present that will respond at a low level (i.e. a primary response) to give help for the production of very low levels of DNP-specific antibody. Therefore, for optimal antibody production the hapten and the carrier must be linked.

requires that the antigen becomes associated with MHC class II molecules, i.e. is **processed**, and is expressed on the cell surface, i.e. is **presented**, in a form that helper T-cells can recognize. This process is known as antigen presentation and is performed by antigen-presenting cells.

Antigen that enters the tissues moves in the lymph flow to the draining lymph node. The antigen may be free in the fluid or carried there by cells that are usually able to present antigens themselves. On reaching the lymph node different types of antigen, depending on their chemical composition, route of entry and physical state, go to different areas and are thus capable of stimulating different lymphocyte populations (Table 4.2) T-independent antigens and antigen/antibody complexes may persist for years on the surface of cells in their native forms whereas those that are taken up by classical macrophages and processed remain only for a few days or weeks. Antigens that enter through the skin may be taken to the lymph node by epithelial Langerhans cells. These cells change their morphology within the lymph node to become interdigitating dendritic cells.

T-cells recognize antigen fragments in association with products of the MHC on the surface of cells. All nucleated cells, except neurons, express MHC class I molecules but class II molecules are confined to cells of the immune system — the antigen-presenting cells. These cells present antigen to MHC class II restricted T-cells (CD4$^+$ population) and therefore play a key role in the induction and development of immune responses.

There are a large number of antigen-presenting cells in the body (Table 4.3) most of which constitutively express MHC class II molecules. Other cells, like T-lymphocytes and endothelium, can be induced to express MHC class II by suitable stimuli such as lymphokines. The relative importance of each type depends on whether a primary or secondary response is being stimulated and on the location. The most studied antigen-presenting cells are the macrophages and dendritic cells. These are the classical antigen-presenting cells of lym-

---

Table 4.2 Antigen-presenting cells in the lymph nodes

Area	Antigen-presenting cell	Antigen
Subcapsular marginal sinus	Marginal zone macrophage	T-independent antigens
Follicles and B-cell areas	Follicular dendritic cells	Antigen/antibody complexes
Medulla	Classical macrophages	Most antigens
T-cell areas	Interdigitating dendritic cells	Most antigens

Table 4.3 Antigen-presenting cells

Group	Type	Location	Expression of MHC class II
Phagocytic cells	Monocytes	Blood	
	Macrophages	Tissues	+
	Marginal zone	Spleen and	↓
	macrophages	lymph node	+ + + +
	Kupffer cells	Liver	
	Microglia	Brain	
Lymphocytes	B-cells	Lymphoid tissue and site of immune responses	+ → + + +
	T-cells		0 → + +
Non-phagocytic constitutive presenters	Langerhans cells	Skin	
			+ +
	Interdigitating cells	Lymphoid tissue	
Facultative presenters	Astrocytes	Brain	
	Follicular cells	Thyroid	0
	Endothelium	Vascular and	↓
		lymphoid tissue	+ +
	Fibroblasts	Connective tissue	

Level of MHC class II expression is indicated by number of + signs: 0 = none present. Arrow indicates that MHC class II is inducible.

phoid organs. However, it has now become apparent that in certain situations B-cells may be important antigen-presenting cells. The relative importance of B-cells becomes greatest during secondary responses, especially if the antigen concentration is low. Here the B-cells can specifically engulf antigen via their surface immunoglobulin. In a primary response specific B-cells are at a low frequency and their receptors are of low affinity. In this situation macrophages and dendritic cells are probably most important.

The key feature of all antigen-presenting cells is that they can ingest antigen and present it, in the context of MHC class II molecules, to T-cells (Fig. 4.7). Since the T-cell receptor binds fragments of antigen, i.e. processed antigen, the antigen-presenting cell must be able to degrade the antigen before it is expressed on the surface in a form that can be recognized by T-cells.

The activation of resting $CD4^+$ T-cells requires two signals. The first is antigen in association with MHC class II molecules and the second is a **co-stimulatory signal**. The generation of the first of these signals, i.e. antigen presentation, has just been outlined and is described in detail in Generation of immune responses (p. 130). The co-stimulatory signal has to be delivered by the same antigen-

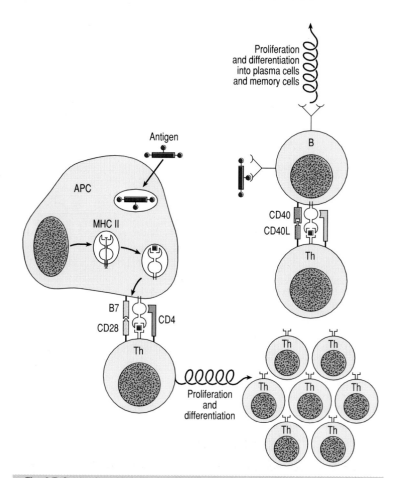

Fig. 4.7 **Generation of help for B-cell activation.**
The antigen-presenting cell (APC), in this case a macrophage or dendritic cell, will engulf antigen via non-specific receptors or as immune complexes using Fc and complement receptors. It is processed intracellularly before fragments associate with MHC class II molecules and return to the cell surface. In this case the antigen has B-cell epitopes (●), equivalent to a hapten, linked to a carrier (■) that contains sequences of amino acids that will generate T-cell epitopes once processed and associated with MHC molecules. CD4$^+$ T-cells (T$_H$) with receptors specific for MHC/antigen complex will bind to APC. This interaction will give the first signal. The APC also expresses B7 which gives the co-stimulatory signal leading to activation of the T-cells. These T-cells will clonally expand and mature to produce cells capable of producing B-cell growth and differentiation factors, i.e. help, and some will develop into memory T-cells. Activated T-cells can then interact with B-cells (B) that have bound specific antigen via their surface immunoglobulin. The B-cell can bind to native, i.e. unprocessed, antigen either free in the surrounding tissues or held on the surface of the antigen-presenting cell. For all these cells and molecules to come together without some kind of focusing would be very unlikely. These interactions are taking place in the secondary

presenting cell that supplied the antigen-specific signal (Fig. 4.7). The best characterized co-stimulatory signals are generated when the molecule B7 on the antigen-presenting cell interacts with CD28 on the T-cell.

If T-cell receptor has been engaged by antigen/MHC in the presence of co-stimulatory signals then biochemical changes occur within the cell, leading to RNA and protein synthesis. The responsive cells progress through the cell cycle from G_0 to G_1. The cells start to express interleukin-2 receptors and produce interleukin-2. Interleukin-2 is a T-cell growth factor and causes the expansion of the responsive T-cell population. After about 2 days interleukin-2 synthesis stops while interleukin-2 receptors remain for up to 1 week if the cell is not re-activated. Therefore, there is a built-in limitation on T-cell growth and clonal expansion. When stimulated, T-cells secrete interleukin-2 which interacts with interleukin-2 receptors to mediate growth. This can be an 'autocrine' fashion if the same cell that released the interleukin-2 is stimulated. If the responding cell is in the vicinity of the producer then the stimulation is in a 'paracrine' manner. Interleukin-2 is not present at detectable levels in the blood therefore there is no 'endocrine' activity involved, i.e. action at a distant site.

The other main type of T-lymphocyte is the $CD8^+$ T-cell. Antigen recognition by these cells is restricted by MHC class I molecules. Again these cells require two signals to be activated: first, antigen fragment associated with MHC class I and then co-stimulatory signal plus interleukin-2 from a T-cell. A cell that 'sees' both these signals responds by clonal expansion and differentiation into a fully active effector T-cell.

Cell interactions for antibody production

The hapten/carrier effect can be explained if we consider the logistics of the required cellular interactions. Antigen from the site of infection enters the lymph node and is taken up into antigen-presenting cells either non-specifically or by specific receptors, such as surface immunoglobulin or Fc receptors. The antigen is then subjected to degradation, probably within phagolysosomes or other specialized organelles, into fragments that can associate with MHC class II molecules. The precise reactions are not known in detail and it is possible

Fig. 4.7 (cont'd)
lymphoid tissues that are specifically designed to facilitate these processes. The B-cell also requires two signals for activation. The binding of antigen via the surface immunoglobulin is the first. The second is the interaction between CD40 on the B-cell and CD40L that is expressed on activated T-cells. Part of the T-cell activation process has been the induction of CD40L. The T_H cells secrete lymphokines (IL-4, IL-5, etc.) directly on to the B-cell.

that various pathways and sites may be involved (described in Generation of immune responses, p. 130). The outcome is that antigen is converted to a state that can fit into the groove formed on MHC class II molecules between the α_1 and β_1 domains. Lymphocytes are continually recirculating and some with the desired specificity will enter the node. Specific $CD4^+$ T-cells recognize this complex and are activated, i.e. proliferate and then mature into cells capable of producing lymphokines (Fig. 4.7). These T-cells are now in a state in which they can 'help' B-cells develop into plasma cells by producing lymphokines, such as B-cell growth and differentiation factors.

The specific B-cells, which have entered the lymph node, will bind free antigen and thus receive one of the two signals necessary for activation (Fig. 4.7). The **co-stimulatory** signal has to come from contact with the specific T-cell and exposure to the lymphokines released by that T-cell. To receive this second signal the B-cell engulfs the bound antigen and presents it on the cell surface in association with MHC class II molecules. The activated T-cell binds the processed antigen. This ensures that a specific T-cell has bound to the correct B-cell. During the maturation process, after it was stimulated by the antigen-presenting cell, the T-cell expresses CD40 ligand (CD40L) and this molecule interacts with CD40 on the B-cell as the co-stimulation signal for B-cell activation. What we now have is the B-cell and T-cell bound together; the B-cell has received both signals (antigen and co-stimulation) and the T-cell releases lymphokines that direct the development of the B-cell into an antibody-secreting plasma cell.

This is probably the sequence of events for a primary response where unprimed T- and B-cells are present at a low frequency. If the B-cell determinant and T-cell determinant were on different molecules then the co-stimulatory signal, i.e. direct contact, could not be generated as the B-cell would not have taken up the correct structure to produce the T-cell epitope, i.e. peptide, to associate with the MHC class II molecule. There is no guarantee that the epitopes recognized by the responding cells will be close together in the same lymph node or even in the same lymph node.

After the first exposure to antigen memory, B-cells will be present at an increased frequency and with high affinity surface immunoglobulin as a receptor. These B-cells can specifically bind free antigen, even at low antigen concentrations, via their surface receptors and, after processing, present it directly to $CD4^+$ T-cells. These two cells will be in intimate contact, i.e. co-stimulatory signals exchanged, therefore the helper factors produced will stimulate the B-cell into antibody production. The need for the hapten to be directly linked to the carrier should be obvious. If it is not directly linked then the B-cell, when it binds the hapten, will not engulf the carrier part and no antigen fragment associated with MHC class II will be generated to activate the T-cell. Since the original experiments were carried out in a secondary response this is the most likely explanation of the hapten/carrier effect (see Fig. 4.6).

In a secondary response memory T-cells bind the processed antigen and are stimulated to release the lymphokines that direct the development of the B-cell into an antibody-secreting plasma cell. In this situation there is therefore a two-way signalling process for the B-cell to receive help. The memory B-cell expressing peptide, in association with MHC class II molecules, also expresses B7. The T-cell receives these two signals and produces the lymphokines necessary to activate the B-cell. The lymphokines alone are not enough but a co-stimulatory signal via CD40 on the B-cell and CD40 ligand on the T-cell is also involved.

Mitogens and T-independent antigens have an inherent ability to drive B-cells into division and differentiation. T-dependent responses rely on T-cells and their products to control the antibody class, affinity and memory. The first cells to be activated are $CD4^+$ T-cells that recognize the antigen in association with MHC class II molecules. These cells respond to the signal of antigen fragment/MHC and produce a variety of lymphokines that act on B-cells and other cell types including macrophages, endothelial cells and T-cells that mediate cytotoxicity. The production of various lymphokines is described in Lymphokine production, p. 124.

As far as B-cell development is concerned the antigen-stimulated cells develop under the influence of interleukin-4 (previously known as B-cell stimulation factor) that is produced by the closely adherent T-cells. Interleukin-5 and interleukin-6 then bring the cells to a state of full activation with terminal differentiation into an immunoglobulin-producing plasma cell. Other factors including interleukin-1, interleukin-2 and gamma-interferon have been reported, in some instances, to activate B-cells. The characteristics of various cytokines involved in B-cell development are shown in Table 4.4. All these cytokines are only active at high concentrations and therefore the producing and responding cells must be close together for effective triggering. Some of the interleukins and a number of other factors are thought to then cause maturation of some B-cells into memory cells and bring about class switch in others. The proportion of the various cytokines present probably controls the differentiation of the B-cells into plasma cells, producing a particular class of antibody. All this will be happening within the environment of a germinal centre of a secondary follicle which has evolved to facilitate the necessary cellular and molecular interactions.

Therefore, for both B- and T-cell activation two stimuli are required. The recognition of antigen makes sure that only those cells that will be effective against the foreign material are recruited since the growth factors produced are antigen non-specific. The provision of the other signal, T-cell help, has evolved to supply growth factors and aid

Table 4.4 **Lymphokines involved in B-lymphocyte activation.**

Lymphokine	Effect on B-lymphocyte*	Other effects
Interleukin-4	Activation Growth Class switch IgG_1 and IgE	Inhibits macrophage activation Growth of mast cells T-cell growth
Interleukin-5	Differentiation to IgA synthesis	Eosinophil growth and development
Interleukin-6	Growth and development	Induces CSF production Release of acute phase proteins
TGF-β	Class switch IgG_{2b} and IgA	Inhibits macrophage activation Activates neutrophils
Interferon-γ	Differentiation to IgG_{2a} synthesis	Activates NK cells Activates macrophages Increases cellular expression of MHC class I and class II molecules

* for mice
TGF-β = transforming growth factor

discrimination of 'self' and 'non-self'. The mechanism for generating diversity in B-cells is random and self-reactive B-cells do exist. These cells are exposed to self antigens all the time and if it were not for the fact that they need a second signal they would damage host tissue. That this does not happen is partly explained by the proposal that the 'help' for these cells is not produced. The possible mechanisms for this tolerance and the consequences of its failure will be discussed later (p. 142).

The multiple cellular interactions and the involvement of molecules that are needed in relatively high concentrations necessitate the development of specialized environments where immune responses can take place efficiently and effectively. Thus the secondary lymphoid tissues have evolved to fulfil these requirements (discussed more fully above, p. 89).

Humoral immunity

Humoral immunity is mediated by antibodies of various different classes. These molecules are produced by cells of the B-lymphocyte lineage in response to stimulation by antigen in the presence of T-cell-derived growth factors. The various antibody classes are found at specific anatomical sites and perform different protective functions.

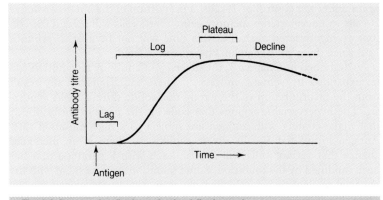

Fig. 4.8 Pattern of antibody production following antigen exposure.
When antibody levels, i.e. titre, are measured after antigen exposure four discernible phases are observed.

Synthesis of antibody

On exposure to antigen, antibody production follows a characteristic pattern (Fig. 4.8). There is a lag phase during which antibody cannot be detected. This is the time taken for the interactions described above to take place and for antibody to reach a level that can be measured. Once the process has been initiated there is a period when there is an exponential rise in the antibody level or titre. This log phase is then followed by a plateau with a constant level of antibody where the amount produced equals the amount removed. The amount of antibody then declines due to the clearing of antigen/antibody complex and the natural catabolism of the immunoglobulin.

If one looks in more depth at what is happening then the outcome can be related to some of the mechanisms that were described previously. On exposure to an antigen for the first time those B-cells that recognize epitopes on the foreign material and receive co-stimulatory signals will proliferate and mature. Some will differentiate into plasma cells and synthesize μ heavy chains which will combine with light chains and IgM is secreted. If the response is to a T-dependent antigen then the B-cells can switch to the production of another isotype, e.g. in a primary response IgM gives way to IgG production. This process is under the control of T-cells since it is not found with T-independent antigens. The class of antibody produced will depend on the signals from the T-cell. If the cell is directed to produce IgG the V_H gene segment is positioned upstream of the γ gene segment. The DNA that was between the original position of the V_H and its new position is deleted. Consequently this cell will be unable to make IgM or IgD in the future. The plasma cell derived from this B-cell will then produce IgG of the same antigen specificity as before. At some point, again under the control of T-cells, a proportion of the antigen-reactive B-cells will develop into memory cells. These cells will react if the epitope is encountered again but this time will not be able to produce IgM since the μ gene segments have been deleted.

As described in Chapter 3, the diversity of antibody recognition can be expanded by somatic mutation. These mutations usually result from the incorporation of the wrong nucleotide during DNA synthesis. The hypervariable regions that code for the parts of the antibody that make contact with antigen are subject to a high mutation rate. Antigen-stimulated B-cells divide rapidly, so there is an increased chance that variant cells will appear, each with a paratope that has been modified by the mutation. Some mutations will be silent with the changed nucleotide not affecting the amino acid used or causing the substitution of a similar amino acid. Other mutations will result in the production of stop codons and subsequent chain termination. Such cells will then fail to produce any immunoglobulin, since they can no longer be stimulated by antigen, and will die.

In some cells the mutation will result in an amino acid substitution within the paratope that changes the affinity of the antibody for its particular epitope. The affinity of the modified paratope for the epitope may be higher or lower than the original and in this case the concentration of antigen will determine if the cells will be activated. At high antigen concentrations both high and low affinity cells will be stimulated. However, when the antigen concentration is low, for example as the antigen is being eliminated by the immune response, only those cells with high affinity receptors will be activated. For this reason, as an immune response develops, the affinity of the antibody being produced will increase with only those cells that can still bind the antigen being activated. Any cells that have undergone somatic mutation to produce a high affinity antibody will be stimulated over a longer period and will have more chance of developing into memory cells. This process leading to increased antibody affinity as a response develops is known as **affinity maturation**.

There are a number of differences in the reaction profile on second and subsequent exposures to an antigen compared to the primary response (Fig. 4.9). There is a shortened lag and an extended plateau and decline. The level and affinity of antibody produced is greatly increased and it is mostly of the IgG isotype. Some IgM will be generated but it will follow the same pattern as in the primary response. The reasons for these differences should be clear when we consider what is happening.

When first introduced the antigen selects the cells that can react against it. However, before antibody is produced the B-cell must differentiate into a plasma cell. For T-dependent antigens this requires T-cell-derived factors and hence T-cells must be activated. All these reactions take time and since only a few cells are initially present a

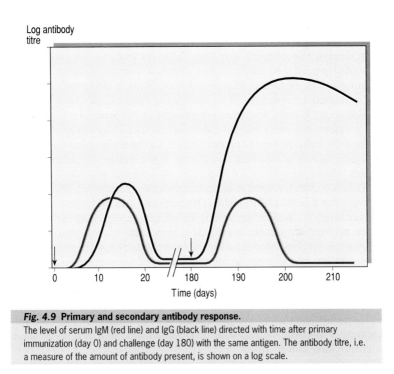

Fig. 4.9 Primary and secondary antibody response.
The level of serum IgM (red line) and IgG (black line) directed with time after primary immunization (day 0) and challenge (day 180) with the same antigen. The antibody titre, i.e. a measure of the amount of antibody present, is shown on a log scale.

great deal of proliferation and clonal expansion must occur. Therefore, there is a considerable lag before antibody can be detected. The B-cells that are stimulated in the primary response will have rearranged their immunoglobulin heavy chain genes so that the V_H gene segment is upstream of the μ constant gene segment; the first isotype produced is therefore IgM. With time, class switch will occur in some of the B-cells leading to the production of other isotypes. Somatic mutations will occur giving rise to affinity maturation through selection of cells bearing high affinity receptors as the amount of antigen in the system falls. Memory cells will also be produced. An equilibrium is reached where there is a balance between the amount of antibody synthesized and the amount used. Then various mechanisms come into play to turn off the response when it is no longer needed (see p. 139). The simplest is the removal of the stimulant, i.e. antigen. The production of antibody is therefore stopped and there is a natural decline in antibody levels.

On subsequent exposure the responding cells are at a different level of activation and present at an increased frequency. Therefore, there is a shorter lag before antibody can be detected. The main isotype is IgG since the memory cells generated on the first exposure to antigen will have undergone class switch and deleted their μ and δ constant gene segments. The level of antibody produced is ten or more times greater than during the primary response. The antibody is present for an extended period and has a higher affinity for antigen due to affinity maturation. As is seen in Figure 4.9, some IgM is also produced during a secondary response. This immunoglobulin is produced by the activation of B-cells that were not present in the lymphocyte pool on the previous exposure but have developed since. The development of these cells follows the characteristics of a primary response and they will give rise to a secondary response if the antigen is encountered again.

This secondary response is maintained at a high level, falling only slowly over a period of months. The response can be boosted to even higher levels by further injections of antigen until a stage is reached when no further increase occurs. It is important to note that once an animal has responded to an antigen, even though exposed to it on only one occasion, the animal retains a **memory** of the antigen so that even after an interval of months or years it is able to react by means of a secondary response with a rapid mobilization of antibody-forming cells. Hence vaccination against infectious agents, such as polio virus, provides many years of useful protection against infection, even though soon after vaccination the level of antibody falls to a low level, since memory has been retained.

It is possible to enhance the natural ability of an antigen to induce an immune response by altering it or mixing it with another substance (called an **adjuvant**). A procedure that is often used is to alter the physical state of the antigen by absorbing it on to mineral gels such as aluminium hydroxide. These alum-precipitated antigens are widely used as immunizing agents for humans. Such particulate forms of antigens seem to be able to initiate antibody production much more effectively than the same antigens in non-particulate form. This effect is not fully understood. It may be that particulate material is more readily phagocytosed by macrophages. These cells have been shown in certain situations to make a contribution by serving as a store of antigen for later release and stimulation of lymphocytes. For a protein antigen a few hundred milligrams is required to stimulate the production of antibody. Above this level the increase in response is small in proportion to the increase of antigen given. At high antigen levels tolerance, i.e. no response, can occur (see p. 149). It is conceivable also that by removing antigen from the circulation macrophages protect the lymphocytes from the effects of excess antigen which would be likely to paralyse the lymphocytes rather than initiate a response. The presence of the adjuvant might cause a localized inflammatory response, which is needed to help induce the production of cytokines that in turn help in the generation of an immune response.

Monoclonal antibodies

When an antigen is introduced into the lymphoid system of a mouse, or any other mammal, then all the B-cells that recognize epitopes on the antigen will be stimulated to produce antibody. If blood is collected from this animal, the serum produced will contain multiple antibodies that react with every epitope (cf. Fig. 3.2). The serum of the immunized animal is known as a polyclonal antiserum since it is the product of many clonally derived B-cells. Even if highly purified antigen is used the antiserum produced will contain a number of antibodies that react to the antigen and others that interact with antigens that the animal encountered naturally during this time. It is extremely difficult to purify the antibodies of interest from this complex mixture but other sources of homogeneous or monoclonal antibodies are available.

Myeloma proteins are antibodies produced by neoplastic plasma cells. These tumour cells grow without the usual controls and there are very large amounts of these immunoglobulins in the patient's serum. If a single B-cell became malignant then the antibodies will all be the same. These proteins have been very useful for studying antibody structure but in most cases their antigen specificity is unknown. However, in 1976 Milstein and Kohler devised a technique for producing antibodies of a single specificity almost at will.

Plasma cells taken from the body will not grow in tissue culture but die within a few days. Myeloma cells, on the other hand, will grow indefinitely in culture. If these two cell types can be fused together the 'hybridoma' that is produced will have the characteristics of both parents. When procedures to generate the required type of myeloma cells were developed monoclonal antibodies could be readily produced.

Myeloma cells were selected to have two important characteristics. They did not produce endogenously coded immunoglobulin and they were defective in an enzyme of the purine salvage pathway (hypoxanthine phosphoribosyl transferase). This latter fact is used to select for hybrids since the unfused myeloma cells die in a medium containing hypoxanthine, aminopterin and thymidine (HAT). Unfused spleen cells die naturally in a few days.

Spleen cells from an immunized mouse are the usual source of the antibody-producing cells. Experimental animals are usually given multiple injections of a preparation containing the structures against which the desired antibody will react. The spleen is removed about 3 days after the final injection at a time when the B-cells will be rapidly dividing. These B-cell blasts are the best cells to use to get successful results. Rats have also been used as a source of B-cells but researchers and clinicians would prefer to use human monoclonal antibodies in patient treatment. For this purpose peripheral blood or easily obtained secondary lymphoid tissue, such as tonsils, have been used. It is impossible for ethical reasons to expose human subjects to most of the antigenic material that would be required to induce useful antibodies. Therefore, cells are only available from patients with certain diseases, such as tumours, infections and autoimmune diseases, or from individuals who have received vaccinations.

Once the myeloma cells have been grown in normal medium and a single-cell suspension has been prepared containing the primed B-cells, the two cell populations are mixed together in the presence of a fusing agent, usually polyethylene glycol (Fig. 4.10). After fusing,

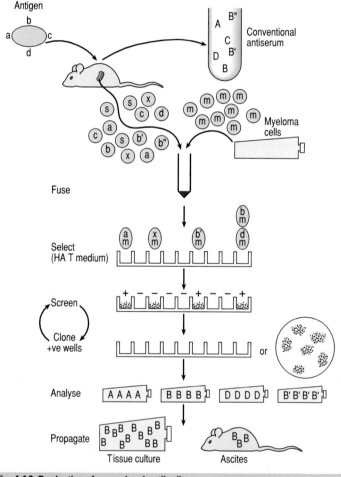

Fig. 4.10 Production of monoclonal antibodies.
Animals, usually mice, are injected with an antigen. In this case the antigen is a microorganism containing four surface molecules (**a b c d**) and we are trying to obtain an

the mixture of hybrids and unfused cells are cultured in the selection medium (HAT). The aminopterin blocks de novo purine synthesis and forces the cells to use the purine salvage pathway. Myeloma cells die because they lack the hypoxanthine phosphoribosyl transferase (HPRT) of the salvage pathway. Normal lymphoid cells die naturally within a few days. The hybridomas, however, survive because the B-cell supplies the HPRT. The cells that grow have the required characteristics of the parents — the ability to grow indefinitely from the

---

Fig. 4.10 (cont'd)

antibody that reacts with molecule b. Each molecule will possess a number of epitopes, e.g. b contains **b b' b"**. The immune system will respond to this antigen and B-cells reactive to the epitopes will be stimulated. The serum of the animal will contain antibodies **A B B' B" C D** derived from all the B-cells that were stimulated, i.e. a polyclonal antiserum.

The first step in producing a monoclonal antibody is to prepare a suspension of the required cells, B-cells and myeloma cells. Within the spleen of the primed animal are B-cells that could be stimulated to produce antibodies that interact with the antigen. If the spleen is removed shortly after antigen challenge, a single-cell suspension can be prepared that will contain stimulated B-cells, **a b b' c d**, and other spleen cells, **s**. No cells reactive with **b"** are present. The spleen cells and myeloma cells, **m**, are centrifuged into a pellet and fused together using polyethylene glycol. After this procedure the cells are added, at a suitable dilution, to the wells of a tissue culture plate. The concentration of cells is such that it is hoped that not more than one hybrid is added to each well. Not all the antigen-reactive B-cells will fuse with a myeloma cell, e.g. **c**, and some hybrids derived from B-cells reactive to other antigens, **x**, will be generated. The cells are cultured in HAT medium to kill the sensitive unfused myeloma cells. Unfused spleen cells die naturally after a few days. Two spleen cells or two myeloma cells can also fuse together but these die in the selection process. Only hybridomas, **am bm b'm dm xm**, survive and proliferate. The wells that show growth are tested for the production of a suitable antibody. In this example the assay is for antibody that binds to the antigen; therefore **xm** will be discarded. The cells in the positive wells are allowed to grow and then they must be cloned to establish that all the antibody is indeed derived from a single cell and is therefore monoclonal. This is achieved by diluting the cells to a level that ensures that only one cell is added to each tissue culture well or by growing diluted cells in soft agar and picking out individual clones. In the illustration this will ensure that **bm** and **dm** are separated. After a number of rounds of cloning it will be established that the cells in each vessel are monoclonal. The hybridomas will be grown in larger amounts and the antibody will be analysed as to its isotype and specificity. The hybridomas that produce antibody with the required characteristics will be propagated in large culture vessels where $1–10 \mu g/ml$ can be obtained. Alternatively the cells can be injected into the peritoneal cavity of a mouse where they will grow to produce an ascites fluid containing up to 1 mg/ml of specific antibody. At all these stages it is important to freeze cells so that they can be retrieved if required. In this example **bm** produced antibody (**B**) that bound to the required epitope with the desired affinity and was of the correct isotype to use in further investigations of the function of the molecule with which it reacts. **A** and **D** interact with other molecules on the antigen and the hybridomas **am** and **dm** will be kept frozen to be used at a later date. **B'** binds to the some epitope as B but the antibody was of very low affinity and not a suitable antibody for the current research. It too may be kept for use in a different assay system where it has the required characteristics.

myeloma and the ability to produce antibody from the B-cell. Cultures producing antibodies of the required specificity have to be identified by a suitable assay, i.e. screened. It is also necessary to establish that the cultures are monoclonal. For this purpose single cells are taken from these cultures and grown so that a clone is produced. This clone, since it is the product of a single cell, will make an antibody of a single specificity. The hybridomas, producing the required antibodies, are then propagated in large culture vessels or they can be injected into the peritoneal cavity of mice. In the latter situation the ascitic fluid produced contains very large amounts of antibody. Hybridoma cells can be frozen and kept for long periods of time before being retrieved and used again.

This technique will give a reagent, a monoclonal antibody, in which all the molecules will be identical. They will have the same isotype, allotype, idiotype, specificity and affinity. In contrast, the antiserum produced by the inoculation of antigen into an experimental animal will be a heterogeneous mixture of antibodies, the majority of which do not even interact with the immunizing antigen. In addition, the same antiserum can never be reproduced, not even when using the same animal. Therefore, monoclonal antibodies are defined reagents that can be produced indefinitely and on a large scale. They provide a standard material that can be used by laboratories throughout the world in studies ranging from the identification and enumeration of different cell types, blood typing and diagnosis of disease. They are also increasingly used in attempts at treating and preventing disease. Recent advances have made it possible to produce antibodies by genetic engineering. Difficulties have been encountered in producing human monoclonal antibodies for use as therapeutic agents. Genetic engineering now makes it possible to humanize rodent monoclonal antibodies so that the molecules are not destroyed by the immune system of the recipient.

Cell-mediated immunity

Cell-mediated responses are difficult to define since the host defences against foreign material involve the co-ordinated action of humoral and cell-mediated reactions. The production of immunoglobulin is dependent on the factors produced by T-lymphocytes and macrophages, and the effector functions of a number of cells are reliant on antibody. Therefore, cell-mediated immunity tends to be used for host defence reactions in which antibody plays a subordinate role.

Specific cell-mediated responses are mediated by two different types of T-lymphocyte. T-cells that have the CD8 molecule on their surface recognize antigen fragments in association with MHC class I molecules on a target cell, causing their lysis. MHC class II restricted recognition is seen with T-cells that have the CD4 marker. These cells secrete biologically active molecules, known as lymphokines, when stimulated by the antigen/MHC class II complex. $CD4^+$ T-cells are involved in two main activities both of which are mediated by the lymphokines they produce: (1) they are involved in cell-mediated reactions because the lymphokines can aid in the elimination of foreign material by recruiting and activating other leucocytes and promoting an inflammatory response and (2) they are involved in the generation and control of an immune response because some of the lymphokines produced are growth and differentiation factors for T- and B-lymphocytes.

Other cell types can participate in cell-mediated defence mechanisms but these do not possess an antigen-specific receptor. In fact, all leucocytes can contribute to the body's cell-mediated defences. Natural killer cells are able to destroy virally infected cells and some tumours. Phagocytes are extremely important in cell-mediated responses. Mononuclear phagocytes perform a central role in immunity and homeostasis. These cells, along with neutrophils, will phagocytose foreign material and can release biologically active molecules. Eosinophils and basophils also produce mediators of inflammation. Specific antibody on the surface of a particulate antigen can opsonize it for phagocytosis but can also lead to antigen destruction by antibody-dependent cell-mediated cytotoxicity (ADCC).

Cell-mediated cytotoxicity

Certain sub-populations of lymphoid and myeloid cells can destroy target cells to which they are closely bound. The stages and process involved are similar for the different cell types although the molecules that mediate the recognition of the target differ.

Cytotoxic T-lymphocytes. Cytotoxic T-cells (T_C cells) are small T-lymphocytes that are derived from stem cells in the bone marrow. These cells mature in the thymus where they acquire an antigen receptor specific for an antigen fragment in association with products of the MHC. Most cells that mediate MHC-restricted cytotoxicity are $CD8^+$ and, therefore, recognize antigen in association with MHC class I antigens. About 10% are $CD4^+$ and, therefore, MHC class II restricted. The most important function of these cells lies in the elimination of virus-infected cells. They will, however, destroy malignant cells and histoincompatible cells, i.e. rejection of tissue grafts. In certain situations they can also destroy cells infected with intracellular bacteria.

MHC-unrestricted cytotoxic cells. A number of partially overlapping cell populations are able to carry out MHC-unrestricted killing. These include the so-called natural killer (NK) cells, lymphokine activated killer (LAK) cells and killer (K) cells. None of these cells kill in an antigen-specific fashion and in addition the mechanisms used may vary between the different types.

Most cells that have the capacity to perform natural killing have the morphology of large granular lymphocytes and have a broad target range. The receptors on the NK cells and the structures that they recognize on the target have not been identified. They will destroy virus-infected cells, tumour cells and allogeneic cells but have also been shown to produce a number of cytokines, including gamma-interferon.

Peripheral blood cells or spleen cells cultured in the presence of interleukin-2 give rise to potent cytotoxic cells. These are probably highly activated NK cells and/or T-cells that no longer show MHC restriction. This type of cell has been used in the treatment of certain tumours. The patient's own T-cells are cultured in vitro with inter-leukin-2 and then returned to the patient. A similar situation can be found when T-cells are cultured with mitogens. T-cells treated in this way exert cytotoxic effects without MHC restriction.

A number of cell types are able to destroy foreign material by anti-body-dependent cell-mediated cytotoxicity (ADCC). As the name suggests a cytotoxic response (toxic — killing: cyto — cell) is mediated by cells and is dependent on the presence of antibody. The cells that carry out this activity have a receptor for the Fc portion of immunoglobulin and are, therefore, able to bind to antibody-coated targets. The mechanisms that lead to target cell destruction by these effector cells, sometimes called killer cells, may depend on the lineage of the cell involved. It appears that a number of cell types can carry out MHC-unrestricted cytotoxicity. The process used, and hence the clas-sification, depends on the signal used to mediate recognition. For example, a large granular lymphocyte could kill a target by ADCC if antibody, bound to the target, mediated the recognition process. However, in the absence of antibody the same cell could destroy the target by natural killing. In the former case the cell would be termed a killer cell and in the latter case a natural killer cell.

Neutrophils are phagocytic cells that usually internalize pathogens and kill them intracellularly. In some situations the target may be too large, e.g. a parasitic worm, to be taken into the cell. If the parasite is coated with antibody then neutrophils can bind to the pathogen by Fc receptors and mediate its elimination by extracellular killing. In this case the neutrophil will be a killer cell mediating ADCC. Eosinophils appear to be very efficient mediators of ADCC against parasitic worms.

Lytic mechanism. Three distinct phases have been described in cell-mediated cytotoxicity: (1) binding to target, (2) rearrangement of cytoplasmic granules and the release of their contents, and (3) target cell death usually by apoptosis (Fig. 4.11).

The close apposition of the target and the effector cell is necessary

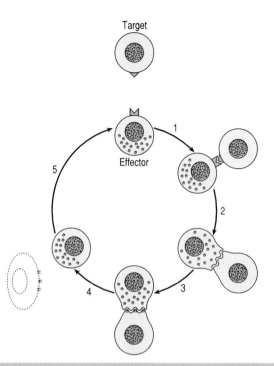

Fig. 4.11 Mechanism of cell-mediated cytotoxicity.
The effector cell has a receptor that is able to bind to a target cell that possesses the appropriate ligand (▼). This could be the Fc portion of immunoglobulin if the effector is mediating ADCC, MHC/antigen for T-cells or alterations in the level of a molecule recognized by a cell capable of natural killing. These structures on the target and effector cells lead to the formation of an effector/target conjugate (1). Following binding to the target the granules of the effector are rearranged and appear to congregate at the membrane adjacent to the target (2). The granule contents are released into the space between the two cells (3) and target cell death ensues (4). The effector cell is undamaged and then proceeds to destroy another target cell (5).

to avoid release of the toxic molecules into sites where they could do damage. Once the effector/target conjugate is formed the cytoplasmic granules appear to become rearranged and concentrated at the side of the cell adjacent to the target. The granule contents are then released into the space between the two cells. There are at least two different types of molecule stored, preformed, within the granules that can cause cell death. T-cells and NK cells contain perforin which is a monomeric protein related to the complement component C9. In the presence of Ca^{2+} the monomers bind to the target cell membrane and polymerize to form a transmembrane pore. At high concentrations this can upset the osmotic balance of the cell and leads to cell death. The granules also contain at least three serine esterases (proteases), known collectively as **fragmentins**, that probably play a role in destroying the target cell. It is thought that in vivo a limited number of perforin pores are formed and serve as a site of entry for fragmentins which are responsible for the induction of apoptosis. A number of other toxic molecules are also produced by cytotoxic cells including tumour necrosis factor-α (TNF-α), lymphotoxin (TNF-β), gamma-interferon and NK cytotoxic factor. The process is unidirectional with only the target cell being destroyed. The effector cell can then move on and eliminate another target cell.

Lymphokine production

The other arm of cell-mediated immunity is dependent on the production of lymphokines from antigen-activated T-lymphocytes. These molecules, produced in an antigen-specific fashion, can act in an antigen non-specific manner to recruit, activate and regulate effector cells with the potential to combat infectious agents.

The first documented reference to the production of lymphokines is credited to Robert Koch in 1880. Koch was studying the cellular response to filtrates from cultures of the microorganisms that caused tuberculosis. Injection of purified antigen (tuberculin) into the skin of immune individuals produced a reaction that peaked within 24 to 72 hours. The response was characterized by reddening and swelling and was accompanied by the accumulation of lymphocytes, monocytes and basophils; in essence an inflammatory response. Because of the time course of the reaction this response became known as delayed-type hypersensitivity (DTH) and the cells responsible were called delayed-type hypersensitivity T-lymphocytes (T_{DTH} or T_D cells). It was soon shown that delayed hypersensitivity reactions were not mediated by antibody but were caused by molecules, lymphokines, produced by activated T-lymphocytes. More recently it has been demonstrated that the majority of cells that produce lymphokines possess the CD4 molecule and, therefore, recognize antigen in association with membrane-bound MHC class II molecules. Although the cells were originally designated T_{DTH} they are identical to the helper T-cell (T_H) subset as far as antigen recognition is concerned. Since T_H cells are CD4$^+$, a cell carrying MHC class II molecules with associated antigen fragments is required to induce/activate them to perform their protective functions. The main cell types involved are therefore macrophages and B-cells. Antigen processing and presentation by these cells has been described above (p. 104). CD4$^+$ T-cells, usually referred to as helper T-cells, are therefore capable of mediating both helper and inflammatory activities by producing lymphokines. The two functions are mediated by different panels of lymphokines. The term delayed-type hypersensitivity should be used only when the inappropriate release of inflammatory lymphokines leads to pathological consequences (Ch. 9).

Table 4.5 Properties of T_H subtypes

	T_H1	T_H2
Cells markers	CD4	CD4
Lymphokines		
Gamma-interferon	+++	−
Interleukin-2	+++	−
TNF-β*	+++	−
TNF-α	++	+
GM-CSF†	++	+
Interleukin-3	++	++
Interleukin-4	−	+++
Interleukin-5	−	+++
Interleukin-6	−	+++
Macrophage activation	++++	+
T-cell activation	++	−
B-cell activation	−	++++

* Tumour necrosis factor
† Granulocyte monocyte-colony stimulating factor

Helper T-cells can be divided into two types on the basis of the lymphokines they produce and therefore the main functions they promote (Table 4.5). T_H1 produce interleukin-2 and gamma-interferon while T_H2 make interleukin-4 and interleukin-5. Both sub-populations secrete tumour necrosis factor (TNF), interleukin-3 and the colony stimulating factor (CSF) that supports the development of granulocytes and macrophages (GM-CSF). These are just some of the many cytokines produced by cells of the immune system. Cytokines are biologically active molecules released by specific cells that elicit a particular response from other cells on which they act. A number of these regulatory molecules produced by lymphocytes (lymphokines) and monocytes (monokines) are shown in Table 4.6. The responses caused by these substances are varied and interrelated. Cytokines can have multiple effects on their own that may vary between different target cells. There are also intricate interactions between different cytokines that depend on the molecules involved and the differentiation state of the responsive cells.

The CD4$^+$ cells that leave the thymus can develop into either of the two subsets of T_H cell. These cells are thought to go through an intermediate stage known as T_H0 before differentiating into either helper or inflammatory T-cells. The factors determining which pathway the cells will go down are not fully understood. The process is controlled

***Table 4.6* Examples of some important cytokines.** Many of the molecules given in this table act synergistically to produce their biological effects.

Cytokine*	Main sources	Effect
Interleukin-1	Macrophages Epithelial cells	T-cell activation B-cell activation Fever
Interleukin-2	T-lymphocytes	T-cell proliferation
Interleukin-8	Macrophages Others	Chemotactic for neutrophils
Interleukin-10	T-lymphocytes Macrophages	Suppresses macrophage function
Interleukin-12	B-lymphocytes Macrophages	NK cell activation Stimulates a T_H1 response
TNF-α[†]	Macrophages NK cells	Local inflammation Increased adherence of leucocytes to endothelium Fever Production of acute phase proteins Cellular catabolism
TNF-β	T-lymphocytes B-lymphocytes	Killing Increased adherence of leucocytes to endothelium Fever
IFN-α[‡]	Leucocytes	Antiviral effect Increased MHC class I expression
IFN-β	Fibroblasts	As IFN-α
Macrophage (M) CSF[§]	Macrophages T-lymphocytes	Monocyte growth and development
Granulocyte (G) CSF	Macrophages T-lymphocytes	Granulocyte growth and development
GM-CSF	Macrophages T-lymphocytes	Growth and differentiation of myeloid cells Macrophage activation

* See Table 4.4 for other examples.
[†] tumour necrosis factor; [‡] interferon; [§] colony stimulating factor.
Macrophages = all cells of mononuclear phagocyte lineage.

by the environment in which the cells first encounter antigen. Both the cytokines present at this time and the amount of peptide/MHC play a role in this process. The presence of interleukin-12 and gamma-interferon leads to T_H1 cell production whereas cells exposed to inter-leukin-4 become T_H2 cells. In addition, activation by low density of antigen/MHC is thought to favour the development of T_H2 cells and high ligand concentration gives rise to T_H1 cells. Other controlling factors include tissue site, type of antigen-presenting cell and availability, and state of activation of responding cells. The demarcations are not complete and in the response to all antigens there will be induction of both types of $CD4^+$ T-cell but it is likely that one will predominate. The development of the correct response can be crucial to the outcome of an infection. In leprosy, the causative organism *Mycobacterium leprae* grows within macrophages. The effective response is to activate the infected macrophages by producing T_H1-derived lymphokines. In individuals where this happens the organism is controlled, few if any bacteria are found and antibody levels are low. However, when T_H2 cells are activated the main response is the production of large amounts of antibody which is ineffective because of the intracellular habitat of the organism. The patient develops lepromatous leprosy in which the bacteria grow to high numbers within the macrophages. This causes gross tissue destruction and is usually fatal.

In addition to the T_H cells whose main function appears to be the production of lymphokines, other cell-mediated reactions lead to the release of cytokines. T-cells that have been activated to carry out cytotoxicity produce various lymphokines, as do B-cells when stimulated by antigen. In general, cytokines control growth, mobility and differentiation of lymphocytes but they also exert a similar effect on other leucocytes and some non-immune cells. Although the division is not absolute, it appears that T_H2 cells are adapted to function as classical helper T-cells for the activation and differentiation of B-cells because of the types of lymphokines they produce (see B-cell activation above and the section on Generation of immune responses, p. 130), whereas T_H1 cells produce molecules that activate macrophages and stimulate T-cell growth.

Role of macrophages

Macrophages are able to carry out a remarkable array of different functions (Fig. 4.12). They play a key role in several aspects of cell-mediated immunity being involved at the initiation of the response, as antigen-presenting cells, and as effector cells having microbicidal and tumouricidal activities. They also produce a number of cytokines (or more precisely monokines) that function as regulatory molecules. These monokines contribute to inflammation and fever and affect the functioning of other cells. Macrophages can also produce various enzymes and factors that are involved in reorganization and repair following tissue damage. However, since they contain many important biological molecules they themselves can cause damage if these enzymes and factors are released inappropriately.

Many of these activities are enhanced in macrophages that have

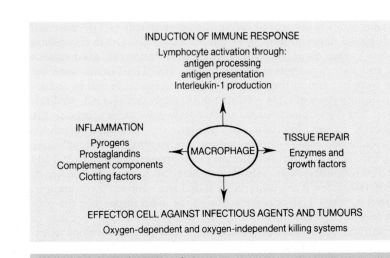

INDUCTION OF IMMUNE RESPONSE
Lymphocyte activation through:
antigen processing
antigen presentation
Interleukin-1 production

INFLAMMATION
Pyrogens
Prostaglandins
Complement components
Clotting factors

MACROPHAGE

TISSUE REPAIR
Enzymes and
growth factors

EFFECTOR CELL AGAINST INFECTIOUS AGENTS AND TUMOURS
Oxygen-dependent and oxygen-independent killing systems

Fig. 4.12 Central role of macrophages.
Macrophages function as effector cells producing molecules that are toxic to
microorganisms, protozoa and tumours. They are important in the inductive phase of an
immune response and contribute to inflammation and tissue repair.

been **activated**. Resident macrophages from the peritoneal cavity of a
mouse show little or no microbicidal or tumouricidal activity.
However, if these cells are exposed to lymphokines produced by
T-cells then they efficiently and effectively carry out these activities.
Macrophage activation is a complex process driven by many different
molecules. It is proposed that the activation process occurs in stages
with different effector functions being expressed at different stages.
The transition between these stages will be controlled by different
molecules. Macrophages from different sites in the body show different characteristics, i.e. they are very heterogeneous, and will have different activation requirements. Blood monocytes are capable of killing
a number of microorganisms. If these cells are cultured in vitro then
some of this ability is lost. Exposure of cultured cells to lymphokines
restores the microbicidal activity and also activates other killing pathways.

A number of morphological and functional cell characteristics
change during activation and the degree of change will vary for different stages of activation. The ability of the cell to spread on a surface,
the cell volume and the level and activity of a number of membrane
molecules and intracellular enzymes are all increased. All these effects
tend to make the macrophages more efficient and effective cells.
Gamma-interferon is a powerful macrophage-activating molecule
which increases the uptake of antigens by enhancing expression of Fc
and complement receptors. This can lead to more uptake and effective
elimination of antigen aided by a rise in the activities of intracellular

enzymes involved in killing. Since gamma-interferon causes an increase in MHC class II expression there will be an enhanced presentation of antigen to CD4$^+$ T-cells. This will lead to the production of more lymphokines and the more effective elimination of the offending material.

The lymphokines that activate macrophages are secreted by CD4$^+$ T-cells; mostly, as we have seen, by T_H1 cells. Therefore, the presentation of antigen by an antigen-presenting cell, usually an infected macrophage, will lead to the production of lymphokines by T-cells with receptors **specific** for the antigen involved (Fig. 4.13). The lymphokines produced will then activate **any** responsive macrophage in the vicinity of the responding cells, including the cell presenting the antigen. The activated macrophages will then resist infection by

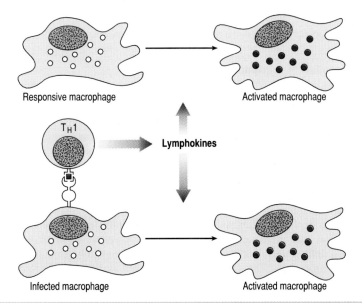

Fig. 4.13 Macrophage activation.
An MHC class II positive cell presents antigen to a T-cell that is then stimulated to produce lymphokines. This interaction is antigen specific since only those T-cells with a receptor that interacts with the MHC class II/antigen complex will be activated. The lymphokines produced then activate any responding macrophage in the vicinity. Thus lymphokines released in response to a particular microorganism may bring about the elimination of a different infectious agent by the activation of macrophages. The inducing microorganism can also be destroyed as the infected macrophage will also be exposed to the lymphokines. It is also probable that since the presenting cell is infected with a particular agent then other cells in the vicinity will be infected with this same microbe. Although a T_H1 cell is shown to be the responding cell, T_H2 and CD8$^+$ T-cells also produce lymphokines capable of macrophage activation when stimulated by antigen.

pathogens, kill intracellular pathogens and destroy tumour cells. The activation process appears to depend on the presence of a number of lymphokines that act synergistically to induce activation. For example, pure interleukin-2, interleukin-4 or gamma-interferon are unable to induce resistance to infection but if gamma-interferon is combined with either of the others then resistance is observed. It should be noted that the lymphokines produced may affect other cell types in addition to macrophages.

Macrophages and monocytes themselves are capable of producing a number of important cytokines. These monokines include interleukin-1, interleukin-6, various colony-stimulating factors and tumour necrosis factor (TNF-α). Tumour necrosis factor and interleukin-1 acting independently and together have effects on many leucocytes and tissues. Tumour necrosis factor is responsible for the tumouricidal activity of macrophages but is also implicated in the elimination of certain bacteria and parasites. It has a synergistic effect with gamma-interferon on resistance to a number of viral infections.

Generation of immune responses

When discussing the structure of lymphoid tissue it was pointed out that immune responses take place in secondary lymphoid tissues, e.g. lymph nodes. The preceding sections have described the characteristics of the acquired immune response and the cells that are involved in these processes. We now need to consider the mechanisms that facilitate the steps between antigen entering the host and the production of the immune effector functions.

Microorganisms that breach the mechanical barriers of the innate defence system enter the tissues and start to multiply. Their numbers increase and an inflammatory response is initiated. Some of these potential pathogens and their products — as well as substances introduced deliberately, such as vaccines — move via the lymphatics to the local lymph node. The antigen may be carried along by the lymph flow or taken there attached to a cell. This cell will most likely be a type of macrophage (tissue histiocyte) or dendritic cell (Langerhans cell of the skin). On reaching the lymph node various antigens move selectively to areas where different populations of lymphocytes are found. Most antigens go to the medulla where they will be taken up by classical macrophages. In an immune individual antigen/antibody complexes tend to accumulate in follicular dendritic cells of the cortex and may persist there for years. Langerhans cells carrying antigens from the skin change their morphology within the lymph node and are found in the paracortex (T-cell area) as interdigitating cells.

As discussed previously the generation of humoral and cell-mediated responses requires the initial activation of T_H cells to produce the required lymphokines. T_H cells, as has been emphasized, only recognize antigen fragments in association with MHC class II molecules. The distribution of MHC class II molecules is limited, in normal situations, to certain cells of the immune system, the antigen-presenting cells. In certain circumstances non-lymphoid cells can present antigens if they are induced to express MHC class II molecules. In order to stimulate a T_H cell the antigen must be taken into the antigen-presenting cell and re-expressed on the surface in association with MHC class II molecules. Since the T-cell antigen receptor recognizes antigen fragments bound to the MHC molecules, the antigen-presenting cell must also be able to process the antigen. Recognition of antigen by both $CD8^+$ and $CD4^+$ T-cells requires antigen processing. The pathways that lead to the association of an antigen fragment with a particular restriction element are only just being unravelled. We now know the overall pathways involved but very few details of the processing in which a particular molecule is degraded to produce the fragments that associate with either MHC class I or class II molecules have been elucidated.

Antigens that become associated with MHC class II molecules, and are therefore involved in the initiation of an immune response by stimulating T_H cells, usually originate from outwith the cell, i.e. are exogenous antigens. These antigens enter the cell and progress down the endocytic pathway. During this process the vesicle in which the antigen is held gradually becomes more acidic and the foreign material is degraded. At some point, before complete destruction of the antigen, peptide fragments are taken to a specialized site, known as the compartment for peptide loading (CPL). MHC class II molecules are produced within the rough endoplasmic reticulum by the protein synthesizing machinery of the cell. The newly synthesized MHC class II molecules pass through the Golgi apparatus and enter the CPL. Here the antigen fragments become associated with the newly synthesized MHC class II molecules and the complex then progresses to the cell surface (Fig. 4.14).

It is known that, in addition to the polymorphic MHC class II α and β chains, an invariant chain is also produced within the endoplasmic reticulum. This invariant chain has only been found to be associated with MHC class II molecules isolated before they reach the surface. It is proposed that this extra chain acts as a mask covering the peptide binding site on the MHC class II molecule until the complex reaches the cellular compartment, CPL, where the processed antigen is to be found. The invariant chain also controls the transport of MHC class II molecules to the CPL. Within the CPL, possibly due to changes in environmental conditions, such as pH, the invariant chain is released and the antigen fragment becomes bound in its place. This complex of MHC class II and antigen fragment is then transported to the cell surface.

The antigen-presenting cell has now produced one of the signals for

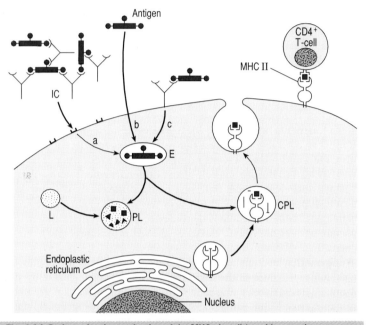

Fig. 4.14 Pathway for the production of the MHC class II/peptide complex.
Exogenous antigen is taken up into a vesicle by a number of pathways depending on the cell type involved. For example, by Fc receptor-mediated uptake of immune complexes (IC) (a), non-specifically (b) or by surface immunoglobulin on a B-cell (c). Once internalized the phagosome (E) joins with a lysosome (L) and degradation of the antigen takes place within the phagolysosome (PL). The mechanisms that ensure that antigen is not completely degraded are not known but at some stage the now processed antigen enters the compartment for peptide loading (CPL). At this site the processed antigen comes in contact with MHC class II molecules. These molecules have been synthesized and undergone post-translational modifications in the endoplasmic reticulum and Golgi apparatus. When first produced the polymorphic α and β-chains are associated with a polypeptide known as the invariant chain (I). This invariant chain is thought to occupy the antigen-binding cleft of the MHC class II molecule. The invariant chain is thought to direct the complex to the CPL where the invariant chain is released and the processed antigen, peptide, binds to the now exposed cleft formed between the α_1 and β_1 domains. The MHC class II with bond antigen completes its journey to the surface and a complex that can stimulate a CD4+ T-cell has been generated.

T_H cell activation, i.e. antigen in association with MHC class II. The co-stimulatory signal, B7, is constutively expressed by certain antigen-presenting cells, such as dendritic cells within secondary lymphoid tissues. In others, such as B-cells and macrophages, expression of this molecule is stimulated by microbial products acting directly on the antigen-presenting cells or cytokines, such as gamma-interferon from NK cells, produced in response to the infection. Responsive T-cells will now have received both signals and will be stimulated into action. The T-cells then start to produce interleukin-2 that will support the growth of itself and other T-cells, i.e. autocrine and paracrine activity. The activated T-cells will in turn produce other lymphokines that can stimulate the differentiation of antigen-triggered B-cells into antibody-producing plasma cells or activate macrophages or lead to the development of other effector T-cells.

Immune responses are generated in secondary lymphoid tissues such as lymph nodes. Since a number of cells and molecules must all interact, the architecture of the secondary lymphoid tissue has evolved for the efficient induction of an immune response. In a secondary immune response the cells involved are at a different stage of activation, i.e. they are memory cells having already been exposed to antigen. Therefore, the growth factor signals may not be so critical but antigen in association with MHC class II molecules is still required. In this situation B-cells are important as antigen-presenting cells.

$CD8^+$ T-cells, as we have seen, recognize antigen fragments associated with MHC class I molecules. Almost all nucleated cells have MHC class I molecules on their surface and would therefore be expected to be capable of presenting antigen fragments to cytotoxic T-cells that are in the most part MHC class I restricted. Some $CD4^+$ T-cells also exhibit cytotoxicity, therefore MHC class II is involved. $CD8^+$ T-cells are mainly involved in the elimination of virus-infected cells. These pathogens replicate within the host cell and therefore their antigens can be considered to be endogenously produced. MHC class I heavy chains, like the class II molecules, are synthesized by ribosomes on the surface of the endoplasmic reticulum. The molecules are produced through the endoplasmic reticulum membrane and then, after formation of the complete molecule, are modified in the Golgi apparatus before being transported to the surface. Only the heavy chain of the MHC class I molecule is coded for within the MHC. This chain is found on the surface of the cell non-covalently attached to β_2-microglobulin. It has recently been shown that fragments of endogenously produced viral peptides, i.e. synthesized with host replicative machinery, become associated with the heavy chain as it associates with β_2-microglobulin within the endoplasmic reticulum. The complete complex, MHC class I with attached peptide fragment, is then transported to the cell surface where it can be recognized by a $CD8^+$ T-cell.

The antigen fragments that associate with MHC class I molecules are derived from endogenously produced molecules that are synthesized in the cytoplasm (Fig. 4.15). Viral and other proteins synthesized in the cytoplasm are degraded by specialized structures known as proteasomes. These multicomponent complexes contain enzymes that generate short peptides from cytoplasmic proteins. At least two of the component parts, LMP-2 and -7 (low molecular weight protein) are

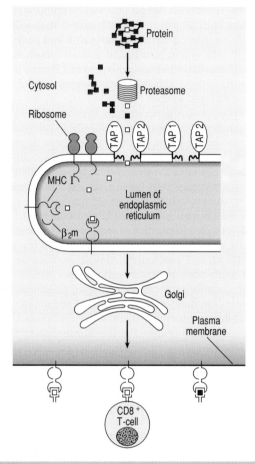

Fig. 4.15 Pathway for the formation of MHC class I/peptide complex.
A protein (■-■-■) synthesized in the cytoplasm contains a T-cell epitope (□). The protein is cleaved by the proteasome and the peptide that is generated is transported into the endoplasmic reticulum by the transporter associated with antigen presentation which is composed of two subunits, TAP-1 and TAP-2. The peptide associates with an MHC class I molecule and is transported to the cell membrane.

coded for by genes in the class II region of the MHC. The peptides that are generated within the cytoplasm have to enter the lumen of the endoplasmic reticulum to combine with the newly synthesized MHC heavy chain and β_2-microglobulin. A transporter molecule composed of two polypeptide chains, called **transporter associated with antigen processing-1 and -2** (TAP-1, TAP-2) carries out this process. Like the LMP-2 and -7 genes the genes for TAP-1 and -2 are found in the class II region of the MHC. This transporter has a similar structure to other transport molecules present in eukaryotic and prokaryotic organisms. These molecules form a family of proteins known as ATP-binding cassettes (ABC) that use the energy from the hydrolysis of ATP to facilitate the movement of various proteins, ions and antibiotics across membranes. Once the processed peptide enters the endoplasmic reticulum it associates with the MHC class I heavy chain and β_2-microglobulin to form the structure that is then transported to the cell surface via the Golgi complex.

The separation of the two pathways of antigen presentation ensures that endogenous antigen associates with MHC class I molecules while peptides derived from exogenous antigens bind to MHC class II molecules (Fig. 4.16). Proteins synthesized in the cytoplasm are processed and transported to the endoplasmic reticulum where they become associated with the newly produced MHC class I molecules. At this site the binding site on the newly synthesized MHC class II molecules is inaccessible due to the presence of the invariant chain. The MHC class I molecules with bound peptide are then taken directly to the cell surface. The MHC class II molecules with attached invariant chain are routed to the compartment for peptide loading where they are exposed to peptides derived from internalized material. Within this compartment the invariant chain is lost and a peptide is bound. The MHC class II molecules are then transported to the cell surface. Thus the site where the antigen is processed determines whether it will associate with MHC class I or class II. Exceptions to these rules have been reported when the site of synthesis or other characteristics result in endogenously produced molecules associating with MHC class II. In the same way exogenous antigen, instead of associating with MHC class II, may reach the site of MHC class I/peptide association and be expressed in the context of MHC class I. This has been described in situations where large amounts of antigen are taken up by antigen-presenting cells. This separation of processing pathways explains why $CD4^+$ and $CD8^+$ T-cells are involved in the destruction of exogenous and endogenous antigens, respectively.

Antigen processing, whether for MHC class I or class II, generates peptides that then associate with the peptide binding groove of the restriction elements, i.e. the MHC molecules. The mechanisms that determine what peptides are produced from a particular protein are not known but some information is available on what constitutes a T-cell epitope. The characteristics of the peptides that comprise the antigen fragments associated with MHC class I and class II differ in a number of respects. From one protein there appears to be a dominant epitope, usually of nine amino acids in length, that binds to a particular MHC class I molecule. For MHC class II the peptides appear to be heterogeneous and slightly larger than the peptides associated with MHC class I.

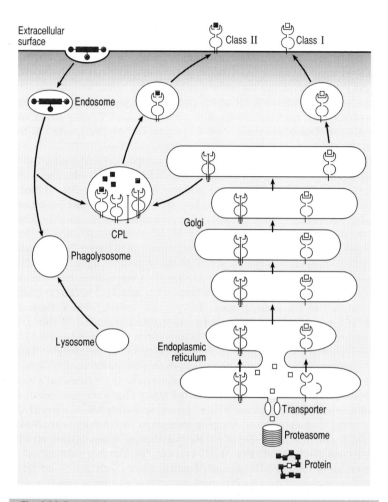

Fig. 4.16 Presentation of exogenous and endogenous antigens.
Endogenous antigens are processed and peptides (□) generated. These peptides associate
with MHC class I molecules and go to the cell surface where they are recognized by CD8[+] T-
cells. Exogenous antigens are endocytosed, partially degraded and the peptides (■) enter
the compartment for peptide loading (CPL). Newly synthesized MHC class II molecules,
produced in the endoplasmic reticulum, interact with the invariant chain (I) which directs the
complex to the CPL. Within this compartment the invariant chain is removed and the peptide
can associate with the MHC class II molecule. After the peptide binds to the MHC class II
molecule the complex is transported to the cell surface where it is recognized by CD4[+] T-cells.

The processing pathways do not provide any mechanism that will
enable the host to differentiate between self and foreign molecules. It
is proposed that many MHC class I and class II molecules appear at

the cell surface with fragments of self molecules attached. It is possible that the density of individual self fragments is too low to trigger a response and that only when a foreign molecule, which is likely to be produced or taken up in large amounts, is present does the specific T-cell see enough antigen on the surface of the cell to be activated. Other mechanisms that lead to tolerance, i.e. non-reaction to self, will be discussed below (p. 142).

The MHC class I and class II molecules are therefore critical for the functioning of T-cells. If a particular antigen does not become associated with these molecules then no T-dependent immune response will be directed against that antigen. Since MHC class II molecules are involved in the initiation of immune responses by presenting antigen fragments to T_H cells, they can control whether a response takes place or not. It has been clearly shown that the level of an immune response to a particular antigen is controlled by the MHC class II molecules. The genes that code for these molecules, i.e. MHC class II genes, have therefore been referred to as **immune response genes** (Ir genes).

It should be obvious that if an antigen cannot associate with the MHC class II molecules of an individual then no immune response will be generated. Since the MHC codes for molecules that are polymorphic, the cells of some individuals will present, and therefore respond to, certain antigen fragments while cells from other individuals will not. Fortunately more than one antigenic fragment can be generated from each pathogen otherwise those who did not respond to the particular sequence would be vulnerable to that microorganism. In addition, individuals can have six different MHC class II genes and therefore an increased chance that some fragments will bind to at least one of their MHC class II molecules. Using a simple antigen containing a single T-cell epitope and inbred strains of mice, responder and non-responder phenotypes can be recognized. This has been shown to be controlled by the MHC class II genes (Ir gene effects). This all or none situation is not seen with complex antigens since many different MHC class II/antigen fragment complexes will be produced. It follows that varying levels and specificity of response will be stimulated in individuals who have different MHC class II molecules and have therefore produced different MHC/antigen complexes on their cells. It is reasonable to expect that a greater response will be generated in a host who has produced many different fragments associated with a number of MHC class II products compared with an individual who has a few antigen fragments associated with only one or two MHC class II molecules.

Immune response gene effects can also be controlled at the level of the T-cell receptor. If an individual does not have a T-cell with a receptor that recognizes a particular antigen/MHC complex then no response will be generated. The T-cell receptor repertoire is generated in the thymus where the genes of the immature T-cells are rearranged to give rise to a functioning receptor. T-cells that cross-react too strongly with self molecules are deleted as are cells whose receptors do not interact with self MHC molecules. Therefore, T-cells that interact weakly with MHC molecules are selected to mature and leave the thymus. When these cells later come across antigen/MHC complex the presence of foreign antigen strengthens the weak T-cell receptor/MHC interaction leading to a stimulatory signal being transmitted to the T-cell. If for some reason T-cells that respond to a particular MHC/antigen configuration have been deleted, suppressed or not formed then no immune response will be generated to that antigen. This is what is known as a 'hole' in the T-cell repertoire.

In the lymph node an antigen-presenting cell processes the antigen and presents it to a CD4$^+$ T-cell in the context of MHC class II. The T-cells that recognize the MHC/antigen complex and receive co-stimulatory signals proliferate and produce interleukin-2 that causes more proliferation and the production of various other lymphokines. These lymphokines will include growth and maturation factors for B-cells and other effector cells. B-cells with surface immunoglobulin that can bind to antigens present in the lymph node will be stimulated by these lymphokines and develop into antibody-producing plasma cells. The antibody produced by these cells will leave in the efferent lymph and enter the blood at the thoracic duct. The blood system will then disperse the antibody throughout the circulation and, depending on the isotype being produced, into the body fluids. The antibody will then interact with any antigen that it comes across and aid in its destruction. Immature effector T-cells that have interacted with antigen in the periphery or in the lymph node will be stimulated to mature into effector cells. They leave the lymph node and return via the blood to the site of infection to help destroy the pathogen.

The necessity for such a complicated recognition mechanism by T-cells may be difficult to understand at first. B-cells recognize free antigen, so why cannot T-cells? The answer probably lies in the fact that T-cells evolved to complement the functioning of the humoral defence system. Antibody is an effective weapon against extracellular pathogens either on its own or in conjunction with other factors (e.g. complement) or cells (e.g. phagocytes). However, if the pathogen can penetrate a host cell and survive then it is reasonably safe from the effects of antibody. T-cells have evolved to combat these intracellular pathogens and therefore need to recognize infected cells. Products of the MHC direct the T-cell onto the surface of the target cell. Hence, although these cells are effective in destroying infected cells, the individual, by recognizing self structures (MHC antigens) run the risk of destroying self. Therefore, in parallel, the requirement for T-cell help as a second signal in the activation of effector cells evolved. This gives the opportunity for the elimination or non-stimulation of strongly self-reactive cells (see Tolerance, p. 142).

The main function of the MHC is to make sure that the T-cell makes contact with antigen on the surface of a cell. These cells cannot destroy extracellular microbes and they would be inhibited in the elimination of intracellular pathogens if they could bind free antigens. In viral infections, after the initial entry of the pathogen when the host replicative machinery is synthesizing progeny virus particles, no infectious agent is present. At this stage antigen fragments associate with MHC class I gene products and are expressed together on the cell surface. Killing of the host cell by a cytotoxic T-cell will prevent production of progeny virions. The cytotoxic T-cell recognizes two features before striking: (1) virus infection by the presence of antigen fragments and (2) cell surface by MHC class I. The T-cell receptor binds to both these entities and eliminates the target cell. It would be inefficient to use these cells to destroy single free virus particles; antibody can do this.

With intracellular bacteria and protozoa, which are capable of independent replication, destruction of infected cells would result in the dissemination of the pathogen. In this situation the effector cells still need to identify infected cells and here too the MHC is involved in the process of identification but a different strategy is used to destroy the pathogen. Macrophages are the usual site of infection so a different restriction element is used. Antigen fragments associate with MHC class II molecules — a signal for the macrophage cell surface — and the CD4$^+$ T-cells produce lymphokines that activate the macrophage to a state where the intracellular pathogen can be killed. If the pathogen does escape because the target cell has been lysed then the lymphokines will have activated other macrophages in the vicinity. Pathogens entering one of these cells will be destroyed because of the enhanced battery of microbicidal molecules.

In the generation of an immune response T-cells must be activated to produce 'helper factors'. B-cells that can produce the antibody specific for the antigen will internalize this antigen through surface immunoglobulin. Again a cell, the B-cell, is the target for the T-cell to recognize and MHC class II is the signal used to stimulate lymphokine production where it is required. Other antigen-presenting cells will carry out a similar function, signalling to the responsive T-cell to produce helper factors in their vicinity within a lymph node since antigen-reactive B-cells are also likely to be close at hand. T-cells must communicate and interact with other cells to make the appropriate immune response and MHC-encoded molecules ensure that the required cellular interactions happen efficiently.

Control of immune responses

An antigen can induce two types of response: immunity or tolerance. Tolerance is the acquisition of non-reactivity towards a particular antigen. The generation of immunity or tolerance depends largely on the way the immune system first encounters the antigen. Once the immune system has been stimulated the cells involved proliferate and produce a response that will eliminate the offending agent. It is then important to dampen down the reacting cells and various feedback mechanisms operate to bring this about.

Role of antigen

The primary regulator of an immune response is antigen itself. This makes sense since it is important to initiate a response when antigen enters the host and once it has been eliminated it is wasteful and in some cases dangerous to continue to produce effector mechanisms. Antigen stimulates the immune system through specific receptors; once this no longer happens the cells will stop being stimulated and die. Memory cells will have been formed to react if the antigen is re-encountered.

Role of antibody

Many biological systems are controlled by the product inhibiting the reaction once a certain level is reached. This type of negative feedback is seen with antibody. Removal of antibody by plasmaphoresis during the course of a response leads to an increase in antibody synthesis. In many cases the injection of preformed antibody markedly depresses the response. The antibody may be acting by blocking the epitopes on the antigen so that it can no longer stimulate the cell through its receptor (Fig. 4.17). In addition, antibody as part of an immune complex may directly inhibit the B-cell. In this situation the simultaneous binding of antigen to the surface immunoglobulin and to Fc receptors on the B-cell surface leads to a negative signal that switches off antibody production.

As antibody levels rise there will be competition between free antibody and the B-cell receptor. The free antibody will mop up the antigen, effectively lowering its concentration. Consequently only those B-cells that have a receptor with a high affinity for antigen will be stimulated and therefore produced high affinity antibody. For this reason antibody feedback is thought to be an important driving force in affinity maturation.

Role of immune complexes

As described above, immune complexes can suppress antibody production by interacting with Fc receptors on B-cells. Sometimes antibody increases the immune response, especially when antigen is in

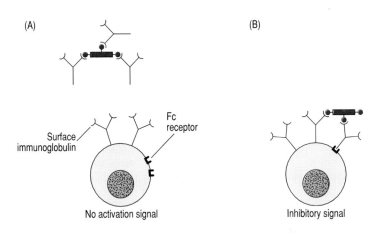

Fig. 4.17 Inhibition of B-cells by antibody.
Antibody can suppress antibody production in two ways. (A) Antigen blocking. Antigen must bind to surface immunoglobulin on B-cells to induce antibody production. If high concentrations of antibody are present immune complexes will form that effectively mask all the epitopes on the antigen and the B-cell will not be stimulated. (B) Receptor crosslinking. If immune complexes are present that bind to Fc receptors when antigen also interacts with surface immunoglobulin then a signal is generated that inhibits antibody synthesis.

excess. This process is dependent on the Fc portion of the antibody and is thought to operate by enhancing the uptake of antigen by certain antigen-presenting cells. It is found that IgM is most efficient in this context, while IgG is usually suppressive. At the beginning of a response IgM is produced and can stimulate immunoglobulin synthesis whereas, as the response matures, the IgG produced will tend to inhibit antibody production.

Regulatory T-cells

T_H cells control the generation of effector cells by producing helper factors. However, the factors that stimulate the expansion of B- and T-cell numbers do not work indefinitely. Maturation factors are also produced that control terminal differentiation into effector cells. Under the influence of these latter lymphokines the action of the proliferation factors is inhibited, mainly by making the effector cell unresponsive to its effects.

Other T-lymphocytes have been described that provide negative signals to the immune system. These T-cells, sometimes referred to as suppressor T-cells (T_S cells), limit the development of antibody-producing cells and effector T-cells. Suppression can involve both the production of soluble factors and direct cell–cell interactions.

Idiotypes

As described in Chapter 3, antibody can stimulate the production of an anti-antibody, an anti-idiotypic antibody. By carrying on this process an idiotype network of interacting antibodies can be generated. These interactions were formulated by Jerne into the idiotype network model that can control immune responses. Since these anti-idiotypic antibodies bind to the variable portion of immunoglobulin they can stimulate or inhibit an immune response in the same way as antigen and antigen/antibody complexes (Fig. 4.18). The exact signals involved in these control processes are not known.

Tolerance

Two forms of tolerance can be identified — natural tolerance and acquired tolerance. The non-response to self molecules is due to nat-

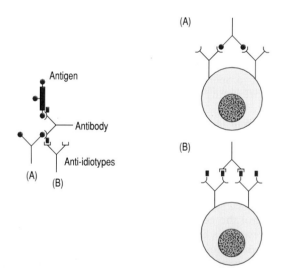

Fig. 4.18 Regulation of B-cells by anti-idiotypic interactions.
(A) Site-associated anti-idiotypic antibody is an internal image of the original antibody and can therefore bind and crosslink surface immunoglobulin on B-cells. (B) Non-site-associated anti-idiotypic antibody generated by the idiotypic network can also crosslink surface immunoglobulin. Both these interactions deliver a signal to the B-cell that, depending on other unknown factors, can be stimulatory or inhibitory.

ural tolerance. If this tolerance breaks down and the body responds to self molecules then an autoimmune disease will develop (see Ch. 9). Natural tolerance appears during fetal development when the immune system is being formed. In experimental animals the introduction of foreign material at the time of birth leads to tolerance. For this state of unresponsiveness to be maintained the foreign material must be continuously present. It is therefore thought that as the cells of the immune system develop those that interact through their surface receptors with a host component will be eliminated so that the host will be unable to respond to that molecule. Acquired tolerance arises when a potential immunogen induces a state of unresponsiveness to itself. This has consequences for host defences since the presence of a tolerogenic epitope on a pathogen may compromise the body's ability to resist infection. In transplant patients and where an inappropriate response is made, e.g. autoimmune diseases, the ability to induce tolerance may be of therapeutic advantage.

Mature T-cells are more susceptible to tolerization than B-cells, although unresponsiveness in immature B-cells is very easy to obtain. T-cell tolerance usually lasts longer than that seen in B-cells. An antigen can induce different effects on the two arms of the immune system. During an infection the host will be exposed to a variety of antigenic determinants on a microorganism. These epitopes will be present at differing concentrations and possibly at different times during the infection. The epitopes can act as either immunogens or tolerogens. Therefore it is possible that the antibody response to a particular antigen may be quite pronounced while the cell-mediated response might be lacking, or vice versa. Alternatively, both arms of the immune response may be stimulated or tolerized.

An antigen can be immunogenic under one set of circumstances but can act as a tolerogen in other cases. Generally, high doses of antigen tolerize B-cells while minute doses given repeatedly tolerize T-cells. A moderate dose of the same antigen might be immunogenic. Protein antigens are more tolerogenic when in a soluble form than in an aggregated or particulate form. This may be because the two forms are processed and presented differently. For acquired tolerance to be maintained the tolerogen must persist or be repeatedly administered. This is probably necessary because of the continuous production of new T- and B-cells that must be rendered tolerant.

Several mechanisms play a role in the selective lack of response to specific antigens. Since each lymphocyte has a receptor with a single specificity the elimination of a specific cell will render the individual tolerant to the epitope it recognizes and leave the rest of the repertoire untouched. Tolerance to self tissues is fundamental to the functioning of the immune system. This mechanism relies on self molecules interacting with the receptor and causing their elimination. It is proposed that during lymphocyte development the cell goes through a phase in which contact with antigen leads to death or permanent inactivation. Immature B-cells that develop in the bone marrow and bind molecules through surface IgM are destroyed; these molecules are likely to be of host origin. The elimination of self-reactive T-cells in the thymus during T-cell maturation is an important step in maintaining a state of tolerance. Tolerance can also be induced by active suppression. Some T-cells are capable of inducing unresponsiveness by acting directly on B-cells or other T-cells. These suppressor T-cells can be antigen-specific and probably produce signals that actively suppress cells capable of responding to a particular antigen.

It was originally thought that unresponsiveness to self was controlled solely by the elimination of all self-reactive cells before they matured. This cannot be true since self-reactive B-cells are found in normal adult animals. These cells survive because elimination of self-reactive cells in the primary lymphoid tissue is not complete; not all self molecules will be produced at these sites. It is thought that these B-cells are controlled by a lack of T-cell help, i.e. T_H have been eliminated. It is thought that Ts cells play a subordinate role acting as a back-up mechanism.

As with B-cells, not all self-reactive T-cells are deleted in the thymus. T-cells with a receptor that can bind to peptides derived from self molecules that are not expressed in the thymus will survive. The requirement for two signals in the stimulation of lymphocytes can give rise to tolerance. In the periphery cells can process these self antigens and express peptides associated with MHC molecules on their surface. These cells will not, however, be expressing co-stimulatory signals. Naive T-cells that recognize the MHC/antigen complex without co-stimulation become anergic. The most important consequence of this is that they cannot produce interleukin-2 and therefore cannot proliferate and develop into effector cells — they are in essence inactive.

In certain situations it may be desirable to suppress the immune system. This will be important in the prevention of graft rejection and the control of autoimmunity. In these situations physical agents (irradiation), antibodies and drugs can be used to modify the immune response. These procedures have a negative aspect in that prolonged immunosuppression increases the risk of contracting infectious diseases or developing cancer since immune surveillance is affected.

Neuroendocrine control mechanisms

Clear evidence is emerging that the immune and neuroendocrine systems behave as an integrated information circuit with common mediators and receptors. Table 4.7 summarises the various pathways and mediators involved. Corticotrophin-releasing hormone (CRH) is a key player and originates both from the pituitary and immune cells. CRH is a major mediator of local inflammation whilst β endorphin when

Table 4.7 Origin of main hormones affecting the activity of the immune system

Hypothalamic Hormones acting on pituitary gland

> Corticotrophin Releasing Hormone (CRH)[*]
> Prolactin Releasing Hormone (PRH)
> Growth Hormone Releasing Hormone (GRLH)
> Thyrotrophin Releasing Hormone (TRH)

Anterior Pituitary hormones and their effects

Adrenocorticotrophin (ACTH)	Adrenal Gland	Glucocorticoids
Prolactin (PRL)	Lymphocytes	IL-2
Growth Hormone (GH)	Lymphocytes	Proliferation
Thyroid Stimulating Hormone (TSH)	T Lymphocytes	B Cells

Hormones produced by cells of the immune system

T Lymphocytes	ACTH, TSH, Endorphins, PRL, GH
B Lymphocytes	ACTH, Endorphins, GH,
Macrophages	ACTH, Endorphins, GH,

[*] CRH can act directly on macrophages resulting in IL-1 release

produced by cells of the immune system by stimuli such as cold shock, can alleviate pain by acting on peripheral sensory nerves. Physical and psychological stimuli lead to production of hormones and cytokines that act on receptors on cells of the immune system that alter immune function either directly or through the induction of other mediators. Cytokines of neural origin appear to act as neurotransmitters and IL-1 produced by electrical stimuli to the brain leads to CRH release from the hypothalamus. The ACTH response that follows, stimulates glucocorticoid release from the adrenals with alterations in metabolism and suppression of the immune system, along with inhibition of synthesis of CRH and ACTH by negative feedback. IL-1 and IL-6 appear to bring about release of hypothalmic and pituitary hormones, IL-1 acts on the pituitary via the release of CRH from the hypothalmus. Receptors for IL-1 are found in the CNS and the pituitary gland. Bacterial endotoxin has been shown to upregulate IL-1 receptors in these tissues with the implication that bacterial infection influences CRH production. It is not clear how IL-1 gains access to the brain but it is believed that it may gain access via the blood-brain barrier, perhaps associated with changes in the vascular endothelium or perhaps from macrophages crossing the barrier.

FURTHER READING

Adams D O, Hamilton T A 1984 The cell biology of macrophage activation. Annual Review of Immunology 2: 283–318

Balkwill F R, Burke F 1989 The cytokine network. Immunology Today 10: 299–304

Butcher E C 1990 Cellular and molecular mechanisms that direct leukocyte traffic. American Journal of Pathology 136: 1–11

Cambier J C, Ransom J T 1987 Molecular mechanisms of transmembrane signalling in B lymphocytes. Annual Review of Immunology 5: 175–199

Childers N K, Bruce M G, McGhee J R 1989 Molecular mechanisms of immunoglobulin A defence. Annual Review of Microbiology 43: 503–536

Cresswell P 1994 Assembly, transport and function of MHC class II. Annual Review of Immunology 12: 259–293

Engelhard V H 1994 Structure of peptides associated with class I and class II MHC molecules. Annual Review of Immunology 12: 181–207

Finkelman F D, Holmes J, Katona I M, Urban Jr J F, Beckmann M P, Park L S, Schooley K A, Coffman R L, Mosmann T R, Paul W E 1990 Lymphokine control of in vivo immunoglobulin isotype selection. Annual Review of Immunology 8: 303–333

Germain R N 1994 MHC-dependent antigen processing and peptide presentation: providing ligands for T-lymphocyte activation. Cell 76: 287–299

Lenschow D J, Walunas T L, Bluestone J A 1996 CD28/B7 system of T-cell co-stimulation. Annual Review of Immunology 14: 233–258

Marrack P, Kappler J W 1993 How the immune system recognizes the body. Scientific American September: 49–55

Mosmann T R, Coffmann R L 1989 Heterogeneity of cytokine secretion patterns and functions of helper T-cells. Advances in Immunology 46: 111–147

Paul W E, Seder R A 1994 Lymphocyte responses and cytokines. Cell 76: 241–251

Reth M, Hombach J, Wienands J, Campbell K S, Chien N, Justement L B, Cambier J C 1991 The B-cell antigen receptor complex. Immunology Today 12: 196–200

Rothbard J B 1994 One size fits all. Current Biology 4: 653–655

Van Bleek G M, Nathenson S G 1990 Isolation of an endogenously processed immunodominant viral peptide from the class I H-2 Kb molecule. Nature 348: 213–216

Weissman I L, Cooper M D 1993 How the immune system develops. Scientific American September: 33–39

York I A, Rock K L 1996 Antigen processing and presentation by class I major histocompatibility complex. Annual Review of Immunology 14: 369–396

Young L H Y, Liu C-C, Joag S, Rafii S, Young J D E 1990 How lymphocytes kill. Annual Review of Medicine 41: 45–54

Immunology in action

5 Infection, immunity and protection

Introduction

In the normal healthy individual, despite popular belief, the relationship between microorganisms and the human body is usually a harmless one. Saprophytic or commensal microorganisms grow and reproduce without apparent damage to either host or microbe. As Lewis Thomas points out in his essay on 'Germs' (*The Lives of a Cell*, Bantam Books), 'we have always been a relatively minor interest of the vast microbial world' and human disease is not 'the work of an organized, modernized kind of demonology, in which bacteria are the most visible and centrally placed adversaries... Most bacteria are totally preoccupied with browsing, altering the configurations of organic molecules so that they become usable for the energy needs of other forms of life'. The normal flora of humans is shown in Figures 5.1 to 5.3 and gives examples of bacteria, fungi and protozoa which are commensals that do not recognize a good situation.

Microorganisms that produce disease are referred to as microbial pathogens. The pattern of disease is closely related to population size. Persistence of a disease is greater if the microbe can survive in the infected individual for some time and if it can be easily transmitted from one person to another. Thus, for such pathogens, a small number of susceptible people are needed to allow the disease to persist.

Measles needs a community of at least half a million people in order to persist. One of the objectives of vaccination policy is to reduce the numbers of susceptible individuals to a number below that required for persistence of the disease. It should be noted that the adaptability of microorganisms by mutation will allow the emergence of variants that have characteristics that can overcome host resistance mechanisms — such characteristics might take the form of more efficient

Nose & nasal pharynx

Staphylococci
Diphtheroids
Neisseria sp
Haemophilus sp

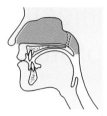

Oropharynx

Staphylococci
Streptococcus sp
Neisseria sp
Haemophilus sp

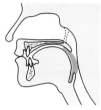

Mouth

Staphylococci
Streptococci
Actinomyces sp
Haemophilus sp
Y easts
Enteric bacteria
Anaerobic bacteria
Spirochaetes

Skin

Staphylococci
Streptococci
Corynebacterium
Propionibacterium
Y easts
Diphtheroids
Enteric bacteria (rare)

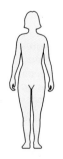

Fig. 5.1 Normal flora of the skin, mouth, nose and nasopharynx, and the oropharynx.
(Reproduced from Blackwell C C, Weir D M 1981 Principles of infection and immunity in patient care. Churchill Livingstone, Edinburgh, p. 53.)

Stomach

Normally sterile

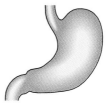

Small intestine

Lactobacilli ⎤
Enterococci ⎟
Diphtheroids ⎟ Small
Y easts (*Candida*) ⎬ numbers
Enteric bacteria ⎟
Anaerobic Gram ⎟
negative bacilli ⎦

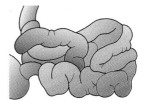

Large intestine

Anaerobic bacteria
  Gram negative
    Bacteroides spp
    Fusobacterium spp
  Gram positive
    Eubacterium spp
    Lactobacilli
    Clostridium spp
    Bifidobacterium
    Streptococci

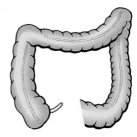

Facultative and aerobic organisms
  Staphylococci
  Enterococci
  Enteric bacteria
  Proteus spp
  Pseudomonas spp
  Y easts (*Candida*)

Fig. 5.2 Normal flora of the gastrointestinal system.
(Reproduced from Blackwell & Weir 1981, p. 54.)

transmissibility or interference with some aspect of the immune defence mechanisms (evasion mechanisms, see p. 154).

Modern medical science has managed to eliminate many of the classical infectious diseases but has also helped to create new ones which

Kidneys and bladder
Normally sterile

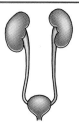

Vagina and cervix
Anaerobic bacteria
  Lactobacilli
  Streptococci
  Bacteroides spp
  Clostridium spp
  Bifidobacterium
  Eubacterium

Aerobic bacteria
  Diphtheroids
  Staphylococci
  Enterococci
  Strep. pyogenes (group B)
  Enteric bacteria

Yeasts
  Candida

Protozoa
  Trichomonas vaginalis
  (10–15% normal women)

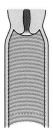

Fig. 5.3 Normal flora of the genitourinary tract.
(Reproduced from Blackwell & Weir 1981, p. 55.)

result from interference with normal host defence mechanisms — consequent upon medical and surgical procedures such as chemotherapy, catheterization, immunosuppression and X-irradiation. Infections that develop in this way are known as iatrogenic (physician-induced) diseases in which host defence mechanisms have been **compromised** in some way (Table 5.1).

It is important to differentiate infection from disease. A host may be infected with a particular microorganism and be unaware of the presence of the microorganism. If the microbe reproduces itself to such an extent that toxic products or sheer numbers of organisms begin to harm the host then a disease process has developed. It is well known

Table 5.1 The compromised host

Predisposing factor	Effect on immune system	Type of infection
Drug or X-rays in immunosuppression Allograft recipients (renal, bone marrow, heart) and cancer therapy	Diminished cell-mediated and humoral immunity	Lung infections, bacteraemia, fungal infections, urinary tract infections
Virus immunosuppression, e.g. rubella, herpes, EB virus, hepatitis virus, HIV	Replication of virus in lymphoid cells with resulting impaired function	Secondary bacterial infections (also fungal and protozal in AIDS)
Tumours	Replacement of cells of immune system	Bacteraemia, pneumonia, urinary tract infections
Malnutrition	Lyphoid hypoplasia Decrease in circulating lymphocytes Decreased phagocytic ability	Measles, tuberculosis, respiratory infections, gastrointestinal infections
Smoking, inhalation of dust particles (e.g. silica, fungal spores)	Inflammatory lung changes, immune complex deposition to fungal spores	Chronic respiratory infections, allergic responses
Chronic endocrine disease (e.g. diabetes)	Decreased phagocytic activity	Staph. infections, tuberculosis, respiratory infections, bacteraemia, etc.
Primary immune deficiency (see Ch. 7)	Diminished cell-mediated and/or humoral immunity	

that certain viruses cause latent infections (e.g. herpes simplex virus) and only cause disease (e.g. cold sores) under circumstances when the host defences are impaired. Other examples are the carriage of potentially pathogenic bacteria in the nose, throat or bowel, e.g. pneumococci, streptococci or salmonellae. This is known as the carrier state and is a source of infection to other individuals. No satisfactory explanation has been given for the persistence of some types of bacteria, viruses, fungi and parasites in their host's tissues. The most popular view is that microorganisms can in some instances conceal their potentially antigenic constituents by covering them with an envelope such as a lipid coat and in the case of viruses by coating themselves with a viral envelope derived from the host cell. This view has led to the suggestion that by removing the envelope with a lipid solvent and reintroducing the treated microorganism into the host the immune response would be generated to the underlying antigens and lead to the elimination of the pathogen.

Evasion of innate and acquired immune mechanisms

Once a microorganism becomes established in the tissues, having escaped the innate defence mechanisms described in Chapter 2, the microorganism can often make use of a number of evasion strategies that protect it from the immune reactions of the host, including interference with phagocytic activity and antibody function.

For example, the pneumococcus secretes large quantities of capsular polysaccharide that repels phagocytes and mops up antibody as it is produced, thus allowing the pneumococcus itself to proliferate unhindered. Trypanosomes appear to change their surface antigenic make-up from one generation to the next, so that the antibody made in response to the antigens of the original organism is inactive against the second generation of organisms.

Many microorganisms, particularly tubercle bacilli, brucellae and viruses, disappear inside tissue cells before sufficient antibody is produced to act against them. Bacteria that invade cells (intracellular bacteria) not only escape the effects of antibody and complement but also have developed mechanisms to avoid intracellular destruction. Some of these bacteria have become so entirely dependent on the intracellular environment that they cannot survive in the extracellular space, e.g. *Mycobacterium leprae*. *Listeria monocytogenes* can only survive in resident macrophages that have not been activated, whilst others such as *Salmonella* spp. and *Brucella* spp. survive because of a resistant glycolipid capsule. *Mycobacterium tuberculosis* secretes molecules that inhibit the fusion of phagosomes with lysosomes and, like other mycobacteria, has a hydrophobic waxy coat with a high lipid content that is very resistant to lysosomal enzymes. Lipoarabinomannan from mycobacteria has been shown to interfere with the protective macrophage-activating effects of gamma-interferon. In the last few years it has been found that leprosy bacilli, which are similar in many ways to tubercle bacilli, have the ability to grow in the thymus-dependent areas of the lymphoid tissues. This affects the development of a cell-mediated immune response against the invading organisms and allows their unhindered proliferation. The same appears to be true for cutaneous leishmaniasis where instances have been described of a loss of cell-mediated immunity. In short, a particular microorganism is pathogenic because in some way it is able to circumvent, at least initially, the immune mechanisms of the host. Table 5.2 gives a list of microorganisms that have been shown to interfere with cell-mediated immune function. In a situation where the host immune defence mechanisms

Table 5.2 **Microorganisms affecting cell-mediated immune function**

Bacteria	Viruses	Fungi
M. tuberculosis	Influenza	Coccidioides
M. leprae	Viral hepatitis	Cryptococcus
Treponema pallidum	Herpes simplex	Histoplasma
Brucella abortus	Cytomegalovirus	Candida
Salmonella spp.	HIV	
	Measles	
	Mumps	
	Rubella	
	Epstein–Barr	

are defective in some way (often called the compromised host) the distinction between pathogenic and non-pathogenic microorganisms becomes unimportant. All microorganisms that are human parasites have the capacity to produce disease in such a defective host. The breakdown of the normal host–parasite relationship then assumes central importance. Restoration of normal immune function is likely to be of more importance in the recovery of the patient than specific antimicrobial drug treatment.

The effects of complement and evasion mechanisms

Microorganisms normally lack the mammalian complement regulatory proteins described on pp. 22–27 and thus are unable to prevent complement deposition and amplification on their surfaces.

The lack of these regulatory molecules, along with the ability of some bacteria to protect C3b from factors H and I, accounts for the ability of most bacteria, viruses, fungi and parasites to activate the alternative complement pathway. Some bacteria and viruses can directly activate the classical pathway in the absence of antibody.

Pathogenic microorganisms have evolved a variety of resistance mechanisms to avoid the damaging effects of complement. Capsules are antiphagocytic as they shield the C3b deposited on the bacterial cell wall from contact with complement receptors on phagocytes. Sialic acid present in the capsules appears to interfere with complement activation, and streptococci, campylobacter strains and *Trypanosoma cruzi* possess surface molecules that interfere with the assembly of C3 convertase. Resistance to destruction by the late complement components is achieved by the presence of a thick peptidoglycan layer. Some viruses, e.g. herpes simplex and Epstein–Barr, produce complement inhibitory factors similar to those used by mammalian cells to prevent their destruction by complement.

Table 5.3 **Some examples of bacterial aggressins and 'impedins'**

Staphylococci	Coagulase
	Leucocidins
	Hyaluronidase
	Protein A
Streptococci	Haemolysins
	Hyaluronidase
	Fibrinolysin
	Leucocidins
Neisseria gonorrhoea	IgA proteases
N. meningitidis	
Streptococcus sanguis	
Pseudomonas aeruginosa	Collagenase
	Elastase

A number of microorganisms use the complement receptors of host cells in order to initiate infection.

Aggressins and impedins

These are a rather ill-defined group of bacterial products (Table 5.3), the presence of which is associated with virulence. If antibody to the aggressin is present, the pathogenicity of the microorganism is likely to be reduced. Aggressins are usually enzymes and many have damaging effects on leucocyte function, for example leucocidins produced by many Gram-positive bacteria. *Staphylococcus aureus* produces at least three separate leucocidins acting on macrophages and polymorphonuclear leucocytes, causing membrane disruption and degranulation. Injection of these substances into experimental animals can lead to leucopenia. The leucocidin diphosphopyridine nucleotidase acts within the phagocyte and destroys it. DNAases and nicotine adenine dinucleotidase have a similar effect. Other aggressins such as hyaluronidase act as spreading factors enabling dissemination of microorganisms through the tissues. Protein A from staphylococci combines with the Fc portion of the IgG immunoglobulin molecule (except the IgG_3 subclass) and prevents complexes of antibody and antigen binding to the Fc receptor on phagocytes. This is an example of what is termed an **impedin**, as are the IgA proteases produced by neisseriae and certain streptococci (Table 5.3). Tables 5.4 and 5.5. show various ways microorganisms can evade immune mechanisms or interfere with induction of immunity.

Susceptibility to infection

Susceptibility to infection is greatest at the extremes of life due to a

Table 5.4 Evasion mechanisms

Microorganism	Product or characteristic	Effect
Staphylococci	Catalase	Protects from phagocyte H_2O_2
	Protein A	Binds antibody and interferes with opsonization
	Peptidoglycan	Inhibition of leucocyte migration
	Capsular material	Interference with opsonization
	Leucocidin	Cytotoxic and leucotoxic
	Haemolysin	Leucotoxic
	Coagulase	? inhibition of phagocytosis
Streptococci	Capsular polysaccharide	Inhibition of phagocytosis, shields C3b from contact with phagocyte complement receptors
	Streptolysins	Cytotoxic, inhibits chemotaxis, inhibition of macrophage migration
	Surface molecule that interferes with assembly of C3 convertase	Resistance to effects of complement
Gonococci and meningococci	IgA proteases	Digest and inactivate IgA
Trypanosomes, malaria parasites	Change membrane components in successive generations	Render immune response to earlier generation ineffective
Intracellular organisms (tubercle bacilli, brucella, viruses)	Ability to survive within cells	Avoid destruction by antibody and intracellular microbicidal agents
Herpes simplex and Epstein–Barr viruses	Complement inhibitory factors	Avoid complement lysis

weak or immature immune system. In the very young individual, infections can spread very rapidly and prove fatal without the clinical and pathological changes seen in adults. Their immature immune systems make the very young highly susceptible to virus infections and their airways are narrower and more easily blocked by secretions and exudates. Loss of fluid and electrolytes have serious effects. In older people latent infections such as varicella–zoster tend to reappear as shingles and their weaker respiratory muscles and reduced cough reflex predispose them to respiratory infections. There are age-related differences in the incidence of infections, with most infections being commoner in childhood because of first exposure whilst sexually transmitted diseases are largely restricted to adolescents and adults.

Recent data have shown increased susceptibility to metazoan and protozoan infections in the elderly. Women living in countries where

Table 5.5 Microorganisms that interfere with induction of acquired immunity

Microorganism	Effect
Measles, rubella, herpes, hepatitis viruses, HIV	Infection of cells of immune system and interference with induction of acquired immunity and expression of cell-mediated immunity
Malaria parasites	Depressed lymphocyte responsiveness to mitogens and some antigens
Leprosy bacilli	Alteration in T:B cell ratio with reduction in expression of complement receptors (? blocked by immune complexes)
	Non-specific impairment of cell-mediated immune response
Schistosomes	Incorporate host antigens and prevent recognition of their antigens
Influenza viruses	Suppress mitogenic responses of lymphocytes
	? Disable macrophages leading to secondary bacterial infection
Herpes simplex and cytomegalovirus	Induce Fc receptors on infected cells that bind and thus inactivate antiviral antibody

malaria is endemic are more likely to become infected when they are pregnant. The parasites localize in the placenta by attaching to chondroitin A and escape the attention of the immune system.

Significant reductions in the numbers and percentages of $CD3^+$ T-cells have been found in studies of aged subjects. An immune response pattern of poor T-cell proliferation, low IL-2 production and high percentages and numbers of $CD8^+$ T-cells has been found to be predictive of higher subsequent mortality. Other studies comparing the immune function of centenarians with individuals of greater than 80 years of age indicates relatively intact immune function in the centenarians suggesting a survival advantage for individuals with good immune function.

Association between certain infections and the blood group status of the individual has been established. Individuals of blood group O are more susceptible than those of other blood groups to cholera. There is also an increased susceptibility if they do not secrete blood group substances into their tissue fluids and mucous secretions (i.e. are non-secretors). Carriers of streptococci tend to be non-secretors. In studies of a Chilean population it was found that people of blood group B had a 50% greater probability than non-B persons of contracting *E. coli* urinary tract infections. Blood group B individuals are more susceptible to gonococcal infections. Non-B persons and non-secretors are more susceptible to rheumatic fever and rheumatic heart disease. In the author's laboratory, blood group B and AB non-secretors have been found to be three times more susceptible to urinary tract infections and non-secretors were much more prevalent amongst cases of meningococcal meningitis in studies carried out with samples from Scotland, Iceland and northern Nigeria. We have also found increased numbers of non-secretors in insulin-dependent (type 1) diabetes and Graves' thyroid disease, both of which may have an infectious basis. Individuals of blood group O are more susceptible to gastric ulcers due to *Helicobacter pylori* (see p. 175) and this too appears be due to the ability of the bacterium to adhere to H blood group substance characteristic of O individuals.

Epithelial attachment and infection

Bacteria

The attachment of a microorganism to an epithelial surface is a prerequisite for the development of an infectious process (excluding entry at sites of trauma). The mucosal surfaces of the respiratory, intestinal and genitourinary tracts are of primary importance as sites of attachment of microorganisms. Certain streptococci that are normal inhabitants of the mouth have been shown to adhere to epithelial cells of the cheek, whilst others preferentially attach to tooth surfaces. Specific attachment of various bacteria to different parts of the intestinal tract may account for the nature of the indigenous flora of the gut. It is suggested that the pathogenicity of *Salmonella typhi* and *Corynebacterium diphtheriae* depends on their ability to attach to the intestinal or pharyngeal mucosa, respectively, and *Neisseria gonorrhoeae* is believed to attach to epithelial cells of the genitourinary tract by means of its 'pili'. This organism at the same time appears to secrete an enzyme that breaks down secretory IgA whilst IgA$_2$ is not affected. The surface of epithelial cells of the respiratory tract of smokers shows an enhanced ability to bind certain potential pathogenic microorganisms and maternal smoking is associated with sudden infant death syndrome. A number of studies have shown that exposure to cigarette smoke is strongly associated with respiratory infection. Respiratory virus infections also appear to induce alteration of epithelial cell membranes so that they are better able to bind bacteria. These epidemiological and laboratory findings have led to the hypothesis that smoking and respiratory virus infections may predispose to colonization with common bacteria capable of producing damaging toxins that under appropriate circumstances can induce production of inflammatory mediators and vascular shock. In young infants with waning maternal antibodies and immature immune systems this could lead to sudden death (cot death).

The portal of entry of microorganisms in a number of infective

Table 5.6 Portals of entry of microorganisms

Route of entry	Cause or result
Ingestion	Food poisoning, cholera, dysentery
Inhalation	Measles, cold, flu
Sexual contact	Gonorrhoea, syphilis, herpes virus, HIV
Iatrogenic	Heart valves, pacemakers and wound infections
Zoonoses	Malaria, salmonellosis, encephalitis, typhus
Self-infection	Urinary tract, eye infection, appendicitis
Accidental	Drug users, motor accidents

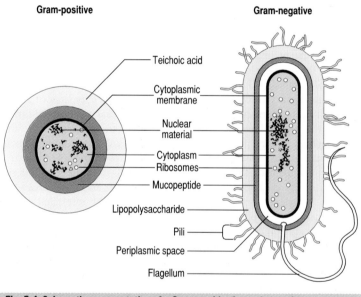

Gram-positive   **Gram-negative**

- Teichoic acid
- Cytoplasmic membrane
- Nuclear material
- Cytoplasm
- Ribosomes
- Mucopeptide
- Lipopolysaccharide
- Pili
- Periplasmic space
- Flagellum

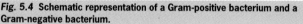

Fig. 5.4 Schematic representation of a Gram-positive bacterium and a Gram-negative bacterium.

states is shown in Table 5.6. Bacteria (Fig. 5.4) have an inner cell membrane and a peptidoglycan cell wall. Outside these basic structures there can be a variety of other components such as proteins, capsules, lipopolysaccharides or teichoic acids. There also may be organelles involved in motility (flagella) or adherence to the host's cells (fimbriae or pili). These are some of the components to which the immune system directs its responses. In general, peptidoglycan is attacked by lysosomal enzymes and the outer lipid layer of Gram-negative bacteria by cationic proteins and complement components.

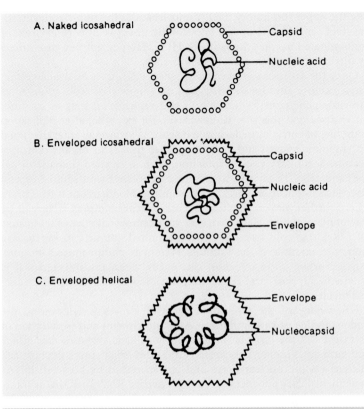

Fig. 5.5 Schematic diagram of three examples of animal virus structure:
the capsid is an outer symmetrical protein shell; when associated with the nucleic acid it is
called the nucleocapsid (C). The capsid protects the nucleic acid, facilitates attachment to
target cell, confers symmetry, usually icosahedral or helical (exceptions are poxviruses and
hepatitis virus that are more complex), and confers antigenicity. Naked viruses (A) have no
envelope. The envelope (B) consists of proteins, lipids and carbohydrates. Retroviruses are
unique and have no envelope but two capsid shells (one as in A and one associated with the
nucleus, i.e. a nucleocapsid — (C). Retroviruses have double-stranded RNA.

Flagella or fimbriae can be recognized and attacked by antibodies.
The capsular material of some bacteria enables them to resist phagocytosis or the shedding of excess capsule will mop up antibodies.
Table 5.4 lists some of the ways in which products of microorganisms
interfere with immune mechanisms.

Viruses (Fig. 5.5)

In virus infections the most common portals of entry are inhalation into the upper respiratory tract (rhinoviruses), ingestion via the intestinal tract (enteroviruses) and injection by insect vectors (togavirus) or contaminated needles (hepatitis B, HIV). Herpes simplex virus enters by direct contact with mucous membranes.

Once the virus has entered the tissues, cells must be available that carry receptor sites for the virus and that allow viral replication. After the virus penetrates its target cells and replicates it may or may not cause disease at this site. Rhinoviruses, for example, after replication at the site of entry, cause localized disease. A virus may enter the blood or lymphatic system and spread to other tissues or organs that may become secondary sites of infection, with associated damage to tissues and cells. Togavirus, transmitted to horses by mosquito vectors, after local replication spreads through the bloodstream to the brain where further viral replication occurs. Herpes simplex is spread by way of nerve tissue. Herpes viruses are examples of viruses that cause infection (e.g. cold sores) and then become dormant, causing disease later, for example if the immune system is compromised in some way. Abortive virus infection can occur when the infected cell is unable to support viral replication but even in this situation disease can result.

Knowledge of the replication cycle of viruses is relevant to the understanding of viral immunity. After attachment and penetration of its target cell the virus is 'uncoated' by cellular enzymes that attack and partially remove viral capsid. Viral DNA then enters the host cell nucleus via the nuclear pores and is transcribed by host cell DNA-dependent RNA polymerase. Viral messenger RNA (mRNA) is transported to the cytoplasm and translated into proteins by cellular ribosomes and tRNA molecules. Viral polypeptides then migrate either to the nucleus or to the cell membrane. At the latter site they become the target of antibody or cell-mediated immunity (see p. 182–186). The site of virion assembly for all DNA viruses (except pox viruses) is the host cell nucleus. Virions are transported to the cell surface and released and this is sometimes associated with lysis of the cell.

Penetration and uncoating of RNA viruses is basically the same as for DNA viruses but replication does not usually involve the host cell nucleus. Replication of RNA viruses varies according to the type of RNA and involves the synthesis of RNA-dependent RNA polymerase. This enzyme is either derived from the parental RNA or brought into the cell by the virions. Retroviruses, in contrast, carry the genetic information for induction of an RNA-dependent DNA polymerase called 'reverse transcriptase' that catalyses the synthesis of double-stranded DNA complementary to the viral RNA. The DNA integrates into the host cell nucleus before synthesis of new infectious virus can occur. This is used as a template for the transcription of RNA that is translated for viral protein production.

Most enveloped RNA viruses are released from the cell by budding through the cell membrane and it is at this stage that they are susceptible to antibody.

The viral-coded antigens (either those inserted into the host cell membrane or associated with the virion) are the ones recognized by the immune system. Viruses can also induce host-coded antigens and, whilst these can serve as markers of virus infection, they are unimportant as far as immunity is concerned. Intracytoplasmic or intranuclear viral antigens are also not accessible to antibody. Some viruses spread from one cell to another cell in contact with it without being released. In this case also the immune system is ineffective.

DEFENCE MECHANISMS

Inflammation

The innate immune mechanisms that protect the individual (mechanical barriers, antibacterial substances and phagocytosis) have been discussed in Chapter 2 and the discussion here is concerned with the protective responses that form a second line of defence. The microorganism, having successfully avoided the innate immune mechanisms, starts to proliferate in the tissues and its toxic products trigger an inflammatory response. The response is initiated by the release of vasoactive amines, principally histamine and SRS-A from mast cells. The resulting increase in vascular permeability leads to an exudation of serum proteins including components of complement, antibodies, blood-clotting factors and phagocytic cells (see p. 35). Phagocytic cells are attracted to the site of inflammation by chemotactic factors generated by interaction of components of the complement system with antibody. C5a acts as a chemotaxin. Anaphylatoxins generated at the same time increase vascular permeability and further encourage exudation of fluid and cells at the site of inflammation. See Chapter 2 for a more detailed discussion of the inflammatory response.

Many types of microorganisms (e.g. staphylococci, streptococci) are effectively dealt with by neutrophils and the intensity and duration of the inflammatory process depends on the degree of success with which the microorganism initially established itself. This in turn depends on the extent of the injury, the amount of associated tissue damage and the number and type of microorganisms introduced. A localized abscess may arise at the site of infection.

Some capsulate microorganisms (e.g. pneumococci) are able to resist phagocytosis and are not dealt with effectively until large amounts of antibody are made. These mop up the released capsular polysaccharide and phagocytosis occurs. If bacteria are not eliminated at the site of entry and continue to proliferate, they may pass via the lymphatics to the regional lymph nodes, causing their enlargement (lymphadenitis). Other microorganisms (e.g. diphtheria, tetanus, cholera) produce exotoxins and are called **toxigenic** organisms. In this situation they can produce their damaging effects without migrating from their site of entry. Immunity in this situation requires the development of specific **antitoxins** (see p. 166).

The types of infection described above are usually referred to as **acute infections** and contrast with protracted or **chronic infection** which is usually induced by microorganisms that are adapted to live within the cells of the host. Included amongst these are mycobacterial infections (e.g. tuberculosis, leprosy), brucella infections and virus infections. In these infections cell-mediated immunity plays a predominant part in the final elimination of the microorganism.

Tables 5.7, 5.8 and 5.9 summarize the roles of phagocytes, antibodies and T-lymphocytes in infection.

Table 5.7 **Phagocytic cells in infection**

1. Attracted to site of infection by chemotaxins
2. Phagocytosis with or without antibody or complement
3. Intracellular killing — oxygen dependent and independent and reactive nitrogen intermediates
4. Extracellular killing with antibody (ADCC)
5. Phagocyte secretions — cytokines
protease enzymes: neutrophils and monocytes

Table 5.8 **Antibody in infection**

Effect	Active against
Opsonization IgG, IgM (+ complement)	Viruses, bacteria and fungi
Neutralization IgG, IgM, IgA ($\pm$ complement) and inhibition of adherence	Viruses, bacteria and toxins
Bacteriolysis IgM (IgG) (+ complement)	Bacteria
Antibody-dependent cell-mediated cytotoxicity IgG, IgE	Virus-infected cells and worm infections
Growth inhibition IgG, IgA with lactoferrin	Mycoplasma and bacteria

Table 5.9 **T-lymphocytes in infection**

1. Major role in recruiting, facilitating and augmenting other effectors by secretion of lymphokines
2. Cytotoxicity — lysis of infected cells

Acquired immunity

The immune system, as has been noted in Chapter 3, has evolved the capacity to respond and react to a large variety of foreign molecules whilst at the same time avoiding self-reactivity. The capacity of the individual to resist infection can be explained in terms of the clonal selection theory of acquired immunity with the production of a specific immune response. The participating molecules and cellular events involved in the generation of an immune response have been described in Chapters 3 and 4. The major histocompatibility complex plays a critical role in determining the level and type of immune response to infection in different individuals. The MHC is a highly polymorphic system of genes that control the expression of the cell surface molecules involved in immune recognition (see Ch. 3).

The existence of such a polymorphic system will inevitably result in individuals with different immunological potentials to respond to a given challenge. Whilst some individuals will be well prepared to resist an infectious agent others will be at risk. It will come as no surprise to find that certain infective states are linked with the MHC, for example the association between viral hepatitis and the HLA-A8 antigen on lymphocytes (see also p. 192). There are many examples of such associations in viral infections of mice.

The evolutionary advantage to a species of such a polymorphic set of determinants of immunity, with its attendant survival value and possibility of adaptation, is clearly an advantage in dealing with unforeseen challenges. Microorganisms have the ability to adapt rapidly to environmental challenges (e.g. development of antibiotic resistance) and are capable of synthesizing a product that interferes with some aspect of the immune response. The most recent example is the AIDS virus (HIV) that appears to have mutated from related viruses infecting monkeys. It has been calculated that as many as 50 mutations accumulate on each lineage each year. The mammalian host has therefore needed to evolve multiple interlocking regulatory mechanisms as extra insurance against adaptable pathogens. The complexity of the cytokine system ensures that interference, by a microorganism, with one component of the system leaves other regulatory cytokines intact. It has recently been established that an important parameter determining the outcome of an immune response to infectious agents is the nature of the cytokines produced by T-cells locally. In experimental models of infection a subset of T-cells (T_H2, p. 125) produces cytokines involved in the pathogenesis of the disease. Interleukin-1 (IL-1) produced by macrophages contributes to the initiation of an immune response by acting as a co-stimulator of T-cells (see p. 107). IL-1 can, however, induce fever, joint and muscle aches, increased sensitivity to pain and lethargy. At higher doses hypotension, gastrointestinal disturbances and haemodynamic shock can be induced. One of the most significant advances in the last few years has been the recognition that different microorganisms trigger the activity of the individual T-cell subsets T_H1 and T_H2. Much of the work has been carried out in murine models of parasite infection and has more recently been studied in humans. The regulatory cytokines produced by the T-cell subsets have now replaced suppressor cells as the main determinants of down regulation. Much effort is now taking place to understand the mechanisms that determine how different microorganisms interact specifically with a particular T-cell subset.

Accumulation of inflammatory cells may in some instances be detrimental to the host, as is shown in experiments in rabbits with bacterial meningitis. Limitation of leucocyte emigration into the CSF was associated with decreased injury and mortality. Whether the procedure (injection of a monoclonal antibody to leucocyte adhesion molecules) will be valuable in human meningococcal disease remains to be established.

Bacterial infection

There are three main forms of bacterial immunity: (1) immunity to bacterial toxins, (2) immunity to extracellular bacteria and (3) immunity to intracellular bacteria.

Antibody-mediated immunity

Antitoxins. Many microorganisms owe their pathogenic abilities to the production of **exotoxins**. Amongst diseases dependent on this type of mechanism are diphtheria, cholera, tetanus, gas gangrene and botulism.

Diphtheria toxin, for example, is a polypeptide chain with a molecular weight of about 62 000 D. The intact molecule is not active but requires the reduction of one disulphide bridge and hydrolysis of the peptide chain to release an active fragment. This is believed to occur on the membrane of host cells, resulting in the entry of the toxic fragment into the cell where it interferes with protein synthesis. The cholera toxin owes its effects to its ability to bind to a specific glycolipid of the intestinal cell wall. A toxin constituent then passes through the cell wall, enters the cytoplasm and irreversibly 'switches on' the adenyl cyclase (the cyclic AMP-making enzyme). The 'activated' cell then proceeds to secrete fluid into the intestinal lumen, resulting in massive fluid loss from the tissues.

Antibodies either acquired by immunization or previous infection, or given passively as antiserum, are able to **neutralize** bacterial toxins. To give protection, antibodies must either be present in sufficient quantity, as they would after administration of antiserum, or be produced faster than the toxin is produced by the microorganism. This would be likely to occur if the individual had previously been exposed to the organism or its products by natural infection or immunization. In such a situation the infected individual would be able to mount a rapid secondary immune response (p. 115). The previously exposed individual can be said to have an **immunological memory** of the toxin, having a population of cells ready and waiting to respond rapidly to the exotoxin. The infected individual with no immunological memory may require to be given antibody prophylactically in order to overcome the first stages of infection until antibody is produced.

Bacterial toxins have been largely identified as enzymatic in nature and the antibody in some way is able to interfere with the ability of the enzyme to interact with its substrate. The antibody is not thought to interact with the active site of the enzyme but the nearer it reacts to this the more effective is its neutralizing power likely to be. The most probable explanation of the inhibitory effect of antibody is that it produces what is called 'steric hindrance', which simply means that it gets in the way and physically prevents the enzyme from coming in close apposition to its substrate. This idea is supported by the finding that antibody is much more effective against enzymes which have high molecular weight substrates than it is against those with low molecular weight substrates.

Immunity to extracellular bacteria. Capsular polysaccharides inhibit opsonization and phagocytosis. *Streptococcus pneumoniae* strains, commonly called pneumococci, are a well-known example of encapsulated bacteria which interfere with phagocytosis by alveolar macrophages. The complex polysaccharide capsules are the main virulence determinants of the species. There are more than 80 serotypes and reinfection with a different serotype is common. Individuals with reduced mucociliary reflexes or macrophage function (e.g. brought about by smoking) are more susceptible to infection.

Group B streptococci are an important cause of neonatal meningitis resulting from colonization of the infant by vaginal flora during parturition. Capsular carbohydrate components are able to block complement activation thus inhibiting this important defence mechanism in infants with their immature immune systems.

The polyribitol capsule of *Haemophilus influenza* is a weak antigen and this respiratory pathogen can cause bronchitis, pneumonia and systemic infection, including meningitis in infants. A conjugate vaccine with diphtheria toxin and outer membrane proteins linked to the polyribitol capsular polysaccharide has been developed for inducing immunity in young children.

Other important encapsulated bacteria are *Neisseria* species, *Klebsiella pneumoniae* and *Bacteroides fragilis*. In *N. gonorrhoeae* and *N. meningitidis* infections the complement system is important in immunity. In *N. gonorrhoeae* infection there is no clear-cut role for anticapsular immunity but in *N. meningitidis* infection group-specific anticapsular polysaccharide antibodies are effective in group A and C infections. The role of specific anticapsular antibodies in *Klebsiella* infections is not clear but such antibodies are active in enhancing phagocytosis and killing *Bacteroides* organisms.

In the case of a microorganism that does not secrete exotoxins, the protection afforded by antibodies depends on the direct effect of antibodies attached to the surface of the microorganism. This can have a number of effects, the most important of which is in encouraging phagocytosis by mononuclear phagocytes and the polymorphonuclear leucocytes. Phagocytic cells have receptors for a site on the Fc fragment of immunoglobulin G (particularly the human IgG_1 and IgG_3 subclasses). There are also receptors for the C3b component of complement. This means that a bacterium coated with antibody and complement will adhere to a phagocytic cell and become susceptible to phagocytosis (see also p. 29). The phagocytic cell in many instances can then digest the ingested microorganism by secreting into the phagocytic vacuole a variety of digestive enzymes carried in the intracellular lysosomes. However, some microorganisms such as the streptococci and *Mycobacterium tuberculosis* are able to resist intracellular digestion. The streptococcus carries, as part of its cell wall, a substance known as M protein, which confers the ability to resist digestion by the enzymes. If immunity exists to the M protein, by previous exposure or artificial immunization, the streptococcus is susceptible to intracellular digestion. Rough (avirulent) strains of salmonellae are susceptible to intracellular digestion whilst the smooth (virulent) strains are able to resist digestion in some way. Some bacterial products, such as muramyl dipeptide and trehalose dimycolate as well as formly-methionyl peptides, activate phagocytes so that they become more efficient at taking up and degrading bacteria. Exotoxins and lipopolysaccharides of Gram-negative bacteria and various carbohydrate polymers (e.g. beta-glucans) found in the bacterial cell wall are also potent activators of macrophages. In the case of enteric infections, such as those due to *Salmonella typhi* or *Vibrio cholerae*, antibodies can be secreted into the intestinal lumen and attack the organism before it invades the intestinal mucosa. These antibodies, secreted by an immune individual, are known as copro-antibodies and are predominantly IgA. The IgA immunoglobulin is selectively produced in intestinal and respiratory mucous membranes (p. 50).

IgA can be detected in many mucous secretions in higher concentrations than found in serum and IgA-producing plasma cells are found more commonly in the lamina propria of mucous membranes than in the spleen and lymph nodes. Various functions have been attributed to such IgA and there is evidence that it acts as an antitoxin together with IgG in protection against experimental cholera infection. Another suggested function of IgA is that by reacting with gut microorganisms it prevents their adherence to the gut wall. This is suggested by experiments in mice in which cholera organisms were prevented from adhering to the gut wall by the presence of IgA. A further function of IgA is suggested by work with IgA fractions of human colostrum, which bind to *E. coli* together with complement. The effect of this on the lipopolysaccharide of the bacterial cell wall is postulated to lead to the exposure of the underlying mucopeptide. This enables the enzyme lysozyme (p. 20) to digest the mucopeptide layer with resulting lysis of the bacterium. Gram-negative organisms such as *E. coli* are normally resistant to the effects of lysozyme (Fig. 5.6). It should be noted that these effects have been shown by in vitro assays and may not reflect what occurs in the intact animal. Other effects of antibody reacting with the surface of the microorganism are cell lysis, brought about by the activation of the complement system, and simple localization of the organism by agglutination or clumping. It is even conceivable that antibody acts by coating growing bacteria so that their daughter cells, when formed, remain in a clump instead of dispersing.

Apart from the clumping effect on the bacteria, agglutination seems to have little effect on the viability or respiratory activity of the organisms, although it is conceivable that the bacteria, at the centre of a large mass of clumped organisms, would be limited in their metabolic activity simply by a lack of sufficient nutrient material. Recent work suggests that antibody can inhibit the uptake of iron by some bacteria and that its lack can inhibit their growth.

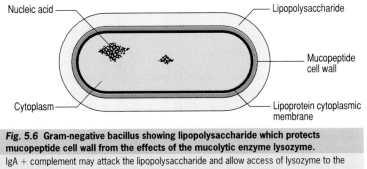

Nucleic acid — Lipopolysaccharide

Mucopeptide cell wall

Cytoplasm — Lipoprotein cytoplasmic membrane

Fig. 5.6 Gram-negative bacillus showing lipopolysaccharide which protects mucopeptide cell wall from the effects of the mucolytic enzyme lysozyme.
IgA + complement may attack the lipopolysaccharide and allow access of lysozyme to the cell wall.

A protective role for IgE has been suggested by the discovery of a similar distribution of this immunoglobulin to that found for IgA in the mucous secretions produced by local plasma cells. IgE is known to attach to the surface of mast cells and on combination with antigen causes degranulation of the mast cells with histamine release. These reactions in the allergic individual lead to hypersensitivity states (Ch. 9). If it occurs on a smaller scale in a localized area it might be helpful in bringing about an inflammatory response with consequent elimination of a microorganism (see also p. 187).

Immunity from infections of this type also depends on IgA production except when bloodstream invasion has occurred. In this situation IgG becomes more important along with effective cell-mediated mechanisms. The cell-mediated immunity is necessary for destruction of salmonellae that have been taken up by macrophages.

Humoral immunity in bacterial infections — summary

1. Antibody can neutralize bacterial toxins from, for example, diphtheria, cholera, tetanus and botulism organisms.
2. Antibody can attach to the surface of bacteria and:
   (a) act as an opsonin enabling phagocytosis, e.g. IgG
   (b) prevent the adherence of microorganisms to their target cell, e.g. IgA in the gut
   (c) activate the complement system leading to bacterial lysis
   (d) clump bacteria (agglutination) leading to phagocytosis
   (e) IgE attached to mast cells interacts with microbial surface to cause histamine release with inflammatory response and elimination of microorganism (if this occurs excessively, it can lead to hypersensitivity — Ch. 9)
   (f) inhibit motility and possibly the metabolic activity of bacteria
   (g) inhibit the uptake of iron by bacteria by preventing bacteria from releasing their iron-binding compounds.

Figure 5.7 summarizes the role of the immune system against bacterial pathogens.

Acquired cell-mediated immunity

Macrophage-dependent cellular immunity. Phagocytosis of microorganisms is a very important effector mechanism for the eradication of infectious agents but the process is frequently used by pathogens to establish infection.

Professional phagocytes represented by macrophages would appear to be an unattractive target for microbial pathogens in view of their large armamentarium of microbicidal factors. They are, however, the preferred target cells for a number of bacterial, fungal and protozoal

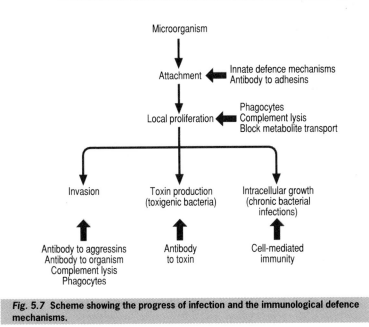

Fig. 5.7 Scheme showing the progress of infection and the immunological defence mechanisms.

pathogens. These pathogens utilize a variety of macrophage surface receptors to gain entry and then resist killing by using various subterfuges. The motility of phagocytes leads to the dissemination of the microbial pathogen throughout the tissues of the host.

Binding of antibody-coated bacteria to the macrophage membrane occurs via surface receptors for the Fc portion of immunoglobulins (FcRs) and triggers the production of reactive oxygen metabolites that are bactericidal. Some bacteria have developed protective mechanisms that neutralize phagocytic bactericidal activities. These intracellular pathogens use the surface receptors to gain entry by activating complement via the alternative pathway and binding to macrophage complement receptors. This not only enables the bacteria to be endocytosed but also avoids triggering the production of the bactericidal oxygen metabolites (in contrast to binding via FcRs). Intracellular pathogens that survive within phagocytes exhibit a variety of mechanisms that resist phagocyte killing. These include interference with oxidative killing (e.g. a phenolic glycolipid of *Mycobacterium leprae* and lipophosphoglycan of *Leishmania donovani* that scavenge oxygen metabolites), resisting the effect of lysosomal enzymes or microbicidal polypeptides and preventing fusion of the endosome with lysosomes (e.g. *Mycobacterium tuberculosis*). Another survival mechanism is to escape from the endosome into the cytoplasm by producing a lysin (e.g. listerolysin of *Listeria monocytogenes*). Recent evidence indicates that *Listeria monocytogenes* is eventually destroyed by both macrophages and neutrophils. Electron microscopic studies indicate that they appear to be able to survive up to between 24 and 48 hours and are then seen to be degraded by the activated phagocytes. *Salmonella typhimurium* in contrast is rapidly killed by the phagocytes. The ability of *Listeria* to induce disease seems likely to be due to its relative resistance to intracellular destruction and its escape into other host tissue cells where proliferation can occur.

Initiation of immunity to pathogens taken up by macrophages depends upon degradation of microbial antigens, probably by lysosomal enzymes. The resultant peptides associate with MHC class II molecules in the late endosomal compartment and the complex is then transported to the surface of the macrophage. The MHC class II/antigen complex is recognized by $CD4^+$ T-cells with the initiation of an immune response. An important element of the immune response is the production by the T-cells of lymphokines (particularly interferon-gamma) that activate the macrophage microbicidal functions (Fig. 5.8).

An additional pathway leading to immunity has recently been recognized that depends upon microbial antigens 'leaking' from the endosomes and entering the cytoplasm of the phagocyte. This leads to association of the microbial derived peptides with MHC class I molecules and the activation of $CD8^+$ T-lymphocytes. These lymphocytes not only can lyse their target cells but also have been shown to produce gamma-interferon and other lymphokines.

The story is further complicated by the finding that $CD4^+$ T-cells also have cytolytic properties. In human mycobacterial infections most of the cytolytic activity found was due to $CD4^+$ T-cells rather than to $CD8^+$ T-cells.

The activity of cytolytic T-cells has been described as a double-edged sword in that whilst lysis of a target cell can result in release of a microbial pathogen from within a cell so that the pathogen becomes susceptible to phagocytosis and destruction, damage to the target cell can also occur such as to a hepatocyte containing intracellular *Listeria* or a Schwann cell containing leprosy bacilli with consequent liver and nerve damage respectively.

Other cells that play a role in cellular immunity to intracellular pathogens are natural killer (NK) cells and a subset of T-cells with a different form of the T-cell receptor ($\gamma\delta$ T-cell receptors) (see p. 74–75) These cells are a relatively minor population of the T-cell compartment (less than 5%) but are considerably expanded by contact with mycobacterial antigens and some streptococcal and staphylococcal strains. Like the majority population of T-cells (with $\alpha\beta$ T-cell receptors) the $\gamma\delta$ T-cells are cytolytic and produce interleukins.

The activation of macrophages as a result of infection by a particular bacterial pathogen is also effective against other bacteria that are taken up by macrophages. For example, infection of mice by mycobacteria

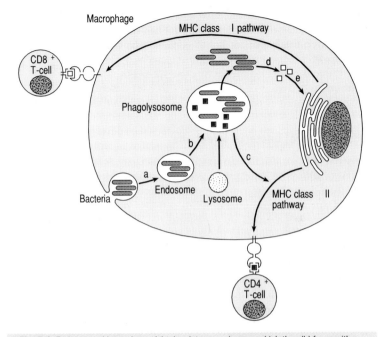

Fig. 5.8 Endocytosed bacteria are (a) taken into an endosome which then (b) fuses with a lysosome to form a phagolysosome. Within this compartment the bacteria are degraded and peptides (■) enter the MHC class II presentation pathway (c). In some instances (e.g. *Listeria* infections) bacteria escape from the phagolysosome and grow in the cytoplasm. Proteins derived from these organisms can be degraded (d) by proteosome and the peptides produced (□) enter the MHC class I presentation pathway (e). CD4+ T-cells recognizing the MHC class II/peptide complex can help initiate an immune response and produce lymphokines that activate the infected macrophage. CD8+ T-cells recognize the MHC class I/peptide complex leading to a cytotoxic response, i.e. cell death, and lymphokine release.

provides resistance to listeria infection by doses of listeria that would normally be lethal.

Inbred strains of mice vary in their susceptibility to infectious agents. This appears to be due to the enhanced ability of macrophages from resistant strains to stimulate T-lymphocytes, probably due to increased MHC class II expression on the macrophage surface.

The higher incidence of tuberculosis and greater difficulty of treatment in black compared with white populations (see p. 17) closely parallels the mouse BCG gene-regulated system in that there is an impaired capacity of macrophages from black subjects to kill intracellular tubercle bacilli. As yet the human equivalent of the mouse BCG gene has not been found. In the mouse the BCG gene locus controls both the growth of the bacteria and the bactericidal activity of the macrophage, although the gene product has not yet been isolated.

Even when macrophages fail to eliminate bacteria they accumulate at the site of infection forming a granuloma and fibrous tissue thus isolating the pathogen and preventing the spread of infection.

The main activities of macrophages in host defences are illustrated in Figure 4.13 and evasion mechanisms are summarized in Table 5.10.

Pathogenesis of bacterial infections

Many bacteria produce toxins both extracellular (exotoxins) and intracellular (endotoxins) and these can act on many tissues and organ systems including the immune system. Bacterial toxins are not only released during natural infection but can also be released from bacteria that have been killed by antibiotics, as in the case of meningitis treatment by penicillin that induces the release of endotoxin that can bring about severe damage.

In septic shock, a severe life-threatening condition induced by the lipopolysaccharide of Gram-negative bacteria, IL-1 appears to play a vital role, along with TNF, as shown by the beneficial effects of blocking its action. Development of such procedures for use in humans is likely to be very valuable in the treatment of Gram-negative bacterial infections. The pyrogenic exotoxin produced by *Staphylococcus*

Table 5.10 Intracellular pathogens and evasion mechanisms

Pathogens	Evasion mechanisms
Bacteria	
Mycobacterium tuberculosis	Prevents phagosome–lysosome fusion and interferes with reactive oxygen metabolites
M. leprae	Escapes from phagosome into cytoplasm and interferes with reactive oxygen metabolites
Listeria monocytogenes	Produces listerolysin and escapes from phagosome into cytoplasm
Listeria pneumophilia	Prevents phagosome–lysosome fusion, inhibits acidification of phagosome and interferes with reactive oxygen metabolites
Fungi	
Histoplasma capsulatum	Interferes with reactive oxygen metabolites and lysosomal enzyme effects
Protozoa	
Leishmania *Toxoplasma*	Interferes with reactive oxygen metabolites and phagosome–lysosome fusion

aureus also causes toxic shock syndrome, which is characterized by fever, hypotension, desquamation of the skin and dysfunction of three or more organ systems. The exotoxin known as TSST-1 is a super-antigen (p. 306) and a potent T-cell activator and binds to MHC class II molecules on antigen-presenting cells (APCs) (p. 107). Stimulation of T-cells follows via specific V_β regions of the T-cell receptor (p. 72). The result is the excessive production of cytokines by these cells and the development of toxic shock, the degree of which depends on the dose of the toxin and the effects of anti-inflammatory agents such as interleukin-10 (IL-10) (p. 126). This interleukin is produced by T_H2 lymphocytes and can be shown in in vitro experiments with human peripheral blood monocytes to substantially reduce the production of cytokines and T-cell proliferation. The glucocorticoid dexamethasone in these same experiments was shown to be even more effective as an inhibitor and holds out hope for its use in toxic shock syndrome. In other experiments in mice IL-10 has been shown to protect the mice from the lethal shock that follows exposure to staphylococcal entero-toxin B.

The pathogenesis of non-invasive bacteria such as *Corynebacterium diphtheriae* and *Vibrio cholerae* depends on their toxin producing ability. Diphtheria organisms grow on epithelial surfaces of the upper respiratory tract and their exotoxin kills mucosal cells. The toxin can enter the bloodstream and lymphatics causing lesions in many organs . The toxin molecule is not active until reduction of one disulphide bridge and hydrolysis of the peptide chain takes place on the membrane of the host cells. Antitoxin antibodies induced by immunization with tox-oid are very effective in preventing disease. Cholera, on the other hand, depends on the production of an exotoxin that acts locally on the mucosa of the small intestine where it binds to a glycolipid so that the toxin component enters the cell cytoplasm and 'switches on' cellular adenyl cyclase so that the activated cells secrete massive quantities of fluid into the intestinal lumen with a resulting watery diarrhoea. Recovery from cholera depends upon the development of IgA against the organism and its toxin. Immunity to the disease follows recovery and is provided by the secretory IgA.

Infections by dysentery-causing bacteria such as shigellae and sal-monellae differ from those just described. The bacteria invade the tis-sues causing mucosal ulceration. In the case of salmonellae, the bacteria may invade the bloodstream thus affecting other organs.

Chronic infection of the gastric mucosa with *Helicobacter pylori* is the most frequent cause of gastroduodenal inflammatory disease, includ-ing gastric and duodenal ulcers. Some strains of the bacteria produce a vacuolating cytotoxin that can be shown to result in gastric lesions in animals. Mucinase production has also been shown to be a virulence factor. IgG is not protective and the bacterium can down-regulate T-cell responses, probably through the induction of IL-10 and by expressing the oncofetal antigen Lewis x induces autoantibodies that cross-react with gastric mucosa. Survival in the acid environment of the stomach appears to be due to urease production by the organism.

Immune complexes in bacterial infections

Antibodies against bacterial antigens can be responsible for harmful as well as helpful effects. Immune complex disease (type 3 hypersensitivity, p. 279) is frequently associated with bacterial infection although it has not been as well studied as in virus infections (see below). Infective endocarditis due to staphylococci and streptococci is associated with circulating complexes of antibody and bacterial antigens and, whilst helpful in diagnosis, can also lead to joint and kidney lesions as well as vasculitis and skin rashes. Other sequelae of acute streptococcal infection, such as rheumatic fever and poststreptococcal glomerulonephritis, are associated with deposition of immune complexes and release of inflammatory mediators (see p. 36). Other examples of bacterial infection where immune complexes may play a role in pathogenesis are leprosy, typhoid fever and gonorrhoea.

Immunity in virus infections

Introduction

Like bacteria, viruses have evolved a multitude of mechanisms for exploiting weaknesses in the host immune system and avoiding, and sometimes actually subverting, immune mechanisms. Such strategies give the virus time to establish itself in the host tissues as exemplified by the long incubation periods of some virus infections, e.g. rabies and hepatitis B. Some viruses are so successful in avoiding host defences that they persist in the host indefinitely, often in a latent non-disease producing form.

One of the most important strategies developed by viruses is to infect cells of the immune system itself (Table 5.11). The effect of this is often to disable the normal functioning of the cell type that has been infected. Many common human viruses infect cells of the immune system including rubella, mumps, measles, certain adenoviruses, most herpes viruses, retroviruses and sometimes hepatitis B virus. The consequences of this type of infection sometimes are a temporary reduction of immunity both to the infecting virus and other microorganisms including bacteria and fungi. Bacterial infections frequently occur following viral infections for this reason. Permanent depression of immunity is a serious consequence leading to susceptibility to otherwise harmless fungi, protozoa, bacteria and viruses.

Other mechanisms used by viruses to escape the immune system include antigenic variation (e.g. the influenza viruses), release of anti-

Table 5.11 **Examples of subvertive effects of viruses on immune function**

Virus	Cells infected	Effects
HIV	T-lymphocytes, B-lymphocytes, monocytes/macrophages, microglial brain cells	Cytopathogenicity, loss of CD4$^+$ T-cells (receptor for virus) Depletion and impaired functioning of infected cells Induce cytokines that activate HIV expression
Lactic dehydrogenase virus (LDV) of mice	Macrophages bearing MHC class II molecules	Depletion of MHC class II +ve cells with depressed antigen-presenting function of macrophages
Herpes simplex 1 & 2 Vaccinia virus Adenovirus 12 Cytomegalovirus	Various cells bearing class I MHC antigens (all nucleated cells)	Reduces expression of MHC class I molecules on cell surface and interference with CD8$^+$ T-cell activities
Epstein–Barr virus	B-lymphocytes (via CR2 receptor)	Polyclonal activation of B-cells Virus produces molecule that mimics IL-10 that inhibits gamma-interferon production
Hepatitis B virus	Liver cells	Release of viral antigen, ? tolerance induction in B-cells with failure to produce antibodies to viral surface antigen Inhibits α-interferon production and blocks response of infected cells to IFN
Lymphocytic choriomeningitis virus (LCM) in mice	T-lymphocytes	Clonal deletion of T-cells with loss of response to virus

Other possible, but as yet unresolved, effects of viruses include production of immunomodulatory substances by viruses with effects on T-cells and on production of cytokines such as interleukins-1 and -2. Some viruses can affect phagocyte function, and immune complexes containing viral antigen can have effects on the immune system.

gens and production of antigens at sites that are inaccessible to the immune system. Reoviruses that infect macrophages use macrophage lysosomal enzymes to initiate uncoating of the virus before replication. This is in contrast to viruses that normally infect mucosa such as poliovirus and rhinoviruses that are rapidly destroyed if they are taken up by macrophages. Viruses that manage to survive within long-lived cells such as macrophages can thus be disseminated in the tissues. Latent virus infections such as herpes simplex or varicella-zoster virus escape attention from the immune system by expressing either none or only limited amounts of antigen on the surface of the cells they infect. Viruses that move from cell to cell without entering the extracellular fluid, such as the respiratory syncitial viruses, escape the effects of antibody.

The most recent example of viral interference with the functioning of cells of the immune system is human immunodeficiency virus (HIV) infection. Studies carried out in response to the emergence of this very serious disease have advanced knowledge to a substantial degree on the mechanisms and consequences of infection by this and a number of other viruses. The consequences of viral infections of cells of the immune system have been categorized as:

1. Infections that cause temporary immune deficiency to unrelated antigens (and sometimes to antigens of the infecting virus, as seen in mouse reovirus, herpes simplex and influenza infections). It is well known that patients who have suffered from virus infections such as influenza, rubella, measles and cytomegalovirus are susceptible to bacterial and other infections. This is sometimes associated with depressed immunoglobulin synthesis by lymphocytes and interference with the antimicrobial functions of phagocytes.

2. Permanent depression of immunity to unrelated antigens (and occasionally to antigens of the infecting virus). The acquired immunodeficiency syndrome is an example of such an effect where the patient becomes susceptible to otherwise harmless protozoa, bacteria, viruses and fungi (see p. 195).

Defence mechanisms in viral infections

The immune response to viral infection, either subclinical or clinical, depends on a variety of mechanisms involving both humoral and cell-mediated immunity. Another important defence mechanism is the production of interferons that have two main functions: (1) inhibition of viral replication and (2) activation of host defence mechanisms.

Interferons

At the time of their discovery in 1957 the term 'interferon' identified a factor produced by cells in response to viral infection that protected other cells of the same species from attack by a wide range of viruses. It is now clear that this activity is mediated by members of a large family of regulatory proteins.

In humans, as in a number of other species, there are two types of interferons (IFN). Type 1, composed of IFN-α and IFN-β is produced by peripheral blood mononuclear cells and fibroblasts respectively. Type II, or IFN-γ, is a lymphokine produced in response to a specific antigenic signal. There is only one gene for IFN-β and one for IFN-γ but there are at least 23 different IFN-α genes coding for 15 functional proteins. All the IFN-α genes are closely related and clustered on chromosome 9, close to the IFN-β gene; the IFN-γ gene is on chromosome 12. The production of interferons is under strict inductional control. Type 1 interferons are produced in response to the presence of viruses and certain intracellular bacteria. Double-stranded RNA may be the important inducer. IFN-γ, which has a much more extensive role in the control of immune responses, is produced mainly from antigen-activated T-lymphocytes.

To exert their biological effects these molecules must interact with cell surface receptors. IFN-α and IFN-β share a common receptor while IFN-γ binds to its own specific receptor. After binding to the cell surface receptors, interferons act by rapidly and transiently inducing or up-regulating some cellular genes and down-regulating others. The overall effect is to inhibit viral replication and activate host defence mechanisms.

The antiviral activity is mediated by the interferon released from a virally infected cell binding to a neighbouring cell and inducing the synthesis of antiviral proteins (Fig. 5.9). Interferons are extremely potent in this function, acting at femtomolar (10^{-15}) concentrations. They can inhibit many stages of the virus life cycle — attachment and uncoating, early viral transcription, viral translation, protein synthesis and budding. Many new proteins can be detected in cells exposed to interferon but major roles have been proposed for two enzymes that inhibit protein synthesis: 2',5'-oligoadenylate synthetase (2,5-A synthetase) and a protein kinase. The activity of both these enzymes is dependent on double-stranded RNA that is provided by viral intermediates in the cell. The protein kinase is responsible for phosphorylation of histones and the protein synthesis initiation factor eIF$_2$. This leads to the inhibition of protein synthesis within interferon-stimulated cells due to inhibition of ribosome assembly. The 2,5-A synthetase is strongly induced in human cells by all three types of interferon and forms 2',5'-linked oligonucleotides of adenosine from adenosine triphosphate (ATP). These oligonucleotides activate a latent cellular endonuclease that degrades both messenger and ribosomal RNA with a resultant inhibition of protein synthesis. The requirement for the presence of double-stranded RNA for the full expression of these effects will safeguard uninfected cells from the damaging effects of these enzymes.

Some effects of interferon are viral specific. The Mx protein induced in mice by IFN-α/β is specifically involved in the resistance to influenza virus infection. There is a related protein in human cells and it is possible that some of the other IFN-induced proteins may confer

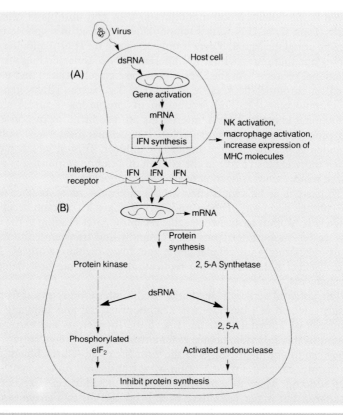

Fig. 5.9 Proposed mechanisms of (A) induction of interferon synthesis and (B) production of resistance to virus infection.
Cell (A) is induced to produce interferon (IFN) by the presence of double-stranded RNA (dsRNA). The interferon (α or β depending on the type of cell) is released and binds to receptors on other cells. This interaction can cause activation of host effector functions and induce an intiviral state in neighbouring cells (B). mRNA = messenger RNA; 2,5-A = 2',5'-oligoadenylate

resistance to specific virus types. Resistance of IFN-γ treated cells to the parasite *Toxoplasma gondii* is associated with induction of the enzyme indolamine dioxygenase, which catabolizes the essential amino acid tryptophan. However, interferons have effects on host cell growth and differentiation. Interferons, particularly IFN-α and IFN-β, are potent inhibitors of normal and malignant cell growth. A number of clinical trials have shown that IFN-α is active against some human cancers, especially those of haemopoietic origin.

Interferons are able to modify immune responses by: (1) altering expression of cell surface molecules, (2) altering the production and secretion of cellular proteins and (3) enhancing or inhibiting effector cell functions. One of the main ways in which interferons control immune responses is by the induction or enhancement of MHC-encoded molecules. Class I MHC genes are up-regulated by all types of interferon, as is the production of β_2-microglobulin. IFN-γ induces and increases the expression of MHC class II antigens. In addition, interferons can induce or enhance the expression of cell surface receptors such as Fc receptors and receptors for a number of cytokines. These activities will increase the efficiency of antigen recognition and lead to a more effective immune response.

Interferons have also been implicated in the control of B-cell responses. When added in vitro or in vivo they can suppress or enhance primary or secondary antibody responses depending on the dose and time of addition. The regulatory effects seem to be on the B-cells themselves, on increased antigen presentation and through an effect on regulatory T-cells.

A number of immune effector cells act by killing infected target cells. The cytotoxicity of macrophages, neutrophils, T-cells and NK cells is enhanced by interferons. IFN-γ produced by T-lymphocytes is capable of activating macrophages to kill intracellular bacteria. This lymphokine has all the activities of the molecule that used to be known as macrophage activating factor (MAF). NK cells are able to destroy a range of syngeneic, allogeneic and xenogeneic cells in a MHC unrestricted fashion (see p. 33). The interaction of NK cells with their target generates the release of IFN-α and IFN-γ. All three types of interferon increase NK cell activity in vitro and in vivo not only by recruiting pre-NK cells to become actively lytic but also by increasing the spectrum of cells lysed. The mechanisms by which interferons make cells cytotoxic are not clear but it is of interest that interferons can stimulate the production of cytotoxins such as tumour necrosis factor (TNF).

Tumour necrosis factor has also been reported to have several antiviral activities similar to IFN-γ but working through a different pathway. However, if both tumour necrosis factor and IFN-γ are added together then a synergistic effect is seen. If tumour necrosis factor is added to cells after virus infection, it can lead to their destruction even though the cells are normally resistant to tumour necrosis factor. This effect is also synergistic with IFN-γ. Certain viruses have been shown to trigger the release of tumour necrosis factor from mononuclear cells and it seems likely that this cytokine is an important host response to viral infections.

Certain cell-mediated reactions are also part of the innate defences against viral infections. In natural killing the structures recognized by the effector cells, termed natural killer cells, are not known but changes in the level of expression of a number of surface molecules on the infected cells may be important. One of the most likely candidates is the transferrin receptor. The formation of a close conjugate between the natural killer cell and the target induces the effector cell to produce toxic molecules that lead to the death of the infected cell. Antibodies that recognize natural killer cells have been used to deplete these cells from mice. It was found that these treated mice were more susceptible to murine cytomegalovirus than were normal mice. Therefore, natural killing may form a first line defence against viral attack before the acquired immune response is generated. Natural killing is increased by interferons, both the number of effector cells and their killing potential, and, therefore, these two innate defence mechanisms appear to work together to protect the host from viral infections.

Antibody-mediated immunity

Virus infections, particularly those caused by enteroviruses, are frequent and severe when humoral immunity is impaired as in inherited immunodeficiency states. In Bruton-type deficiencies (see p. 287) poliomyelitis may develop after vaccination; meningoencephalitis, caused by echovirus and Coxsackie virus, may also be seen. In a variety of mouse experimental models the administration of immunosuppressive drugs has shown that antibody is essential for recovery from a number of virus infections, including influenza and Coxsackie viruses. Antibody appears to operate through opsonization followed by ingestion by macrophages or by neutralization of virus haemagglutinins.

In many situations viruses seem to be able to escape these protective mechanisms of the host and remain infective, even when complexed with antibody. Some viruses become latent, e.g. the herpes group, and are reactivated despite the presence of circulating antibody, passing from cell to cell without entering the bloodstream. Other escape mechanisms, such as that of the influenza virus, are discussed below. Complement can take part in the neutralization of viruses by opsonizing virus particles or directly lysing enveloped viruses. Retroviruses have a protein that can act as a receptor for C1q and other viruses have been found to activate the alternative complement pathway.

Bloodstream or surface protection. In virus infections the efficiency of antibody depends largely on whether the virus passes through the bloodstream in order to reach its target organ. A well-known example of a virus which follows such a route is the polio virus. This crosses the intestinal wall, enters the bloodstream and passes to the spinal cord and brain where it proliferates. Small amounts of antibody in the blood can **neutralize** the virus before it reaches its target cells in the nervous system. A number of other viruses behave in the same way and pass through the bloodstream on their way to their target organ; examples are the viruses of measles, mumps, rubella and chickenpox. Disease caused by these viruses is characterized by a **prolonged** incubation period.

In comparison, in another group of virus diseases with a **short** incubation period, such as influenza and the common cold, the viruses do not pass through the bloodstream, as their target organ is their site of entry to the body, namely the respiratory mucous membranes. In this type of infection even a high blood level of antibody will be relatively ineffective against these viruses in comparison with its effect on the blood-borne viruses. For this antibody to act on such respiratory viruses it must pass through the mucous membranes into the respiratory secretion. Examination of the antibody content of mucous secretion has shown that in contrast to the blood there is very little IgG antibody and often no IgM and it thus appears that the mucous membranes are not very permeable to antibodies of these classes. However, it has been found that the predominant immunoglobulin in these secretions is IgA manufactured by plasma cells in the lamina propria of the mucous membranes. IgA present in nasal secretions has been shown to be responsible for most of the neutralizing activity against common cold viruses. One conclusion which can be drawn from this is that conventional immunization methods designed to produce high blood levels of antibody are unlikely to be effective against viruses which attack the mucous membranes and some effort is being directed at developing methods for stimulating local antibody production of IgA type in the mucous membranes themselves (see p. 217). An example of this is the intranasal administration of a live attenuated influenza virus which has been used extensively in the United States and the former Soviet Union and is now available in Britain.

The best way to achieve protection against a viral disease is to use a live virus vaccine and it is clear that natural infections of humans by influenza virus confer more complete and long-lasting protection than does vaccination. There is evidence that cytotoxic T-lymphocytes may be as important as immunoglobulins in this protection. Inactivated influenza vaccines and subunit vaccines result in antibody production but are much less efficient in inducing cytotoxic T-lymphocytes. The neutralizing antibodies generated in influenza infection are highly specific for the haemagglutinin of the infecting virus. In contrast, cytotoxic T-lymphocytes appear not to discriminate between different type A influenza viruses. Thus for efficient long-term T-cell immunity live vaccines appear to be preferable to inactivated vaccines.

The high degree of immunity provided by the live oral polio vaccine seems likely to be due in part to locally produced antibody in the gut neutralizing the virus even before it reaches the bloodstream. The presence of IgA antibody against polio virus has been demonstrated in the faeces, in duodenal fluid and in saliva. The nasopharyngeal antibodies have been shown to persist for at least 300 days, which is consistent with the long-term protection that the oral vaccine affords. It is of some interest that the levels of IgA antipolio antibody were found to be lower in children who had their tonsils and adenoids removed. Furthermore, primary vaccination in such children produced lower levels of these specific antibodies than in children who had not had their tonsils removed. Virus infections can be particularly dangerous when humoral immunity is impaired. In Bruton-type deficiencies (p. 287) poliomyelitis may develop after vaccination with the live virus and meningitis may develop after echovirus or Coxsackie virus infections.

'**Antigenic drift**'. In those virus infections in which repeated attacks occur, e.g. influenza and the common cold, fresh infection is due to different strains of the virus which are relatively insusceptible to the antibodies induced by previous infection by other strains. Evidence for a persisting immunity to a virus comes from studies in the Faroe islands where successive measles epidemics were separated by intervals of 65 and 31 years. Only those who had not been previously infected developed the disease.

Influenza epidemics have occurred at 2–3 year intervals over the last 40 years and type B virus outbreaks tend to alternate with type A epidemics. Type A virus is responsible for pandemic influenza infections. Type C influenza virus rarely, if ever, gives rise to epidemics and no variants have been reported since it was first isolated in 1950. The main viral antigen responsible for inducing immunity is the haemagglutinin (HA). It is sometimes called the 'V' antigen and is thought to be located on the spikes projecting from the viral envelope. Influenza viruses types A and B have different HA antigens and within these two types are a number of distinct families with HA antigens which differ markedly from one another. Antigenic differences between HA antigens form the basis for classification of the viruses into families of the same type. In type A infection, the families A, A_0, and A_2 have appeared successively, and each in turn has dominated the epidemic history of influenza for periods of 10–15 years and is then displaced by later antigenic variants. It is believed that this 'antigen drift' from one virus family to another is one of progressive mutation and that immunity against earlier strains becomes obsolete once further antigenic variants have appeared. The consequence of antigenic drift is that new strains do not react well with antisera against older strains. Antigenic drift is probably due to selective pressures brought about by antibody that favours the emergence of mutants expressing surface antigens sufficiently different as to be unable to combine with existing antibody.

There is a danger that mutants responsible for 'antigen drift' may emerge and dominate as a result of widespread use of vaccination procedures directed against strains responsible for epidemics. In this situation such insusceptible mutants would be 'selected' from the virus population and replace the previously dominant strain.

The phenomenon of 'antigen drift' is not limited to influenza virus and the argument outlined above has been used for not instituting nationwide vaccination as a means of protecting cattle from foot and mouth disease virus. The same difficulties stand in the way of the development of common cold vaccines and vaccines against HIV. The latter may be mutating at a rate five times faster than the influenza virus. Viruses with RNA genomes are known to have the ability to mutate particularly frequently. It is also likely that viruses with altered nucleotide sequences emerge during the course of infection. Isolates of the same virus from the same patient can be shown to be distinguishable.

Antigenic shift involves major antigenic variations and is shown in type A influenza. The changes that have been identified have occurred three times in the haemagglutinin antigen and twice in the neuraminidase antigen. These changes have been found in influenza viruses responsible for epidemics spread over the last 70 years.

Cell-mediated immunity in virus infections

Viral antigens, like other antigens, are presented to CD4$^+$ T-cells by macrophages and other antigen-presenting cells in association with MHC class II molecules. Cells that are supporting viral replication express viral antigen fragments in association with MHC class I molecules. Association of viral antigens with MHC class II molecules leads to initiation of an immune response whilst association with MHC class I molecules leads to lysis of the infected cell by CD8$^+$ T-cells.

The humoral immune response is probably the predominant form of immunity responsible for protection from reinfection by viruses. For this reason immunization procedures aim at producing circulating or mucous membrane antibody. In the case of primary virus infections the position is not very clear but it seems likely to involve some form of cell-mediated immunity. It is known that children with congenital hypogammaglobulinaemia (p. 288) can recover from virus infections without producing any virus-neutralizing antibody. Although it is possible that these children are producing small amounts of neutralizing antibody sufficient to provide immunity, it is significant that the capacity to resist virus infection is associated with normal cell-mediated immune reactions. These subjects are able to develop normal T-cell reactions to bacterial and viral antigens and contact sensitivity to simple chemicals (p. 285). In patients with Swiss-type agammaglobulinaemia (p. 288), who have an additional cell-mediated immune deficiency, susceptibility to virus infection is very great and death often follows the development of severe generalized vaccinia after routine inoculation with live smallpox vaccine.

A laboratory model is available that has enabled the detailed study of the role of cell-mediated immunity in virus infection. Mice infected with lymphocytic choriomeningitis (LCM) virus at birth or in utero become lifelong carriers in most of their organs including the thymus. These carrier mice show no detectable T-cell responses to the virus (but normal responses to other antigens). This appears to be due to 'clonal deletion' of the virus-specific cytotoxic T-lymphocytes within the thymus. Continuous infection with LCM virus is necessary to maintain the tolerant state. In contrast B-cells produce anti-viral antibody. Adult mice infected with LCM virus, which itself is not damaging to cells (non-cytopathic), develop clinical signs (e.g. meningitis) with the onset of an immune response to the virus. If this response is prevented by means of immuno-suppressive agents (e.g. antilymphocyte serum, cytotoxic drugs, irradiation or thymectomy) then the disease does not develop. If an infected animal treated in this way is then given spleen cells from an untreated virus-infected animal, the pathological changes characteristic of the disease develop in the recipient.

Further evidence that cell-mediated immune reactions are involved in resistance to viruses comes from the finding that, just as in the case of intracellular bacterial agents such as tubercle bacilli and brucellae, cell-mediated reactions leading to lymphokine release (p. 124) can be demonstrated after many types of virus infection. The best known example of this is the reaction soon after revaccination with vaccinia virus where there is an accelerated reaction (compared to primary vaccination) reaching its maximum at 72 hours with a minimum of tissue damage and a rapid elimination of the infective agent.

Many viruses, such as polioviruses and papillomaviruses, replicate and produce infectious particles inside cells. They are then liberated from the infected cell as it disintegrates and go on to infect other cells. In an immunized individual, antibody can provide immunity by attacking free virus. Virus-derived peptides are also found at the surface of an infected cell in association with MHC class I and class II molecules and can act as recognition sites for $CD8^+$ T-cells and $CD4^+$ T-cells. In some situations viral antigens are found on the cell surface and antibodies directed against these molecules can act in conjunction with cells bearing Fc receptors in antibody-dependent cell-mediated cytotoxicity (p. 122). Some viruses appear on the cell surface in enveloped form, e.g. budding heptadanoviruses and paramyxoviruses.

Recognition of viral antigens associated with MHC class II molecules by T-helper cells, in conjunction with co-stimulation signals, leads to the production of growth and differentiation factors for T- and B-lymphocytes, inducing an immune response as previously described (Fig. 4.7). Cytotoxic T-lymphocytes, both CD8 and CD4 T-lymphocytes, generated in this way recognize viral antigens associated with MHC class I and class II molecules respectively and release toxic substances that destroy the infected cell (p. 178). There is increasing evidence that cytokines can contribute directly to the elimination of viruses by antiviral effects. Interferon-gamma plays an important defensive role by up-regulating the expression of MHC class II molecules on antigen-presenting cells thus enabling them to present viral antigen to CD4 T-cells.

Pathogenesis of viral infections

In the mouse model described above the pathological changes appear to be brought about by a cytotoxic effect of the transferred spleen cells interacting with infected cells of the recipient. A variety of cytokines are generated in this infection. Interferon-γ possesses antiviral activity but other cytokines may contribute to the tissue damage as in subacute sclerosing panencephalitis (SSPE). The consequences of this immune response can thus be seen to be twofold: (1) virus-infected cells are destroyed by stimulated spleen cells with the likely elimination of the virus and (2) host cells are themselves damaged and this is responsible for the pathological manifestations of the disease. Whether or not the pathological changes in any human virus infections depend on mechanisms of this type is not clear at present. However, some in vitro experiments in which cells infected with measles or mumps virus are destroyed by incubation with spleen cells of a virus-immunized animal suggest that such phenomena may take place in the disease state itself. In volunteers infected with influenza virus a correlation was found between cytotoxic T-cell activity and diminished shedding of virus. MHC restriction (p. 185) applies to the action of T-cells in virus infection, the $CD8^+$ cells recognizing viral antigen associated with MHC class I molecules on infected cells.

Immune complexes in viral infections

Formation of immune complexes between microbial antigens and antibodies leads to the neutralization and clearance of many pathogens by phagocytes. This is brought about by interaction of Fc receptors on the phagocyte with exposed Fc regions of the antibody molecule. In certain circumstances, such as when complexes are formed in antigen excess (i.e. with fewer Fc sites available as well as being small and soluble), or in antibody excess when also small and soluble, clearance is less effective and the complexes may be deposited on filtering membranes (e.g. kidney glomeruli or choroid plexus in the brain) and at sites of turbulence and high pressure in the vasculature (e.g. aortic area). In other situations complexes may themselves be formed on cell surfaces by antibody bound to cell surface antigens that may be endogenous, as in autoimmune disease (p. 295), or exogenous and derived from a microorganism such as viral antigens inserted into a cell membrane. This will lead to cytotoxic effects due to antibody-dependent cellular cytotoxicity (ADCC) (see p. 122). Large complexes formed near equivalence (p. 316) not only express Fc regions of the antibody molecules but also fix complement, thus leading to effective uptake and clearance by cells of the mononuclear phagocyte system with Kupffer cells of the liver playing a predominant role.

In infectious disease, formation of local complexes is rare but circulating complexes can be deposited at various sites, such as the kidney glomeruli, the intima of arteries, synovial membranes of joints and the choroid plexus. This can lead to the release of inflammatory mediators resulting from activation of the complement cascade and by binding of complexes to Fc receptors on platelets, mast cells, monocytes and neutrophils. The enzymes released from the latter two cell types include elastase, collagenase and neutral proteases with damaging effects on connective tissue and activation of the coagulation system.

In viral infections, immune complexes are frequently produced and can lead to serious complications in infections such as hepatitis B and dengue virus infections in humans, and in mice in lymphocytic choriomeningitis infection. The pathogenesis of the latter infection is relatively well understood (p. 185) and immune complexes in neonatal mice can be identified in the kidneys, heart, liver, spleen and central nervous system of transplacentally infected mice. The pathogenesis of such neonatal infections contrasts with that in adults where the damage is primarily due to cell-mediated cytotoxicity. The immune complex form of the disease in neonatal mice varies from strain to strain and may be related to the amount of C1q (p. 22–27) that binds to the complexes.

In infections of humans by hepatitis B virus the surface antigens are shed into the bloodstream and form complexes with antibody. Persisting levels of hepatitis B antigen can lead to immune complex mediated damage such as polyarteritis nodosa and glomerulonephritis. In acute infections vasculitis, skin rashes and polyarthritis can occur as prodromal symptoms. Whilst the major hepatic damage in the disease is cell mediated, immune complexes are sometimes found in the hepatic sinuses but are probably not responsible for liver damage. Complexes in the synovial membranes with associated depletion of complement components can lead in a proportion of cases (up to one-third) to a self-limiting polyarthritis resembling rheumatoid arthritis. Another way that complexes can contribute to persistence of hepatitis B infection is by blocking ADCC-mediated killing of virus-infected cells. The complexes, by attaching to the Fc receptor of the phagocyte, prevent it recognizing antibody on the surface of the virus-infected cells.

Dengue haemorrhagic fever is a disease widespread in southeast Asia and found in the Caribbean, the Pacific islands and Africa. Antibody has been implicated in the pathogenesis of a severe illness associated with dengue virus infection. This is the most prevalent arbovirus disease of humans and it is normally a mild disease with fever and a maculopapular skin rash. However, occasionally a more severe form of infection can occur with a haemorrhagic fever and shock called the dengue shock syndrome. This form of the disease is usually seen in children who develop a haemorrhagic rash (purpura) with extensive bleeding and death occurs from hypotensive shock in 10–30% of cases. There are four serotypes of dengue virus and primary infection with one of the serotypes produces an immune response that eliminates the virus. However, there is antigenic overlap between the different serotypes and antibodies produced against the first serotype can react with a subsequent infection. This cross-reactive antibody is non-neutralizing and leads to the formation of immune complexes and subsequent complement activation and shock. The presence of the antibody-coated virus leads to its ingestion by macrophages where it replicates; because of the enhanced uptake, viral replication is more extensive than in the primary infection. The exact role of antibody in the pathogenesis of dengue shock syndrome will have to be determined before a vaccination programme can be instigated.

Other virus infections in which immune complexes may play a role in the pathogenesis of the disease process are flavivirus infections including yellow fever and West Nile virus infections. In Epstein–Barr virus infections viral antigens have been found in immune complexes in the kidneys of patients with Burkitt's lymphoma. Complexes deposited in various tissues may be responsible for some of the symptomatology of many acute virus infections. Deposition of complexes in the choroid plexus has been suggested as underlying behavioural disorders in asymptomatic virus infections.

Viral depression of the immune system

Babies with congenital rubella infection have been shown to excrete virus for periods up to 18 months of age. Such infants can be shown to possess high levels of IgM antirubella antibody, which indicates that they have not developed neonatal tolerance (p. 142) to the virus. Their cell-mediated immune mechanisms seem, however, to be defective due to a direct effect of the virus on lymphocytes. Lymphocytes taken from such an infant do not respond normally to the plant mitogen PHA (p. 102) and normal leucocytes infected in vitro with the virus can be shown to become defective in the same way. **Depression of lymphocyte reactivity** has been associated with a number of virus infections, e.g. rubella, herpes, Newcastle disease virus (causing fowl pest) and hepatitis virus. Certain viruses are able to **replicate** in **macrophages** (e.g. arboviruses, murine hepatitis virus, lactate dehydrogenase virus and herpes simplex virus) and others do so in **lymphocytes** (e.g. lymphocytic choriomeningitis virus, leukaemia viruses and Epstein–Barr virus).

The effects on the activity of the immune system brought about by viral infection have been studied with murine leukaemia viruses. Infection of mice with these viruses usually results in depression of the activity of the immune system affecting both humoral and cell-mediated immunity. In some instances (e.g. Friend virus infection) there is selective depression of a particular class of immunoglobulin (IgG) suggesting an effect on particular populations of lymphocytes. Graft rejection was found to be profoundly depressed in animals infected with Gross leukaemia virus. The mechanisms underlying these effects are not clear. Amongst the proposed mechanisms are virus-induced changes in the uptake and processing of antigens, destruction of cells of the immune system, and antigenic competition by the virus preventing the host response to other antigens. A number of viruses (herpes simplex 1 and 2, vaccinia virus, adenovirus 12 and cytomegalovirus) are able to reduce the expression of MHC class I molecules on the surface of infected cells, thus reducing the possibility of recognition by T cytotoxic cells. The interferons and tumour necrosis factor (TNF) cytokines have been recognized as mediators of local and systemic antiviral responses but recent work indicates that certain cytokines may actually promote viral replication. For example, HIV replication appears to be dependent on the state of activation of the host cell with increased cytokine production. TNF-alpha and IL-6 up-regulate HIV expression. A soluble factor capable of suppressing T-cell function is induced by HIV-1 infection of $CD4^+$ T-cells and is recognized by antibodies directed against epitopes of p15E and gp14. These highly conserved amino acid sequences have been incorporated into a synthetic peptide termed CKS-17 and has been shown to have strong immunosuppressive influences on immune assays. The effects include reduction of the levels of IL-2, IL-12 and IFN-gamma and augmentation of IL-10. Dysregulation of IL-10 and IL-12 is believed to contribute to immunological disturbances in patients. IL-10 inhibits HIV replication in macrophages but not in T-cells whilst IL-12 enhances HIV replication in peripheral blood mononuclear cells but not in macrophages. (see also p. 195).

A gene present in Epstein–Barr virus codes for the protein that mimics IL-10 and its expression leads to inhibition of IFN-gamma production by human peripheral blood mononuclear cells. Human T-cell leukaemia virus type-I modifies the expression of a number of cellular genes including those for cytokines. The abnormal or inappropriate expression of cytokines in viral infections may underlie some of the clinical manifestations of viral disease.

The clinical implications include persistence of virus in the absence of a protective immune response, the development of immune complex disease (p. 187), and potentiation of tumour growth as a result of depressed immunological capacity and thus of immune surveillance mechanisms (p. 259).

Other viral host reactions

Recent studies have indicated that the lesions associated with virus infections cannot be explained simply by the cytopathic effects of the virus on cells. The immune response of the host to the viral antigen appears to play a role in producing tissue damage due to the immune complexes (see p. 187) formed by virus and antibody.

Cytotoxic T-lymphocytes will kill histocompatible target cells (see p. 244) infected with a variety of viruses, e.g. LCM and influenza. $CD8^+$ cytotoxic T-cells play a central role in antiviral immunity but there are exceptions. The importance of $CD4^+$ T-cells in protection from measles virus has been shown in experiments in rats. In contrast $CD4^+$ T-cells are not required as long as $CD8^+$ T-cells are present in cytomegalovirus infections. Most $CD8^+$ T-cells express cytolytic activity and produce interferon-γ but it is still not certain which of these activities is essential for protection. Another protective mechanism operates through Fc receptor-expressing cells such as macrophages that will lyse antibody-coated virus-infected cells. This is called antibody-dependent cell-mediated cytotoxicity (ADCC). The mechanism has been shown to be effective against mumps, herpes simplex, vaccinia and influenza virus-infected cells. Another lymphocyte population that cannot be identified as either T- or B-cells by their surface markers are the so-called natural killer cells or NK cells. These can destroy cells infected with a number of viruses — Epstein–Barr, Coxsackie, and LCM — and this ability of NK cells seems to be potentiated by interferon.

Epstein–Barr virus infection is usually a self-limiting disease of adolescents characterized by fever, pharyngitis, lymphadenopathy, splenomegaly and fatigue. The serological response is dominated by rising antibody titres to the virus capsid antigen and atypical lymphocytes can be found in the blood. The condition usually resolves within 1 to 3 months with disappearance of the atypical lymphocytes. Chronic symptomless carriers of the virus are found and occasionally chronic symptomatic cases of the disease have been reported.

If macrophages are rendered inactive by injections of silica, herpes simplex infections have been shown to be potentiated. Macrophages can restrict replication of hepatitis virus in the mouse; this is genetically controlled. The ability of macrophage cultures to resist viral replication in vitro is correlated with in vivo susceptibility or resistance to the virus.

Another way in which a virus can initiate destruction of host cells is by virus-induced changes in the surface antigens of the host cell. The altered surface antigen stimulates an immune response with subsequent destruction of the cell by antibody and complement and possible concomitant release of pharmacologically active mediators of inflammation. Such a phenomenon is not necessarily detrimental only to the host cells as these are virus-infected cells and their elimination would lead also to destruction of the virus. In conclusion it can be seen that the outcome of a virus infection is the result of the **interplay** between **protective** and **hypersensitivity** mechanisms, the balance usually settling in favour of protection. Figure 5.10 is an attempt to summarize these complex interrelationships.

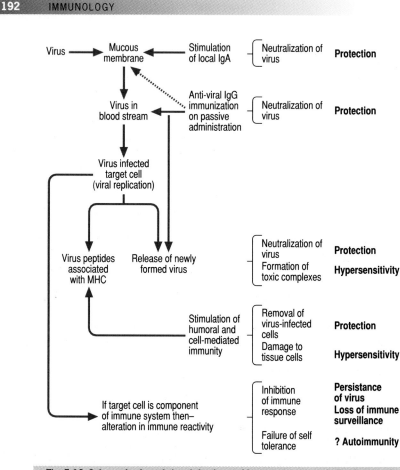

Fig. 5.10 **Schematic view of virus infection and immune response, indicating some possible consequences.**

Susceptibility to virus infections and the role of the major histocompatibility antigens

One of the valuable roles of interferons in antiviral immunity is to increase the expression of class I MHC antigens. This is likely to facilitate the interaction between virally infected cells and cytolytic lymphocytes ($CD8^+$ cells). A possible mechanism the viruses might use to circumvent immune surveillance by $CD8^+$ cells is to reduce the expression of the class I antigen. Adenoviruses have the ability to diminish messenger RNA levels for class I antigens and also produce a glycoprotein that forms complexes with class I antigens that interfere with their intracellular transport. There appear to be differences in the strength of interaction between the glycoprotein and different HLA types of class I antigen, suggesting that the pathogenicity of the virus may be dependent on the HLA type of the infected individual.

In Chapter 4 consideration is given to the genetic control of the immune response by a specific group of genes called **Ir genes**. These have been shown to be closely related to those genes controlling the major antigenic determinants of graft rejection (MHC genes). Gene products associated with the MHC genes involved in cooperation between T- and B-lymphocytes, leading to an immune response, have been described on page 137. This phenomenon is of interest in view of the known relationship between histocompatibility antigens (determined by the MHC gene complex) and susceptibility to certain virus-induced leukaemias in mice. The susceptibility of mice to lymphocytic-choriomeningitis virus (p. 185) and humans to the SV40 virus may also be determined in this way. The response in vivo in humans to certain viral antigens appears to be under HLA control as judged by the response to live vaccines. Poor responses to influenza vaccine have been found in HLA-Bw38 and Bw39 individuals whilst HLA-Bw55 and Bw56 individuals produced high titres to rubella vaccine. In vitro lymphocyte responsiveness to tetanus toxoid, vaccinia, PPD and streptococcal antigen show association with HLA, for example B5 persons tended to respond poorly to tetanus toxoid and Cw3 individuals to vaccinia. With increased knowledge of the gene complex controlling histocompatibility antigens and various functions of lymphocytes associated with the immune response, it should be possible in the next few years to elucidate some of the factors that determine susceptibility to virus diseases.

The role of the MHC in graft rejection was the first evidence that the control of the immune response depended on activities of the genes in that area (see p. 243). It later became apparent that T- and B-lymphocyte interaction and macrophage T-lymphocyte co-operation also required compatibility between the MHC regions of the cell types involved. In this instance surface molecules (Ia antigens) determined by I region genes are those involved and thus are important determinants of immunity: (1) to intracellular bacterial infections and (2) in control of cellular interactions in antibody production. The H-2K and H-2D regions control surface molecules involved in cytotoxic T-lymphocyte (CD8$^+$) activities and thus determine protective immune responses to viruses as well as graft rejection.

Since viruses can infect a large variety of different cell types the ubiquitous distribution of H-2K and H-2D antigens enable CD8$^+$ cells to deal with virus infections of all cell types. In contrast Ia antigens are more limited in distribution, being found mainly on cells of the immune system including a proportion of macrophages, other inducer cells and B-lymphocytes. They are important in generation of protective responses to intracellular bacteria, acting as receptors for signals leading to T-cell generated signals for B-cell differentiation, such as switching on of Ig production and changes from IgM to IgG (see Ch. 4).

Examples of immunity in virus infections

Measles. Measles virus is an enveloped paramyxovirus with a single-stranded DNA genome. One strain with minor antigenic variations is of clinical importance. The rash results from the host cellular immune response to the virus. The presence of IgM antibody to the virus confirms the diagnosis. Protective immunity is directed at the envelope proteins (the fusion and haemagglutinin proteins). The virus markedly depresses cellular immunity and is sometimes associated with reactivation of tuberculosis. The antibody response can also be reduced, indicating that the virus may affect both B- and T-lymphocytes. Patients with defective cellular immunity are likely to develop progressive infection. Protection by antibodies resulting from infection persists for life whilst antibodies induced by immunization (particularly before 1–2 years of age) may not persist as long. Control of the disease by vaccination with live attenuated virus is important as the disease is highly infectious and can lead to pneumonia, otitis media and viral encephalitis. Children should be vaccinated unless they suffer from a congenital immune deficiency. A small proportion of individuals may later (years) develop a chronic progressive neurological disorder — subacute sclerosing panencephalitis. The activated T-lymphocytes, macrophages and astrocytes present in the brain lesions are associated with the production of IFN-γ and TNF-α that are believed to be responsible for the progressive tissue damage.

Respiratory syncitial virus. This is a single-stranded RNA enveloped virus with one serotype with minor envelope protein variations. It causes bronchiolitis and pneumonia in infants and upper respiratory infections in adults. The severity of the bronchiolitis correlates with the finding of mast cell products in secretions and it is possible that this indicates IgE involvement. Recovery from infections is complete and depends upon both humoral and cellular immunity. No vaccine is available but a nucleotide analogue (ribavirin) can accelerate recovery.

Hepatitis B. This virus is a non-enveloped DNA virus with a surface (HBs) and a core (HBc) antigen that replicates in hepatocytes. The surface antigen is produced in large amounts and is found in the blood. Persistent infection is associated with a high risk of hepatic carcinoma. The virus is transmitted by intravenous drug abuse, sexual contact and blood products, and may be passed from mother to infants. Chronic carriers may remain infectious for life. A useful diagnostic test is IgM antibody to core antigen as this is found only in acute infections. Liver damage depends upon the cellular immune response to the virus and this response normally eliminates the virus.

Immune complex disease can result from complexes of surface antigen and antibody and causes fever, skin rashes and arthritis. Alpha-interferon and a nucleoside analogue vidarabine, or alpha-interferon alone, have been used for therapy, and pooled human gamma-globulin and more recently an HBV vaccine are used for protection. The virus is able to inhibit alpha-interferon production and block the response of infected cells to interferon.

AIDS. The acquired immunodeficiency syndrome (AIDS) was first described in 1981 and the HIV virus characterized a few years later. Virus infection results in an acquired defect in immune function, especially involving cell-mediated immunity. The initial infection is usually asymptomatic but results in a progressive disease with opportunistic infections, certain cancers and general debilitation, sometimes with central nervous system degeneration.

Research into HIV has resulted in a massive stimulus to investment and research in virology and collaboration with immunologists in an attempt to understand the interaction of the virus with the immune system. HIV is a retrovirus in the lentivirus family whose reverse transcriptase allows the synthesis of a DNA copy of the viral genome. The lentivirus family is characterized by a long latency period between infection and the onset of clinical symptoms. Other members of the family cause progressive neurodegenerative disease in sheep and goats. A variant HIV-2 is the major cause of AIDS in West Africa.

The env, gag and pol structural genes code for viral envelope proteins, core protein and reverse transcriptase respectively. The presence of six other genes in HIV is a feature unique among retroviruses and they include regulatory genes, e.g. tat, which can accelerate HIV replication, and vif, which increases viral infectivity.

A variety of cell types can be infected by the virus and the prominent immunological feature is a reversal of the CD4:CD8 T-lymphocyte ratio resulting from progressive depletion of $CD4^+$ T-cells. Monocyte/macrophage cells provide a reservoir of virus and the infected cells secrete an inhibitor of interleukin-1 (IL-1), a cytokine that is important for T-cell proliferative responses. Elevated levels of IL-6 are found in the plasma of HIV-infected individuals. This cytokine plays an essential role in the differentiation of B-cells to immunoglobulin-secreting cells and thus might be responsible for the polyclonal B-cell activation found in AIDS patients. Transforming growth factor-β (TGF-β) is also increased in HIV-infected individuals. This is an immunosuppressive cytokine that inhibits lymphocyte function and deactivates macrophages, thus contributing to immune dysfunction. It seems likely that the immune dysfunction resulting from HIV infection is a consequence of viral effects on both T-cells and MHC class II expressing, antigen-presenting cells such as macrophages (discussed on p. 190). Infection of multinucleated giant cells, mostly of monocyte/macrophage origin, in the brain possibly underlies the neurological symptoms.

Some individuals show the clinical features of acute infection and this usually appears within 2–6 weeks after exposure to the virus. Symptoms include fever, myalgia and arthralgia, lethargy, lymphadenopathy, pharyngitis, nausea, headaches, photophobia and rashes. At this stage high titres of virion-associated RNA are detected in the blood and a relatively homogeneous population of genetic variants are found. With the onset of an HIV-specific immune response the RNA titres decline. The first antibodies to appear (2–12 weeks after infection) are IgM anti-p24 (core) and anti-gp41 (transmembrane) whilst antibodies against pool gene products appear later. The virus itself may be detected in culture or by the polymerase chain reaction (PCR). Antibody screening is usually done using an ELISA test (p. 330) and confirmation by a Western blot assay in which purified viral proteins are electrophoresed in polyacrylamide gel and transferred to a nitrocellulose membrane. The viral proteins are then detected using a serum containing antibodies to HIV.

The AIDS syndrome may appear years later during which time the population of genetic variants diversifies due to mutation and repetitive cycles of viral replication and recombination events. Early symptoms usually show as opportunistic infections that include *Pneumocystis carinii* pneumonia, toxoplasmosis, mycobacterial infection, herpes simplex and cytomegalovirus infections. In time the immune system becomes compromised and eventually the patient succumbs to HIV-related infections and neurologic and neoplastic complications. The rate of progress is highly variable and useful markers of resistance are relatively stable $CD4^+$ numbers and low levels of HIV-RNA.

Therapeutic measures include prevention of viral entry into target cells using soluble recombinant CD4, interference with reverse transcriptase by zidovudine, inhibitors of regulatory proteins, e.g. tat inhibitors, interference with HIV translation and assembly, e.g. ribavirin, and interferons to prevent virus budding from infected cells. Therapeutic intervention during the primary infection when there is a relatively limited distribution of distinguishable genotypes is likely to be more effective than later in the disease when mutation is likely to have resulted in variants resistant to therapy.

New developments that show promise, particularly if given early after infection, are the protease inhibitors that act to block HIV reproduction by preventing the assembly into mature virus particles. These include Saquinivir, Ritonavir and Indinavir and a number of others under development. They are usually given in combination with AZT. The viral load can be shown to show a remarkable decrease and T-lymphocyte levels improve substantially but it is not clear if the virus has been eliminated entirely from within cells and for how long the new drug combinations will be effective before resistant variants arise. Unfortunately these new drugs are expensive and are unlikely to be available for general use in developing countries.

Vaccines against the virus are proving difficult to develop despite detailed knowledge of the virus and its genome. The high degree of glycosylation of the envelope glycoproteins, variability between strains and the possible antigenic relationship with the host CD4 antigen may be responsible for these difficulties.

The envelope gene from the AIDS virus has recently been inserted into the vaccinia virus (p. 218) so that it makes the envelope proteins, including one called gp4l that appears to be conserved. It is hoped that a vaccine made from the altered vaccinia virus might be able to give protection from the HIV virus. The situation may be complicated by the possibility suggested by some virologists that AIDS patients are infected by several strains of HIV and that the virus can change its envelope proteins in successive generations. This possibility is supported by recent evidence that some of the virus genes show up to 30% divergence from their common point of ancestry about 20 years ago (see also p. 165). If this is the case the production of an effective vaccine is likely to be difficult. The existing strains of the virus are fortunately not easily transmissible but with its high mutation rate a new strain may emerge that is much more contagious.

PARASITE IMMUNITY

Introduction

Parasites have evolved to be closely adapted to the host and have developed a variety of escape mechanisms to avoid the immune response (Table 5.12).

The large size of parasites compared with bacteria or viruses means that they carry more antigenic epitopes and because of their complex life cycles (Table 5.13) some antigens are specific only for certain developmental stages.

Most parasite infections are chronic and often show specificity for a particular host species. The plasmodia of malaria are different for humans, birds and rodents and cannot complete their life cycle in the wrong species. Tapeworms can, however, cross species and the pig tapeworm can infect humans.

Infections caused by protozoa and helminths

Introduction

Parasites in this category affect many millions of people in tropical parts of the world and are responsible for severe and debilitating disease. Malaria affects some 200 million people and at least 1 million children die of the disease every year. The World Health Organization esti-

Table 5.12 Parasite escape mechanism

Escape mechanism	Parasite
Intracellular habitat	Malaria parasites, trypanosomes and *Leishmania*
Encystment	*Toxoplasma gondii* and *Trypanosoma cruzi*
Resistance to microbicidal products of phagocytes	*Leishmania donovani*
Resistance to complement lysis	*Entamoeba histolytica* (under stress conditions)
Masking of antigens	Schistosomes
Variation of antigen	Trypanosomes and malaria parasites
Suppression of immune response	Most parasites, e.g. malaria, *Trichinella spiralis*, *Schistosoma mansoni*
Interference by antigens Polyclonal activation	Trypanosomes
Sharing of antigens between parasite and host — molecular mimicry	Schistosomes
Continuous turnover and release of surface antigens of parasite	Schistosomes
Exposure to very small numbers of parasites at intervals (trickle infection) so that strong immune response does not develop	

mates that more than 107 million people contract malaria each year around the world. Research is being carried out to find if HIV infection affects the course of this disease (in the same way as it increases susceptibility to tuberculosis). Schistosomiasis and filariasis fall into the same category as malaria and are responsible for enormous morbidity and mortality.

Malaria

Four species of mosquito-borne malaria parasite can infect humans: *Plasmodium falciparum*, *P. vivax*, *P. malariae* and *P. ovale*. There are several kinds and combinations of *Plasmodia* and *Anopheles* resulting in different physiological and ecological patterns of disease. The major combination is *Plasmodium falciparum* transmitted by the extremely efficient and persistent *Anopheles gambiae* complex of mosquito vec-

Table 5.13 Parasite infections

Disease	Features
Malaria	Sporozoites from mosquito develop in liver, progeny (merozoites) in erythrocytes, cyclic chills–fever–sweat syndrome. IgG to merozoites protective. Antigenic variation of parasites. Gradual long-term resistance develops. Transplacental IgA protects.
Toxoplasmosis	Infection (through gastrointestinal tract) usually asymptomatic. Clinical disease with lymphadenopathy and/or CNS infection. Fetus (2nd & 3rd semester) and immunocompromised host vulnerable. Reservoir unknown. Encysted parasites survive. Macrophages + Ab + C′ can kill trophozoites. γ-IFN activates macrophages.
Amoebiasis	Pathogenic strains cause ulceration of intestinal mucosa with systemic spread. Liver abscesses. Depressed CMI to amoebic antigens. Macrophages — deficient release of oxygen intermediates and not cytotoxic. CD8 lymphocytes can kill parasite.
Leishmaniasis	Sandfly vector. Obligate intracellular infection of macrophages, skin and viscera. Different species and strains produce large variety of pathological and immunological consequences (anergic or allergic responses). CMI and Ab may provide protection in cutaneous form. Delayed hypersensitivity may protect in visceral form.
Trypanosomiasis (sleeping sickness)	Tsetse-fly vector. Many varieties. Evasion by antigenic variation prominent, increased non-specific IgM not protective. Specific antibodies may protect. Immunosuppression to unrelated antigens. Multiple variants acts against vaccination.

tors. Those most at risk from malaria are young children, pregnant women, people moving from non-malarious to malarious zones and those from industrialized countries who visit malarious areas and return home with the disease. In each instance lack of immunity underlies the infection risk. In many parts of the world the parasites have become resistant to some of the major drugs used for treatment, including chloroquine and its derivatives except for central American countries where by 1994 chloroquine resistance had not been recorded. Newer drugs include mefloquine, halofantrine and artemisinin.

Each of the malaria parasites has a similar life cycle. After infection by inoculation of sporozoites by anopheline mosquitoes these extracellular forms circulate in the blood for about 30 minutes before penetrating liver parenchymal cells. After asexual multiplication merozoites are released and, after a short extracellular period, infect erythrocytes where a second asexual multiplication cycle occurs. The merozoite becomes a trophozoite that in turn becomes a schizont containing merozoites. Rupture of the infected erythrocyte releases merozoites that go on to infect other erythrocytes. Some merozoites develop into male and female gametocytes that initiate the next phase of the life cycle if ingested by the appropriate mosquito, leading to the sporozoite stage and start of a fresh cycle. In pregnant women the parasites can localize in the placenta by attaching to chondroitin A.

Trypanosomiasis

The parasites are flagellate protozoa that appear in different morphological forms in their life cycle. Trypomastigotes are found in mammalian blood and epimastigote and amastigote forms may also occur. The parasite undergoes a complex cycle of development in the tsetse fly before appearing as an infective trypomastigote in the fly's salivary glands. In humans the tsetse fly bite is sometimes associated with the development of a swollen vesiculate lesion (chancre). The patient goes on to develop an acute febrile illness with lymphadenopathy and splenomegaly. The late stage of the disease involves the CNS with increased CSF protein and cells. Progress of the disease is accompanied by anaemia, leucopenia, muscle wasting and myocarditis. The trypanosome population induces humoral immunity that reduces parasite numbers. Survival is ensured by antigenic variation, the continual switching of the variant surface glycoprotein (VSG). This glycoprotein is the only antigen on the surface of the parasite that is accessible to antibody. At each stage only one VSG is expressed and it acts to block access of antibodies to other surface molecules. Recent increased understanding of trypanosome biology is likely to lead to the development of drugs that interfere with replication and may provide a more effective means of control than attempts to produce a vaccine are likely to achieve.

The South American trypanosome *T. cruzi* causes Chagas' disease, which lies in third place after malaria and schistosomiasis affecting 16–18 million people in the region. The disease is transmitted to humans by vectors (Triatomine, 'kissing bugs') that live in the cracks of mud huts. The trypomastigotes derived from faeces of the vector enter the skin through scratches and infect both smooth and striated muscle, where they transform into amastigotes. The heart muscle may be affected and also the muscle of the alimentary tract. The disease usually begins as an acute infection in childhood followed by a slow chronic inflammatory process which in around a quarter of those infected damages the autonomic nervous tissues of the heart. No treatment is available for the chronic forms of the disease whilst nifurtimox and benzidazole are used for the acute forms of the disease but have unpleasant side affects. The life cycle of the parasite is completed in the vector after it feeds on the blood of an infected person. An important difference between the South American and African trypanosomes is that the former are intracellular and thus immunity depends upon oxygen dependent and independent phagocytic defences rather than antibody and complement for the African variety.

Control of blood banks is important as the prevalence of *T. cruzi* infected blood is higher than that of hepatitis or HIV and screening of blood banks is compulsory in Argentina, Bolivia, Brazil, Columbia, Honduras, Uruguay and Venezuela. Control measures include the use of insecticides in paints, fumigant canisters, housing improvement and health education.

Leishmaniasis

Leishmania parasites (around twenty different types) are transmitted by sandfly vectors and induce at least five distinct diseases with different symptoms: cutaneous leishmaniasis appears as lumps under the skin that develop into a large sore and is self-limiting after a few months; diffuse cutaneous leishmaniasis is rare but more serious when the immune system fails to react to the infection; mucocutaneous leishmaniasis begins with the skin and spreads to the mucous membranes of the nose, mouth and pharynx with ensuing unpleasant tissue destruction; visceral leishmaniasis (kala-azar) is the most serious form manifesting as weight loss, fever, enlarged liver and spleen, this form has a high mortality unless treated; the post-kala-azar dermal form may develop in treated patients and the nodules may last for years. The parasites invade the host macrophages and treatment has been based on compounds of antimony.

Lymphatic filariasis and onchocerciasis

Filariasis affects about 300 million people and is transmitted by mosquitoes (and for some species, horse flies and black flies). The parasites, as adult worms, live in the lymphatics and cause obstruction, inflammation and swelling of the arms, legs and genitals (elephantiasis). The most dramatic form of filariasis is river blindness caused by the worm *Onchocera volvulus*, transmitted by the black fly. The worms can reach half a metre in length and can live for up to 15 years, producing millions of embryos that invade the skin and eyes.

The most widespread filarial parasite is *Wuchereria bancrofti* that affects about 106 million people in the tropical areas of Africa, India, south-east Asia, the Pacific islands and South and Central America. India has by far the most cases. The *Anopheles* mosquitoes of the same genus that transmits malaria is the responsible vector in rural areas, particularly in Africa, whilst in cities the *Culex* mosquito species that lives in latrines, sewage and ditches is the main vector. In the Pacific region a mosquito (*Aedes*) that can also transmit yellow fever and dengue transmits the filarial parasite.

River blindness is the most dreaded form of filarial disease and is due to *Onchocera volvulus*. It affects some 17 million people in Africa and a smaller number in Central and South America. The parasite vector is *Simulium* blackflies that breed in fast flowing rivers. Grape-sized nodules form in the skin and the female produces millions of microfilariae that, rather than settling in the lymphatics and the blood, invade the eye and skin.

Drug treatment with ivermectin has proved very effective, particularly if combined with diethylcarbamizine (DEC). This can reduce microfilaraemia in the lymphatic form by 95% two years after treatment. DEC-medicated salt has been introduced in India and is used in China. This has proved to be an effective means of eliminating the disease. River blindness is mainly treated with ivermectin alone.

Schistosomiasis (bilharzia)

This disease is the result of infection by schistosome trematode worms. The female of the species lays eggs that can remain in the body for up to 35 years. Some eggs are trapped around the liver and bladder where they are attacked by the immune system, forming a granuloma that destroys neighbouring cells. Around half the eggs are excreted in the urine and faeces and pass into freshwater snails where they develop into free-swimming cercariae that can penetrate human skin. Around 200 million people are infected with the parasite. Of these some 20 million suffer clinical morbidity or disability, mostly in Africa but also to a lesser extent in Brazil, China and Egypt. In highly endemic regions three out of four children are infected and the debilitating effects of the disease create a problem of major public health importance. *Schistosoma mansoni* is the most widespread species, which affects the bowel and is prevalent throughout Africa, the Middle East and parts of South America. Three other species infect humans, two infecting the intestine and the other the urinary system. Effective drug treatment is available using praziquantel combined with the anti-helminthic albendazole.

Immune defence mechanisms

Introduction

The life cycles of organisms in this category, as noted above, are complicated and the immune response, to be effective, has to interrupt the cycle at a stage when the parasite is accessible to the immune processes.

The physical barrier of the skin provides protection against invasion by many parasites but can be side-tracked by blood-feeding insects such as mosquitoes or by schistosomes that have the ability to penetrate skin. Individuals with the sickle cell trait are resistant to malaria because of a genetic defect in their haemoglobin molecules. As the parasite attaches to red blood cells by the Duffy blood group antigen, individuals who lack this antigen are also resistant. Like bacteria and viruses, parasites are susceptible to phagocytosis or attack by monocytes/macrophages, neutrophils and NK cells working as we have seen in conjunction with antibodies acting as opsonins and with the complement system.

Both humoral and cell-mediated immune mechanisms are involved in immunity to parasites with the cell-mediated form being most effective for intracellular parasites in the same way as for intracellular bacteria or viruses. The form of immunity that provides protection will vary with different stages in the life cycle of parasites.

The specific immune response to parasite antigens is a T-cell dependent process and leads to the production of the different antibody isotypes and activated cell-mediated mechanisms. IgE and IgA are of particular importance in relation to intestinal parasites. Parasite antigens crosslink IgE on the surface of mast cells and cause degranulation followed by attraction of eosinophils. The eosinophilia (and the increase in mucosal mast cells) characteristic of many parasite infections is a T-cell dependent phenomenon and the lymphokines that induce the production of eosinophils also bring about their activation. Mediators produced by mast cells bring about a local inflammatory response with vasodilation and increased vascular permeability. Inflammatory cells migrate to the site of infection and eosinophils, which play a particularly important role, are induced to degranulate by the presence of antibodies and complement on the surface of the parasite, resulting in the production of toxic molecules that can destroy the parasite. Platelets also contain molecules that are toxic to various parasites (e.g. schistosomes, *T. cruzi* and *T. gondii*) and the cytotoxic capacity of platelets is enhanced by gamma-interferon and tumour necrosis factor.

Role of antibody

Antibody, by reacting with parasite surface antigens, can neutralize the parasite by interfering with essential functions and block attachment to its target cell as, for example, with antibodies to the merozoite stage of *Plasmodium* spp. that can block infection of red blood cells by the parasite. Agglutination by IgM antibody, as with bacteria and viruses, can limit the spread of parasites in the tissues and their toxins can be neutralized by IgG. Complement lysis can also occur and antibody can act as an opsonin to facilitate phagocytosis, particularly in plasmodium and trypanosome infections.

T. cruzi, *T. spiralis*, *S. mansoni* and filarial worms can be killed by antibody-dependent cytotoxicity mechanisms. The effector cells bind to the antibody-coated parasites via the phagocyte Fc receptors and the toxic products released from the phagocyte damage the parasite target. Major basic protein from eosinophils damages the tegument of schistosomes and other worms causing their death. Eosinophils are more effective at killing newborn larvae of *T. spiralis* than other phagocytes whereas macrophages are very effective against microfilariae.

Cell-mediated mechanisms

Experiments with mice whose T-lymphocytes have been depleted have shown the importance of T-cell dependent immunity in protection from malaria and trypanosome infections. The transfer of spleen cells from immune animals can restore protection. CD4$^+$ T-cells transfer protection against *L. major* and *L. tropics*, which cause cutaneous leishmaniasis, and also protect against *Giardia muris*, which inhabits the gut of mice. Cytotoxic T-cells appear to be able to destroy *Theileria parvum* in cattle and are effective in mice against malaria parasites during the liver stage of infection whilst CD4 cells are active for the blood stage. The latter cells, as has been noted, not only assist B-cells to produce antibody but secrete colony-stimulating factors to enhance production of granulocytes as well as other lymphokines that enhance the activity of effector cells.

Macrophages play an important role in many parasite infections, particularly after activation by lymphokines, as well as acting as antigen-presenting cells. These mechanisms are the same as already described for intracellular bacteria and viruses involving their oxygen dependent and independent digestion mechanisms along with nitric oxide.

Polyclonal activation of B-lymphocytes and the production of high levels of non-specific immunoglobulin are common findings in parasite infections and can give rise to autoantibodies against, for example, red blood cells and DNA. Host antigens incorporated into the parasite have also been found to induce autoimmunity. Presumably the host antigen attached to a parasite carrier molecule can break T-cell tolerance to the host antigen. In Chagas' disease about 20% of individuals develop progressive cardiomyopathy and neuropathy of the digestive tract that is believed to be autoimmune in nature. Immune complex formation, as with viruses and bacteria, can lead to pathological complications and has been described in malaria, trypanosomiasis, schistosomiasis and onchocerciasis.

Immunopathogenisis of parasitic diseases

This involves hypersensitivity reactions, which are described in Chapter 9. IgE antibodies and eosinophilia are the hallmark of parasitic disease and are associated with type I antibody-mediated hypersensitivity (p. 272). Type II autoimmune reactions, directed at antigen on a cell surface with resulting lysis, are frequently found. Blood group substances incorporated into the tissues of the parasite can result in the development of autoantibody against host tissues. Type III immune complex-mediated disease occurs in malaria, trypanosomiasis, schistosomiasis and onchocerciasis. Delayed hypersensitivity type IV reactions are found in toxoplasmosis, leishmaniasis and South American trypanosomiasis. The liver, renal and cardiopulmonary pathology of schistosomiasis is related to cell-mediated responses to the schistosome eggs (see p. 208).

Examples of immunity in parasite infections

Malaria

Malaria infections are initiated by sporozoites and at this stage there is recognizable immunity. The discharge of merozoites from the liver into the peripheral circulation leads to antibodies that are readily detectable in the serum, increase until the crisis 7 to 10 days later and then slowly decline. Because these antibodies are able to get access to the parasite only during a relatively short period of its life cycle, immunity is incomplete and the host usually fails to eliminate the parasite completely. This state in which the organisms persist in small numbers in the tissues in the presence of an immune reaction is called ***premunition*** by parasitologists.

The IgG class of immunoglobulin is the major antibody class involved in acquired resistance to malaria and there is a considerable rise in the levels, and rate of synthesis, of this isotype. However, if serum from an infected individual is incubated with parasitized erythrocytes, only a small quantity of the IgG antibody is absorbed. The major part of the IgG probably represents antibody to soluble malarial antigens and seems unlikely to play a role in protection except perhaps when it is directed against toxic malarial products. Parasitic growth within erythrocytes is unaffected by the presence of immune serum in the culture medium, but invasion of new red cells by merozoites and subsequent parasite multiplication is inhibited. IgG antibodies can bind to Fc receptors on macrophages and it seems likely that phagocytosis of antibody-coated merozoites is an important mechanism of acquired immunity. There is evidence that antibody may act on mature intraerythrocytic forms of the parasite, possibly due to expression of parasite antigen on the surface of the red cells that renders the red cells susceptible to attack by antibody-dependent cell-mediated cytotoxicity.

Considerable experimental evidence exists showing that malarial infection is associated with **immunosuppression**. Depressed responsiveness of T-lymphocytes to PHA (p. 339) and B-lymphocytes to bacterial lipopolysaccharide can readily be demonstrated, as can diminished antibody responses to certain antigens. In a recent study of a group of patients infected with *Plasmodium falciparum*, peripheral blood lymphocytes, when tested in a lymphocyte proliferation assay, were shown to be unresponsive to antigen prepared from the parasite and in 37.5% of the patients this persisted for more than 4 weeks. The existence of unresponsiveness was present in all patients and was not related to the degree of parasitaemia or severity of the clinical illness. Suppression of lymphocyte reactivity was also found to an unrelated antigen but was much less profound and only seen in patients with moderately severe disease or with cerebral malaria. The depressed lymphocyte reactivity was associated with a loss of both $CD4^+$ and $CD8^+$ T-lymphocytes from the peripheral blood. Once the parasite was cleared from the blood the responses returned to normal. Cytokines are responsible for some of the lesions in malaria. In human cerebral malaria tumour necrosis factor (TNF) levels in the serum are correlated with severity. Overproduction of TNF is dependent on gamma-interferon and monoclonal antibody to the interferon can prevent experimental malaria. The findings indicate that malaria pathology is dependent on the T_H1 subset of T-cells (Table 4.5) as they produce gamma-interferon (and IL-4).

Trypanosomiasis

The efficacy of the immune mechanisms against trypanosomes is complicated by the fact that the parasites can change their surface antigenic constitution from one generation to the next. The number of variants which can be produced by a single strain is at least 20. It is not yet clear how the organism controls the generation of the variants but variation is thought to arise by selection of mutants from a heterogeneous population of parasites.

This complication means that the immune response has great difficulty in keeping up with the antigenic changes in the parasite and, in the case of the trypanosomes responsible for African sleeping sickness, the parasite does not induce an effective immunity. The infected subject develops a progressive infection with invasion of the central nervous system leading to death. Trypanosomiasis is associated with high levels of IgM immunoglobulins in both the blood and CSF. It is not certain if this is due to the repeated new antigenic stimuli resulting from changes in the organism or if the parasite in some way influences directly the cells of the immune system. Increased immunoglobulin production is a common finding in protozoal infections and often affects all classes of immunoglobulins. Because usually less than 5% of the total immunoglobulin appears to react specifically with the inducing parasite, it is probable that protozoa stimulate the lymphoid cells in a non-specific way to overproduce immunoglobulins (i.e. polyclonal B-cell activation).

This type of evidence has turned the attention of immunologists away from a direct role for antibody in protection in protozoal infections towards antibody-independent cell-mediated immunity. This, as has been noted, takes three forms: direct cytolysis by T-lymphocytes, soluble lymphocyte products from T-lymphocytes and natural killer cell (NK) activity. Recent evidence points to a central role for T-cell cytolytic reactions in an important tick-borne cattle disease, theileriasis, caused by several species of *Theileria* prevalent in several parts of Africa and for *T. cruzi* infections that parasitize heart cells.

In summary, immunity against protozoal infections seems to be dependent largely on antibody, particularly against those parasites that live in the bloodstream or have a bloodstream phase as part of their life cycle, e.g. malaria or trypanosomes. The effects of antibody are the same as those against other microorganisms including lysis with complement, opsonization, phagocytosis, antibody-dependent cell-mediated cytotoxicity and limitation of spread (Table 5.14). Protection against parasites, once they have become intracellular, in the same way as for intracellular bacteria, depends upon the oxygen dependent and independent microbicidal activities of phagocytes and nitric oxide. This in turn depends upon the enhancement of these functions by lymphokines derived, as already described, by stimulation of $CD4^+$ T-cells by antigen-presenting cells and the subsequent elaboration of lymphokines.

Helminth infections

Helminths, like protozoa, go through a complex life cycle and protective immune mechanisms appear to act only at an early stage in the cycle. The main stimulus appears to be due to antigens derived from the adult worm and the immunity derived from this acts on new parasites entering the body. A noteworthy feature of these infections is the appearance of IgE with associated pulmonary eosinophilia and it

---

Table 5.14 Humoral defence mechanisms against parasite infections

Mechanism	Effect	Parasite
Neutralization	Block attachment to host cell	Protozoa
	Act to inhibit evasion mechanisms of intracellular organisms	Protozoa
	Bind to toxins or enzymes	Protozoa and worms
Physical interference	Obstruct orifices	Worms
	Agglutinate	Protozoa
Opsonization	Increase clearance by phagocytes	Protozoa
Cytotoxicity	Complement-mediated lysis	Protozoa and worms
	Antibody-dependent cell-mediated cytotoxicity	Protozoa and worms

seems likely that IgE-mediated release of mediators from mast cells is involved in the pathogenesis of helminth infection.

Schistosomiasis

In *Schistosoma mansoni* infections the pathogenesis appears to be largely due to an **inflammatory granulomatous reaction** around the **schistosome eggs** trapped in the host tissues with a periovular area of necrosis surrounded by inflammatory cells, including many eosinophils. The most severe lesions occur during early infection. The adult schistosome (like other helminth parasites) does not replicate in the human host. The number of eggs produced (and thus the immunopathology) depends on the number of adult worms that mature within the human host and on the lifespan of these worms. The factors that determine morbidity include the intensity of infection, duration of infection, host genetic differences, parasite strain differences, concomitant infection and host nutritional status. Mice in experimental schistosomiasis infections reject 70 to 80% of new infections 12 weeks after their first infection. In baboons a significant reduction in the damage done by the parasite to the host organs was found in pre-immunized animals. The experimental findings suggest a gradual waning of egg hypersensitivity but the mechanism is not understood. In the murine model of schistosomiasis it has recently been found that T_H1 cells are stimulated by larval antigens and T_H2 cells by egg antigens. The induction of the T_H2 responses is associated with down-regulation of T_H1 responses and thus inhibition of potentially protective T_H1 responses. This inhibitory effect is due to the production of IL-10 by the T_H2 cells. The tissues commonly affected are the liver, which shows chronic portal inflammation, the lungs, the kidneys and the spleen. The renal and splenic lesions are not directly related to the presence of worms or eggs but may in part be due to immune complexes between worm antigens and antibody. In *Schistosoma haematobium* infection the urinary tract is the primary target and calcification of the bladder can occur in advanced cases. Migration of larvae into the lungs is sometimes associated with eosinophil infiltration and pneumonia, which can be fatal.

So far no vaccine is available. Immunity can be shown to develop to new schistosome infections whilst leaving established worms unaffected. This appears to be due to the worms acquiring host-derived macromolecules and the deployment of various enzymes to interfere with the host's immune response. When worms are transferred from mice to monkeys that are immunized against mouse red blood cells, the worms are killed by an antibody-mediated reaction directed at the surface of the parasite. In humans the host antigens acquired by the worms appear to be A, B and H blood group substances (Ch. 6) and possibly the Lewis antigen. Work is in progress on various subcomponent vaccines, particularly directed at the schistosome worm to reduce worm load and thus egg production.

Like murine schistosomiasis *Trichinella spiralis* infections also show that T_H1 cells play a central role in resistance and T_H2 cells in susceptibility to infection. The role of T_H1 versus T_H2 lymphocytes has been studied in patients with filariasis with similar conclusions to those in murine infection. Work of this type has led to clinical trials using recombinant cytokines (IL-2 and IFN-γ) particularly in patients with leishmaniasis. Treatment for three weeks with IFN-γ resulted in lesions smaller than in controls. IL-2 treatment resulted in an influx of $CD4^+$ T-cells and plasma cells into the lesions. The number of parasites was significantly reduced and the lesions became sterile in some patients. The objective of these strategies is to develop therapeutic procedures that induce resistance but minimize disease pathology.

In many helminth infections there is an association between increased levels of eosinophils in the blood and high IgE levels. If eosinophils are experimentally depleted in mouse schistosome infections, immunity to the parasite is decreased. It is likely that lymphokines produced by T-lymphocytes control the IgE and eosinophil response and that mast cells at the site of infection release mediators including eosinophil chemotactic factor of anaphylaxis (ECFA). Eosinophils in conjunction with IgG, and probably IgE, adhere to the schistosomula and eosinophil enzymes and proteins are released, destroying the parasite. Figure 5.11 illustrates the series of interactions involved. The eosinophil products include peroxidase and a basic protein, which are likely to be involved in the destruction of the parasite as well as enzymes that inactivate the mast cell products histamine and slow-reacting substance of anaphylaxis (SRS-A) (see also p. 34). Table 5.12 summarizes some of the mechanisms used by parasites to avoid the immune response.

Leishmaniasis

A high titre of antibody to the intramacrophage parasite is found and there is suppression of the cell-mediated response to *Leishmania* antigen as seen by negative skin tests. The response is restored after successful drug therapy. In experimental models of the disease in mice it appears that the parasite causes the expansion of the T_H2 subset of $CD4^+$ T-cells and these release soluble factors that interfere with the expansion of antigen specific T_H1 cells leading to failure to control the spread of the disease. Vaccines have been developed using killed parasites with BCG. Recombinant vaccines (*mycobacteria*, *salmonella* and *vaccinia*) carrying various leishmanial genes are under active investigation.

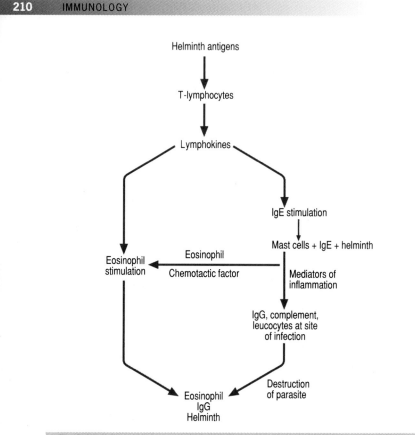

Fig. 5.11 Scheme showing the role of IgE and eosinophils in helminth immunity.

Filariasis

The immune response to filarial antigens has been shown to be correlated to the microfilaraemic status of the mother during pregnancy. Infants of infected mothers appear to be less capable of mounting an immune response to the parasite, indicating tolerance induction during development. Cytokine responses to filarial antigens in microfilaraemic but asymptomatic individuals appear to be skewed to the T_H2 type (high IL-4, IL-5, IL-10 anti-inflammatory type).

Diagnosis

The immunodiagnosis of parasitic infection involves the detection of antibody to current or past infection. The availability of commercial antigens has led to exploitation of immunological procedures such as ELISA (p. 330), fluorescent antibody tests (p. 327) and radioimmunoassays (p. 330).

Fungal infections

Fungi are eukaryotic organisms whose cell walls are different from mammalian cells in that they contain ergosterol, which is the target for the anti-fungal agent amphotericin B. There are three main forms of fungal infection: superficial and cutaneous mycoses, subcutaneous mycoses and systemic invasive mycoses. The superficial mycoses are not exposed to the influence of antibodies or cell-mediated immunity whilst cutaneous infections induce delayed hypersensitivity. Immunity to cutaneous and systemic forms of the mycoses is mainly dependent on neutrophils, macrophages, lymphocytes and perhaps NK cells. Most fungi are not able to be killed by antibody and complement. Individuals with neutropenia or defective neutrophil function are susceptible to candidiasis, aspergillosis and zygomycosis whilst defective cell-mediated immunity predisposes to candida infections of the mucosa, systemic cryptococcosis, histoplasmosis and coccidioidomycosis (Table 5.15). Like other microorganisms, fungi may exist as opportunist pathogens such as *Candida albicans* or *Aspergillus fumigatus*, or as pathogens such as *Histoplasma capsulatum* or *Coccidioides immitis*.

Table 5.15 **Systemic invasive mycosis**

Disease	Features
Blastomycosis	Pulmonary inhalation, remains localized or spreads to skin, bone, genitourinary tract, islands of suppuration and granulomas
Coccidioidomycosis	Pulmonary inhalation localized or disseminated infection to skin, subcutaneous tissues, bones, joints, meninges
Histoplasmosis	Pulmonary inhalation localized or disseminated infection to reticuloendothelial system, mucosal surfaces, adrenal glands
Paracoccidioidomycosis	Pulmonary inhalation, localized or disseminated infection to skin, mucous membranes, reticuloendothelial system, adrenal glands
Candidiasis (opportunistic)	Superficial infection (e.g. thrush), deep local invasion (e.g. oesophagitis), haematogenous dissemination (e.g. eyes, skin, kidneys, brain)
Cryptococcosis (opportunistic)	Pulmonary inhalation, localized or disseminated to meninges, skin, bone, eyes, prostate
Aspergillosis (opportunistic)	Pulmonary inhalation, localized or disseminated infection, particularly in immunocompromised patients. Bronchial ulceration, parenchymal invasion, widespread metastatic infection. *Aspergillus* spp. produce toxins. Aflatoxin linked to hepatocellular carcinoma, gliotoxin destroys macrophages and cytotoxic T-cells

Susceptibility to superficial fungal infections such as those due to *Candida albicans* is usually the result of an alteration in the mucous membrane defence mechanisms, commonly following the use of antibiotics that disturb the normal flora or as a result of hormonal changes. Studies in the author's laboratory have shown that individuals who are non-secretors of blood group substances tend to be more susceptible to infections by *Candida albicans* (see p. 158). It seems likely that the Lewis blood group substance is involved in binding of the organism to its target cells. Fungi often enter the host after phagocytosis by macrophages and, like many intracellular pathogens, use the complement receptors on the macrophage membrane. This depends on their ability to activate the alternative complement pathway. Binding to complement receptors (as distinct from the receptors for immunoglobulin) does not trigger production of reactive oxygen metabolites and thus antimicrobial activity.

Alterations in the host's immune response, for example as a result of immunosuppressive therapy, are the usual cause of systemic fungal infections. Cellular immune mechanisms appear to be important in defence against such systemic infections.

Allergic alveolitis and anaphylaxis

A few examples of pulmonary hypersensitivity to inhaled fungal antigens have been reported. The existence of a state of immunity has been confirmed by the finding of precipitating antibodies in their serum. The first of these disorders to be recognized was **farmers' lung** disease in which precipitating antibodies could be demonstrated against antigens derived from mouldy hay. The antigen has since been found to be *Micromonospora faeni*. Subsequently, work in Edinburgh has demonstrated precipitins, i.e. antibodies, against *Aspergillus clavatus* in **maltworkers** exposed to high concentrations of *A. clavatus* spores from contaminated barley. Antibodies against *Caniosporum corticale* have been found in the serum of maple bark strippers.

It is likely that following exposure to high concentrations of any of a variety of fungal spores individuals would produce precipitating antibodies and thus this form of pulmonary hypersensitivity may be more widespread than has so far been identified. The hypersensitivity reaction induced by the presence of precipitating antibodies would be of the toxic-complex (type III) form inducing a diffuse pulmonary interstitial pneumonitis which has been termed allergic alveolitis. Some of the antigens responsible for this form of hypersensitivity can also provoke in susceptible individuals the anaphylactic (type I) response exemplified by pulmonary asthma. If growth of the fungus should occur in the lungs, as in the case of *Aspergillus fumigatus*, the metabolic products of the organism will cause further immunization and increase in precipitating antibodies with the development of an accumulation

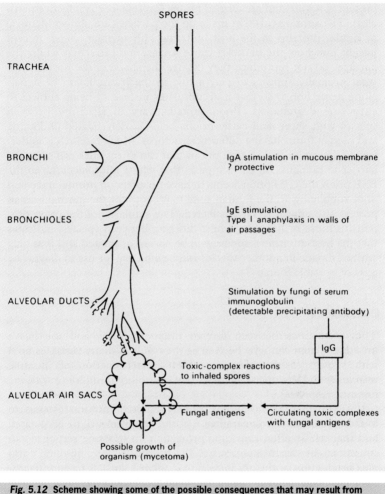

SPORES

TRACHEA

BRONCHI — IgA stimulation in mucous membrane
? protective

BRONCHIOLES — IgE stimulation
Type I anaphylaxis in walls of
air passages

ALVEOLAR DUCTS — Stimulation by fungi of serum
immunoglobulin
(detectable precipitating antibody)

IgG

Toxic-complex reactions
to inhaled spores

ALVEOLAR AIR SACS

Fungal antigens   Circulating toxic complexes
with fungal antigens

Possible growth of
organism (mycetoma)

Fig. 5.12 Scheme showing some of the possible consequences that may result from the inhalation of fungal spores.

of inflammatory cells at the site of infection. Figure 5.12 illustrates some of the possible consequences of a fungal respiratory infection.

Unusual infections

Scrapie, bovine spongiform encephalitis (BSE) and Creutzfeldt–Jakob disease (CJD) agents have proved to be something of a biological puzzle as unlike other infective agents they manage to reproduce without containing either DNA or RNA. The infective particles turn out to be protein in nature and are termed prions (proteinaceous infective particles). The amino acids that make up the particles are almost identical to similar proteins in the host, differing only in their shape. Recent insight into how the particles cause disease indicates that whilst the particles do not reproduce they change the shape of the host protein (that normally appears to play a role in the transmission of signals along nerve fibres) so that it accumulates instead of being subject to enzymatic degradation. Prion proteins vary in structure between species with sheep and cattle prions being closely related and cattle and human forms having differing structures. Much research is underway to determine if BSE type prions that can infect mice can cross the barrier to humans. So far it appears that whilst mice succumb to the BSE prion the CJD prion seems to have no effect on normal mice and mice supplied with the human gene that codes for the normal human protein also appear to be unaffected. The similarity of the prion proteins to those of the host, whilst differing between species, indicates that the host immune response will be absent or limited and that only antibody made in another species will be effective for use in diagnostic tests or possible therapy.

Conclusions

The interactions between foreign microorganisms and the host's immune system can now be seen as the result of many variables both with respect to the host (e.g. MHC determination of immune response) and the microorganism (e.g. its ability to interfere with the immune response).

It is clear that the development of an acquired immune response to a microorganism is no guarantee that the organism will be eliminated and that whilst often providing protection an immune response can sometimes be disadvantageous to the individual (e.g. immune complex production or the production of cytokines such as tumour necrosis factor that is involved in the pathogenesis of cerebral malaria (p. 206)).

Table 5.16 and Figure 5.13 are attempts to summarize the protective activities of the immune system with general application to the various types of microorganism discussed in this chapter.

COMMON VACCINATION PROCEDURES

Efficacy and hazards

It is generally accepted that one effective way of controlling the spread of infectious disease is by immunization with antigens derived from the appropriate organism. The isolation and bulk preparation of the

---

Table 5.16 **Summary of immune response to organisms**

Induction stage

1. Microbe breaks through innate immune mechanisms and is taken up by antigen-presenting cell (macrophage, dendritic cell)

2. Microbial-derived peptides associate with MHC class II molecules for presentation to $CD4^+$ T-cells

3. The production of co-stimulatory signals induces $CD4^+$ T-cells to produce receptors for interleukin-2 and also interleukin-2

4. B-lymphocytes can also present antigen to $CD4^+$ T-cells

Effector stage — humoral and cell-mediated immunity

1. Interferon produced induces antiviral state and stimulates natural killer cells that attack virus-infected cells and prevents viral infection of contiguous cells

2. T-cells kill cells infected with intracellular pathogens

3. T-cells produce lymphokines that destroy microorganisms and stimulate other defence mechanisms

4. Antibody kills microorganisms with complement, brings about opsonization and phagocytosis and coats the virus-infected cell so that cells with Fc receptors (e.g. macrophages and killer cells) can destroy the infected cell (IgG, IgM). IgA prevents adherence of microorganisms to mucosal surfaces and IgE recruits inflammatory cells by releasing mediators from mast cells

5. Regulatory mechanisms dampen down response

Note: excessive production of cytokines and inappropriate stimulation of T-cells can bring about tissue damage, e.g. IL-1 can induce haemodynamic shock, cytotoxic effects on insulin-producing β-cells of the pancreas, arthritis and osteoporosis. TNF along with IL-1 results in the production of collagenase in joint fluids that can damage cartilage. Cytolytic T-cells can damage hepatocytes containing listeria and Schwann cells containing leprosy bacilli. TNF appears to be involved in the pathogenesis of cerebral malaria.

---

particular antigens which confer protective immunity is a major difficulty but success in this field with a number of potentially dangerous microorganisms has radically altered the chances of them causing widespread disease in the population. The use of diphtheria toxoid (inactivated diphtheria toxin) is a noteworthy example. In Scotland, notifications of diphtheria averaged about 10 000 cases annually before 1940 when widespread immunization was instituted. The incidence of the disease rapidly decreased thereafter and, with the exception of an outbreak in 1968 involving six cases, none of whom had been fully immunized, the disease can be said to have been virtually eradicated. Sporadic outbreaks of meningococcal meningitis have caused anxiety in the last few years, particularly cases infected with the B15 strain that appeared in 1970. Unlike the A- and C-type meningo-

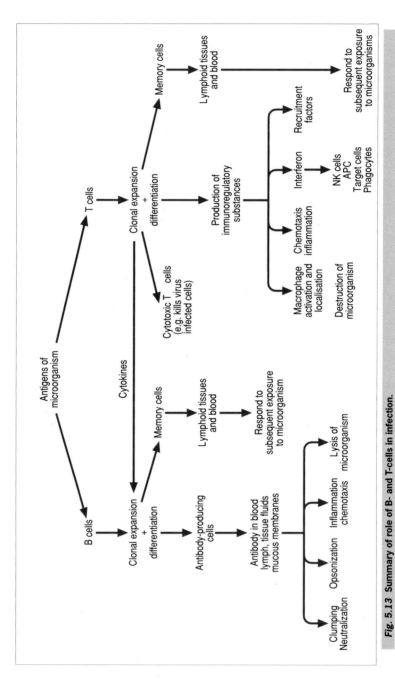

Fig. 5.13 Summary of role of B- and T-cells in infection.

cocci B strains are not readily immunogenic and a suitable vaccine has only recently been developed and is undergoing trials.

Immunization procedures are clearly not the only factor contributing to the decreasing morbidity and mortality from infectious disease. The combined death rate for scarlet fever, diphtheria, whooping cough and measles from 1860 to 1965 for children up to 15 years of age shows that nearly 90% of the total decline over the intervening century had occurred before widespread immunization and the use of antibiotics. Improved environmental conditions and, in particular, higher host resistance due to improved nutrition are probably major factors underlying the decline.

Much consideration has been given to the safety of vaccines and it is generally agreed that the greatest danger arises from the introduction of infection at the time of administration of the vaccine. Complications such as encephalitis after smallpox vaccination, febrile convulsions after whooping-cough vaccination and neurological complication after rabies vaccination are extremely rare phenomena. The risk is by far outweighed by the protection that immunization can give from the disease itself. Now, however, the risk of vaccine-induced problems is beginning to be of concern. Much of the rationale for developing new vaccines is to eliminate this problem. The development of a cell-free pertusis vaccine is an attempt to overcome problems associated with the whole-cell vaccine. The development of new more successful vaccines depends upon an improved understanding of the complex immunoregulatory mechanisms that determine protective immunity, unresponsiveness and tissue damage. Several cytokines normally associated with resistance to a pathogen are also responsible for tissue damage and sometimes with enhanced viral replication (see p. 190). These factors will need to be taken into account in the future development of vaccines.

New developments

Most infectious diseases are encountered through the mucous membranes that are protected by locally produced antibodies rather than those produced systemically. At present most vaccines are administered systemically rather than orally, largely due to the problem of enzymatic degradation in the gut. New developments have been directed at overcoming this problem and make use of the fact that oral immunization provides a disseminated IgA response at mucous surfaces of the respiratory tract and other areas associated with the mucosal immune system. One of the most useful approaches is the use of encapsulation of antigens within biodegradable particles such as poly-D,L-lactide-co-glycerol copolymers. The particles protect the antigen after ingestion and target its delivery to the Peyer's patches. Different rates of biodegradation of the particles can be achieved so that a secondary response can be generated by antigen released at a later stage. This has potential value in developing countries where booster immunization is achieved less readily than in more developed areas of the world. Other developments include the coupling of antigens to the B subunit of cholera toxin that attaches to the GMI ganglioside that is expressed on nucleated cells and the use of attenuated strains of bacteria as vectors for bacterial and viral antigens introduced by incorporation at the appropriate coding genes. Two inactivated oral cholera vaccines consisting of inactivated bacteria alone or in combination with the B subunit of cholera toxin each conferred 50% protection over 3 years in a field trial in Bangladesh. An engineered live oral cholera vaccine, strain CVD 103-HgR has been shown in extensive clinical trials to be well tolerated and highly immunogenic after a single oral dose. Another approach under development is the incorporation of antigen in lipophilic immune-stimulating complexes (ISCOMS) that form spontaneously on mixing cholesterol and saponin. Protective immunity has been induced in a variety of species to several viral diseases (e.g. equine influenza) and toxoplasmosis. They can be used for oral immunization to protein antigens and the saponin appears to act as an adjuvant to enhance the immune response. Combined parenteral and oral immunization is under investigation as a way of inducing systemic and mucosal immunity.

Other vaccines under development include subunit vaccines in which polypeptides are isolated from the infective material (e.g. hepatitis B, influenza), recombinant DNA vaccines in which antigens are synthesized by prokaryotic cells (e.g. *E. coli* or yeasts) or lower eukaryotic cells (e.g. mouse fibroblasts), recombinant infectious vectors in which the genome of the infective agent (e.g. HSV, hepatitis B, HIV) is inserted into a vector such as vaccinia or BCG, internal image idiotypes in which anti-idiotypic antibodies are produced that mimic the antigenic determinants of the required immunogen (e.g. reovirus, sendai virus, polio type II and HBs antigen), and finally synthetic peptides produced by synthesizing sequential antigenic determinants (e.g. cholera toxin, polio). An interesting approach for immunization against *Salmonella* infections has been the use of non-reverting mutants with a requirement for certain metabolites such as aromatic metabolites. A mutation of *Salmonella typhi* with deletions at Aro A and pur A requires aromatic metabolites and adenine. Ingestion of this bacterium caused no adverse effect in trials and induced both cellular and humoral immunity. Two new vaccines against typhoid fever (oral Ty21a and parenteral Vi polysaccharide) have been licensed in a number of countries and others undergoing trials are recombinant attenuated strains and Vi polysaccharide-carrier protein conjugate vaccines. As well as holding promise for protection against typhoid fever, bacillary dysentery and cholera, non-reverting live bacterial vaccines, with defined deletions of two or more genes, have been suggested as possible vectors for the delivery of antigenic epitopes of other microorganisms such as *Helicobacter pylori*, *Neisseria gonorrhoeae*, *rotavirus* and perhaps other viruses.

Viruses

Hepatitis B virus (HBV) cannot be propagated in laboratory animals or cell culture. In order to obtain sufficient viral material to use as a vaccine, gene cloning has been used with HBV derived from human plasma. Recombinant plasmids have been prepared for the expression of the surface antigen (HBs Ag) in *E. coli* and the yeast *Saccharomyces cerevisiae*. The best yields are obtained from the yeast and the antigen obtained resembles the natural material in physical and biological properties. Even larger amounts of viral antigen have been produced by inserting viral genetic material into a virus that infects caterpillars (Baculovirus). Insect cells infected with the altered virus are stimulated to produce large amounts of the hepatitis viral antigen that is at present undergoing clinical trials. In another approach, resulting from the sequencing of the amino acids of the HBs Ag, synthetic antigenic material has been prepared adsorbed onto alum and this is being increasingly used for individuals at risk of infection by the virus, particularly those who come into contact with contaminated blood.

Immunization against influenza viruses has proved to be a difficult problem because of the variety of subtypes of the virus that exist (p. 184). Disrupted or split influenza A vaccine preparations contain the haemagglutinin and neuraminidase but have proved to be less effective than whole virus vaccines. Protection, however, is of much shorter duration (about 1 year) than is achieved by natural infection (4 or more years). As with the hepatitis antigens, amino acid sequencing techniques have led to the availability of synthetic oligopeptides and it is hoped that common sequences might be found to be present in the different viral subtypes so that cross-reactive immunity could be induced.

Malaria

The strategy underway for developing a malaria vaccine is to identify the protective epitopes that will stimulate either inhibitory antibodies or activated T-cells. Evidence is accumulating indicating that T-cells play an important role in immunity to malaria not just as helper T-cells but as effector cells and by activating macrophages and producing lymphokines. One of the procedures under investigation is the insertion of circumsporozoite antigen genes into salmonellae. Mice immunized in this manner show protective T-cell immunity in the absence of antibodies. A similar approach is under development using *vaccinia* virus engineered to contain seven leading malaria candidate antigens. The importance of the spleen in immunity to malaria with the development of protection of reticulocytes from infection has recently been recognized but the mechanisms underlying this are not understood.

Much effort is being devoted to the development of a sporozoite vaccine for malaria. The identification and purification of plasmodial antigens has been considerably helped by the use of monoclonal antibodies. Identification of protective antigens should lead to their large-scale production and use as a malaria vaccine. As in the case of viral antigens referred to above, the use of recombinant DNA technology and the development of synthetic peptide vaccines is underway. Recent phase III trials of a Columbian Spf66 peptide vaccine (containing 45 amino acids forming three blood-stage epitopes linked by two identical sporozoite-derived sections) claimed to show that the vaccine reduces the numbers of first malarial fevers in children by around a third. More recent trials have failed to confirm this finding. A number of problems remain to be solved, such as the cost of vaccine production, the possible requirement of adjuvants to enhance the immune response (a problem with many vaccine preparations) and the level of immunity required for individuals exposed to infection. Even if only partial immunity was achieved in a population, it is likely that the level of transmission of malaria would decrease.

Another approach involving prevention of transmission is based on recent work in mice immunized with a protein (Pfs25) that is produced by a parasite stage (ookinete) that develops in the gut of the mosquito. The antibody can block the transmission of the parasite to a new host. If such an antibody can be induced in humans it would be taken up by the mosquito in the blood meal along with the parasite. The antibody to the Pfs25 protein blocks the ookinete from forming a cyst in the mosquito gut and thus prevents further transmission. Such a vaccine does not, of course, protect the infected individual but protects the community by preventing transmission. Another approach under development uses an artificial gene precisely designed to destroy the mosquito's capacity to transmit the malaria parasite that if released into mosquito populations would be likely to spread over several decades and diminish transmission.

Leprosy

Knowledge of the molecular biology and genetics of mycobacteria is much less advanced than for many other microorganisms. The genome of *M. leprae* consists of one big chromosome that is too large to allow direct cloning and subsequent genetic analysis. A cosmid library has recently been achieved by transfection of different fragments of the genome into *E. coli* and it is hoped that this will aid the development of new diagnostic and therapeutic tools. The development of genetically engineered mycobacterial vaccines containing protective antigens has not yet been achieved. Much effort is being expended in cloning T-cells from patients with leprosy who show resistance to the disease (i.e. the tuberculoid form) and from individuals vaccinated with a vaccine made in armadillos. The cloned cells from both groups appear to be able to recognize two antigens in particular but whether or not these antigens are responsible for cell-mediated immunity against the disease has yet to be determined. As about 12 million people suffer from leprosy throughout the world, recognition of the immunizing antigens and the production of a vaccine using recombinant techniques is much needed. The BCG vaccine has some effect against leprosy but attempts to find a specific vaccine have not yet met with success at levels that are useful in practice. A vaccine may arise from work in armadillos, a species in which the bacteria can be grown.

Drug treatment appears to be the most effective approach for the control of leprosy and drugs such as Ofloxacin (which targets DNA gyrase) and macrolides such as Clarithromycin (which inhibits bacterial protein synthesis by linking the 50 S ribosomal subunit, thereby preventing elongation of the protein chain) are under extensive clinical trials in 15 countries.

Cholera

Cholera vibrios (and *E. coli* responsible for endotoxin-induced diarrhoea) do not invade the intestinal tissue but remain in the lumen or attached to the epithelium. Thus, secretory IgA provides the main protective role and can be shown to protect mice from intestinal challenge. Research is required to identify the epithelial target material for such microorganisms, which seem likely to be carbohydrate in nature, such as fucose associated with blood group substances. The parenteral whole-cell cholera vaccine gives only 50–70% protection for 3 to 6 months whilst clinical illness provides protection for several years. Vaccination efforts against cholera are directed at stimulating mucosal immunity with non-toxic preparations that contain appropriate protective immunogens such as a combined vaccine containing toxoid and somatic antigens.

Work in Australia in which genes from typhoid and cholera bacteria are cloned in harmless bacteria is hoped to produce more effective and less toxic vaccines than the existing ones derived from dead bacteria. Mutants of *Vibrio cholerae* defective in intestinal colonization abilities have been constructed and after trials have been completed may prove to be useful for vaccination purposes. Attenuated strains lacking the genes for cholera toxin have also been produced. These strains, with further development, may prove to be useful vaccine candidates.

Trypanosomes

The future development of vaccines against trypanosomes has been aided by studies of *T. cruzi* (responsible for Chagas' disease affecting 10–12 million people in Central and South America). The disease is transmitted by blood-sucking insects and blood transfusion (3% of donors in Sao Paulo in Brazil harbour the disease and 10 000–12 000 new cases arise each year as a consequence of blood transfusion). Amongst the glycoprotein surface antigens of the organism, one appears to be involved in the penetration of human cells by a mechanism that depends on the recognition of *N*-acetyl-D-glucosamine. The production of monoclonal antibodies to these various surface antigens and their systematic screening for their ability to inhibit internalization of the parasite should lead to recognition of the protective material for use in recombinant DNA technology and vaccine production.

Other developments

One of the most exciting new developments involves the use of vaccinia virus recombinants that express genes introduced from other infective agents. Tests in mice indicate that protection can be achieved with influenza, herpes, rabies and vesicular stomatitis viruses and against hepatitis B virus in chimpanzees.

Genetic immunization with DNA-based vaccines has been recently introduced and results in in vivo synthesis of vaccine immunogens thus avoiding the need to produce and purify protein antigens. The procedure has been shown in animal models to be protective against influenza, malaria, hepatitis B, Leishmania, mycoplasma and rabies infections. Plasmids encoding viral membrane and core antigens or parasite glycoproteins are used along with appropriate promoters to provide suitable levels and persistence of antigen expression. It is likely that this approach will be developed for human use.

Immunization services are among the least expensive and most effective of all health services. Estimates of the costs of providing a fully immunized child can be as low as (US) $5 when the coverage is extensive. About 50% of the costs are for personnel salaries, whilst the vaccine itself accounts for about 14%. The remaining costs are for equipment, training and operating costs.

Antigens of microorganisms

Bacterial and viral antigens are in common use in medical practice as a means of inducing immunity to infectious diseases such as smallpox, diphtheria, measles, poliomyelitis, typhoid fever and many others. There are four main types of conventional antigen preparations or **vaccines**.

Toxoids

These are the soluble exotoxins of bacteria, such as diphtheria and tetanus bacilli, which have been modified and rendered less toxic by the addition of formalin or gentle heating. They are administered either in solution or precipitated on alum. Many years of useful immunity can be achieved by these procedures.

Killed vaccines

Killed vaccines are cultured organisms killed by heat, usually 60°C for 1 hour, ultraviolet irradiation or chemicals such as phenol, alcohol or formalin. Protection against whooping-cough, poliomyelitis and perhaps cholera can be achieved in this way.

Antigens isolated from infectious agents (subunit vaccines)

An example of these is the capsular polysaccharide of the pneumococci. A diffusible factor of *B. anthracis* and a cell wall preparation of haemolytic streptococci have been shown to induce immunity but such preparations are not in general use in medical practice.

Attenuated living vaccines

These are made from strains of organisms that have lost their virulence by growth in culture (e.g. Pasteur's chicken cholera vaccine, p. 6) or in animals when the conditions are not favourable for the growth and proliferation of the virulent strain. Strains emerge which, whilst not able to produce disease, can induce immunity; such strains are known as **attenuated** organisms. The BCG vaccine (Bacille Calmette-Guérin) for tuberculosis and the cowpox vaccine for smallpox are the outstanding examples of this type of vaccine. The oral administration of a strain of poliomyelitis virus induces a powerful immunity without producing the disease. The virus spreads from one individual to another and so is able to produce immunity in a community. An attenuated strain of yellow fever virus has been developed, obtained from the original virulent material by prolonged cultivation in tissue culture. Attenuated strains of measles virus are also used and rubella virus vaccination has reduced the hazard of congenital abnormalities developing in the infants of mothers infected with virus.

In veterinary medicine successful vaccines have been produced against canine distemper, canine hepatitis and Newcastle disease (fowl pest) of chickens.

Routine procedures

The determining factors in the selection of immunization procedures for a particular population must depend on local environmental con-

Table 5.17 UK schedule for vaccinating children

Age	Vaccine	Notes
From 2 months	DPT (diphtheria, pertussis, tetanus), oral polio, Hib	Pertussis may be omitted if contraindicated; 3 doses at intervals of 4 weeks
3–4 months	DPT, Polio, Hib 2nd dose	
4–6 months	DPT, Polio, Hib 3rd dose	
12–18 months	MMR (mumps, measles, rubella)	Live vaccine
5 years	Diphtheria, tetanus (booster), polio (booster)	
10–14 years	Rubella	For seronegative girls only (may be phased out with use of MMR)
Girls and boys at about 13 years	BCG (tuberculosis)	Not earlier than 3 weeks after rubella vaccine; for tuberculin-negative children or contacts at any age
School leavers	Tetanus, diphtheria (booster)	

ditions and epidemiological considerations. In Britain, a child is immunized during its first year of life with a vaccine containing diphtheria and tetanus toxoids in combination with a killed suspension of whooping-cough (*Bordetella pertussis*) organisms. This is known as **triple vaccine** and its efficacy as an immunizing agent is in part due to the adjuvant effect of the pertussis component. Oral polio vaccine is given at the same time. At 15 months of age the mumps, measles, rubella (MMR) vaccine is given and will eliminate the need to give the rubella vaccine to seronegative girls at 10–14 years. Table 5.17 shows the UK vaccination schedule.

In the USA the official recommendation for childhood immunization comprises three primary doses of DPT vaccine and oral polio vaccine at intervals of 4 to 6 weeks, beginning at the age of 2 or 3 months. A booster is given 1 year after completion of the primary course.

Live vaccines should not be given to persons whose ability to respond to infection is reduced as, for example, after radiotherapy, immunosuppressive drugs, steroids or in patients with immunodeficiency states. If a subject has had a local or general reaction to a vaccine, there is a risk of even more marked reactions to the next dose. For full details of current vaccination programmes and contraindications the reader is referred to the *British National Formulary* current edition.

Timing of vaccinations

At birth the level of maternal IgG in the infant is the same as maternal levels and provides protection against bacterial toxins. By 2–3 months the level is less than half that at birth even though the infant is beginning to produce its own IgG. IgM produced by the infant (none is passed via the placenta) is present before birth and reaches nearly adult levels by the end of the first year. IgA in contrast rises only slowly, reaching near adult levels only after age 14. The newborn infant can produce antibody to some antigens such as toxoids, inactivated polio virus and attenuated polio virus but not against pertussis vaccine, which fails to induce a protective response and may result in an impaired response to the vaccine given later. Maternal antibody can also result in an impaired response to vaccination, e.g. enough maternal IgG to measles antigens persists in the infant up to the end of the first year to interfere with a response to the vaccine. Giving the vaccine by the respiratory route avoids this complication. New strains of measles vaccine have been developed which, if given in appropriate doses, even at 6 months of age avoid the inhibitory effect of maternal antibody. Children of less than 2 years of age respond poorly to bacterial polysaccharides such as those of *Haemophilus influenzae* type b, meningococci group B and *Streptococcus pneumoniae* serotypes.

Special circumstances

Protective immunization can be performed in situations where a particular hazard exists such as to the fetus if rubella occurs in pregnancy, the infectious hazards of travelling abroad and the occupational hazards of acquiring certain infections. Table 5.18 shows situations when such immunization procedures may be adopted.

Immunization against rubella

All seronegative girls should be immunized just before puberty with

---

Table 5.18 Diseases against which protective immunization may be provided in special circumstances

Hazards to the fetus	Hazards associated with occupation or other special circumstances
Rubella	
	Anthrax
Hazards to travellers	Influenza
Enteric fever	Mumps
Yellow fever	Plague
Cholera	Q fever
Smallpox	Rabies
	Tularaemia
	Typhus
	Hepatitis A and B

the live attenuated virus. This avoids the risk of their contracting the disease subsequently when they are pregnant, as rubella in pregnancy may lead to malformations of the fetus.

Female school teachers, nursery staff, and nurses and doctors caring for children in hospital and in clinics may be exposed to rubella. Staff working in antenatal clinics may acquire the infection and pass it on to patients in the early stages of pregnancy. These groups should be offered rubella vaccination if preliminary serological tests are negative. However, as the vaccine should not be given during pregnancy, assurances must be sought from women in these groups that they are not pregnant and that they will take precautions against becoming pregnant for at least 2 months after taking the vaccine.

Immunization of travellers

Travellers are exposed to infectious hazards that vary from country to country. There are national and international regulations which make vaccination against yellow fever and cholera statutory for persons travelling to and from countries where the diseases are endemic or where an epidemic has recently occurred. As the regulations are subject to change, a traveller who is visiting any country where the diseases have occurred in recent years should check with the relevant embassy what certificates of vaccination are necessary, if any.

The traveller is often well advised to seek immunization against other diseases that may be encountered (Table 5.18). Travellers may be unaware that poliomyelitis, diphtheria, tetanus and tuberculosis are still significant risks in some countries; medical students volunteering for work in developing countries should bear these special occupational hazards in mind. International certificates for yellow fever vaccination are valid for 10 years and become valid 10 days after primary vaccination. In contrast, cholera vaccination certificates are valid for only 6 months, becoming valid 6 days after primary vaccination. All non-immune children over 10–12 months going to live in the tropics should be vaccinated against measles.

Occupational hazards

Immunization against the various infections considered above and also against hepatitis B, mumps, Q fever, plague, tularaemia and typhus may be offered to laboratory workers and others at special risk.

In view of the success of the WHO smallpox eradication programme, vaccination against smallpox is no longer routinely required.

High titre hepatitis B immunoglobulin is available for the temporary passive protection of clinical and laboratory workers who sustain a skin-penetrating injury under circumstances associated with a risk of the transmission of the hepatitis B virus. Prophylactic immunization is now available using synthetic antigens or those prepared by recombinant DNA techniques (p. 218).

An anthrax vaccine is recommended for those who handle animal hides and bones, etc. Vaccination has similarly been practised against brucellosis and leptospirosis in humans but the protective value of available vaccines against these two occupational hazards is not established.

THE IMMUNE SYSTEM AND VACCINES

Stimulation of an immune response is one of the most effective ways of protecting an individual from potentially infective microorganisms and much effort has gone into producing effective vaccines. Recent developments in understanding the complex relationships involved in initiating an immune response have contributed to the safety and efficacy of current vaccines.

Vaccines in use for travellers

Enteric fever. TAB vaccine provides useful protection against typhoid fever but its protective value against the paratyphoid fevers has not been proved. Tourists, business people and others who travel from countries in northern and western Europe and North America to Mediterranean countries, Africa, Asia and Latin America are advised to be immunized; this is obligatory for members of most armed forces. The paratyphoid components are omitted from **typhoid vaccine** and this is less likely to give the local and systemic reactions that are quite common with TAB vaccine.

Yellow fever vaccine. A preparation of live attenuated virus is given by injection and one dose confers immunity for 10 years for travellers to tropical Africa and South America.

Cholera vaccine. This vaccine is a preparation of killed cholera vibrios. Two subcutaneous injections with an interval of about 4–6 weeks give a degree of protection against *V. cholerae* and *V. eltor* that is unfortunately only transient. Patients travelling to a country where cholera exists should be warned about dangers even after vaccination. The best protection is good hygiene and avoidance of contaminated food and water.

Meningitis. Meningococcal polysaccharide vaccine is indicated for travellers to the meningitis belt of Africa, New Delhi, Nepal and Mecca. Whilst vaccines are available for groups A, C, Y and W135 there is no vaccine against group B.

Rabies vaccines. A human diploid cell vaccine is now in use and may be offered prophylactically to individuals at risk, e.g. animal handlers, veterinary surgeons and those working with quarantine animals. Post-exposure treatment involves a course of injections on days 0, 3, 7, 14, 30 and 90 but may be discontinued if it is proved that the patient is not at risk. In cases of severe exposure, passive immunization with rabies antiserum may also be advisable.

Hepatitis. Persons eating and drinking under poor hygienic conditions have a rate of hepatitis A infection of 20/1000 per month. Seroprevalence of hepatitis A antibodies increases with age and screening may eliminate the need for vaccination in about 40% of adults. The duration of protection following vaccination with current vaccines has yet to be established. Inactivated hepatitis A vaccines are more potent than the current hepatitis B vaccines. Plasma-derived and yeast-derived recombinant hepatitis B vaccines have gained an acceptable record of efficiency although poor responses can occur even in healthy individuals. Combined vaccines (recombinant or attenuated forms) are likely to replace existing vaccines.

Q fever. Cardiothoracic surgical teams operating on patients with cardiac complications of Q fever endocarditis can be protected by an inactivated whole-cell vaccine.

Passive immunization

Passive immunity against some diseases can be conferred by injecting specific antibodies obtained from the serum of a convalescent patient or from a previously immunized animal. The extra circulating antibodies, added to those that might be naturally produced, may help to curtail an infection or neutralize a toxin and so moderate the illness. Passive immunization has the disadvantages that it provides only temporary protection and, if an animal serum is used, it is liable to provoke hypersensitivity reactions that range from a minor upset to severe anaphylaxis.

In practice, passive immunization has been most effectively exploited in the prophylaxis or treatment of infections caused by bacteria that produce exotoxins, such as diphtheria, botulism, tetanus and gas gangrene. Antisera against other bacteria have been prepared; effective antipneumococcal sera became available just before the introduction of sulphonamides, which proved to be much more effective, less hazardous and cheaper. Today, except for the antitoxic sera, the use of antisera is limited. Passive immunization may be more useful in the future, especially for the prevention or treatment of conditions for which no effective antibiotic therapy is available. Infectious diseases, in which human immunoglobulin can be used in prophylaxis, include hepatitis A and B, rubella, measles, varicella-zoster, tetanus and rabies. The amount of antibody required is relatively small and is usually provided by alcohol precipitation of an appropriate serum or pool. The protection offered by the intramuscular injection of these preparations lasts between 3 and 6 months and should be given either before exposure or at least early in the incubation period. In severe septicaemia, patients have been successfully treated with large doses of normal human immunoglobulin given intravenously. Much effort is being directed at improving this form of therapy and identifying the protective bacterial antigens so that appropriate antisera can be selected.

Passive immunization: mother to fetus

Human milk contains a number of factors that have effects on microbial agents, enhancing desirable gut flora and inhibiting others. Inhibitors include lysozyme, lactoferrin and interferon. IgA, 80% of which is secretory IgA, is found in high concentration in the colostrum — about 600 mg/dl at day 1 but falling off to less than 100 mg/dl by day 4. IgG and IgM are also present at about 80 and 125 mg/dl respectively but decrease substantially by day 4. These immunoglobulins have been shown to contain antibodies to pathogenic intestinal bacteria and viruses. Low birthweight infants whose mothers cannot produce colostrum may be fed IgA and IgG derived from human serum.

Reactions and contraindications

In general, active immunization with any vaccine should be postponed if the patient is temporarily unwell. If more than one live vaccine is to be given, there should be an interval of at least 3 weeks between them. Live vaccines should not be given to patients whose defences are compromised by malignant disease, severe chronic disease or immunodeficiency. This includes those receiving steroid therapy or cytotoxic drug therapy. Live viral vaccines, and especially rubella vaccine, should not be given during pregnancy.

Patients should be asked if they have previously reacted adversely to a vaccine and such a history should be taken into account before administering the vaccine again. This is of special importance in relation to pertussis vaccine and in cases of reactions to passive immunization with heterologous antisera when there may be a danger of serious anaphylaxis.

Local erythema and tenderness at the injection site are common minor reactions. Fever, headache and malaise for a day or so occur in some people, especially after endotoxin-containing vaccines such as TAB or after a prolonged series of doses of cholera vaccine. Immune adults tend to react adversely to diphtheria immunization. Children with a history or a family history of neonatal cerebral irritation, a tendency to convulsions or epilepsy, or a previous reaction to pertussis vaccine should not receive the pertussis component of triple vaccine and should be given only the diphtheria–tetanus toxoids.

FURTHER READING

Arya S C 1994 Human immunisation in developing countries: practical and theoretical problems and prospects. Vaccine 12: 1423–1435

Blackwell C C, Weir D M , Busuttil A 1995 Infectious agents, the inflammatory responses of infants and sudden infant death syndrome (SIDS). Molecular Medicine Today 1: 72

Bloom B, Oldstone M B A 1991 Immunity to infection. Current Opinion in Immunology 3: 453

Capron A, Locht C, Fracchia G N 1994 Safety and efficacy of new generation vaccines. Vaccine 12: 667–669

Coleman R M, Lombard M F, Sicard R E 1992 Acquired immune deficiency syndrome. Fundamental immunology, 2nd edn. W M C Brown, Dubuque

Department of Health 1992 Immunisation against infectious disease. HMSO, London

Edelman R 1993 Vaccines: new technologies and applications. Vaccine 11: 1361–1364

Eskola J 1994 Epidemiological views into possible components of paediatric combined vaccines in 2015. Biologicals 22: 323

Frank M M 1989 Evasion strategies of microorganisms. Progress in Immunology 7: 194

Haraguchi S, Good R A, Day N K 1995 Immunosuppressive retroviral peptides: cAMP and cytokine patterns. Immunology Today 16: 595

Kaye P M 1995 Costimulation and the regulation of antimicrobial immunity. Immunology Today 16: 423.

Ken-ichi A, Lee F, Miyajima A, Shoichiro M, Yokota T 1990 Cytokines: coordinators of immune and inflammatory responses. Annual Review of Biochemistry 59: 783

Langer R 1990 New methods of drug delivery. Science 249: 1527

Levine M M, Noriega F 1993 Vaccines to prevent bacterial enteric infections in children. Pediatric Annals 22: 719

Lindberg A A 1995 The history of live bacterial vaccines. Developments in Biological Standardization 84: 211

Mandell G L, Bennett J E, Dolin R (eds) 1994 Principles and practice of infectious diseases, 4th edn. Churchill Livingstone, Edinburgh

Mekalonos J J 1994 Live attenuated vaccine vectors. International Journal of Technology Assessment in Health Care 10: 131

Pawelec G, Adibzadeh M, Pohla H, Schaudt K 1995 Immunosenescence: ageing of the immune system. Immunology Today 16: 420

Phair J P, Wolinsky S 1996 Recent developments in the biology and natural history of HIV infection. Current Opinion in Infectious Diseases 9: 1

Playfair J H L (ed) 1990 Immunity to infection. Current Opinion in Immunology 2: 345

Roitt I M 1997 Essential immunology, 9th edn Blackwell Scientific Publications, Oxford

Scott P, Kaufmann S H E 1991 The role of T-cell subsets and cytokines in the regulation of infection. Immunology Today 12: 346–348

Shalaby W S 1995 Development of oral vaccines to stimulate mucosal and systemic immunity: barriers and novel strategies. Clinical Immunology and Immunopathology 74: 127

Stites D P, Terr A I (eds) 1994 Basic and clinical immunology 8th edn. Appleton and Lange, Norwalk, Conn.

WHO Tropical Disease Research 1995 Twelfth programme report. World Health Organization, Geneva.

6 Immunohaematology

Knowledge of blood groups in humans and animals has been very closely associated with the development of the science of immunology. Differences between the red blood cells of animals were first noted in goats as early as 1900 when Ehrlich and Morgenroth immunized 'a strong male goat' with nearly a litre of blood obtained from three other goats. The serum which they obtained from the immunized goat lysed the cells of all but one of the nine goats they tested. However, to Ehrlich the most important finding was that the cells of the immunized goat itself were completely unaffected. This proved to him that an animal would not produce autoantibodies against its own tissues and so destroy itself. It was left to Karl Landsteiner, who made the same observations in humans, to take up the detailed study of these antigenic differences. Landsteiner's important work on the immunological determinants of antigenic specificity stems from this period and still stands today as of fundamental value to our understanding of antigens (Chapter 3).

Studies in blood group serology have led to the development of a large variety of techniques which have wide application to immunological problems outside this field. Notable amongst these is the antiglobulin test devised by Coombs and his associates, by means of which enormous advances have been made in many branches of immunology. Study of the development of blood group antibodies in serum has thrown light on the mechanisms underlying the formation of natural antibodies. Apart from these contributions to the understanding of immunological problems, information on blood groups has important implications in genetics and in forensic studies.

As has been noted in Chapter 5 (p. 158), blood group status appears to be associated with susceptibility to infections such as cholera (blood group O), gonorrhoea (blood group B) and *E. coli* infections of the urinary tract (groups B and AB). The reasons for these associations are not clear but may be related to cross-reactions between isohaemagglutinins or isoantibodies (see p. 300) and cell wall antigens of various microorganisms. Such natural antibodies may act by blocking attachment of the bacterium to its target cell (see also p. 158–159).

Blood groups

ABO antigens and isoantibodies

The ABO blood group system was described as a result of Landsteiner's demonstration of four distinct groups of agglutination reaction between human red blood cells and normal human serum. The differences in agglutination were due to the presence or absence of two antigenic determinants A and B on the red cell membrane. The four combinations which result from this are: (1) the presence of A determinant in the absence of B — group A cells, (2) the presence of B determinant in the absence of A — group B cells, (3) the presence of both A and B determinants — group AB cells, and (4) the absence of both A and B determinants — group O cells.

The sera of certain individuals also contain antibodies able to react with, and agglutinate if present in sufficient concentration, the cells of other individuals of different blood group.

These natural antibodies or **isoantibodies** are formed shortly after birth and appear to be stimulated by A and B antigenic determinants present on the normal bacterial flora of the gut. Antigens with blood group specificity are widely distributed in nature.

From a consideration of the phenomenon of immunological tolerance and the fact that an individual is tolerant to 'self' antigens (Ch. 9), it can be seen that an individual will respond only to an antigen to which he is not already tolerant. Thus an individual with blood group A cells will be tolerant to the A determinant and will therefore respond only to the B determinant on the gut flora. The same holds for blood group B individuals who can respond only to the A determinant.

Thus individuals of blood group A will have isoantibodies of blood group B specificity, i.e. anti-B antibodies, and blood group B individuals will in the same way have anti-A isoantibodies. Blood group O individuals whose immune system will not have developed tolerance to either A or B antigens will have, as would be expected, both anti-A and anti-B isoagglutinins.

The blood group antigens A and B occur not only in the red cells but are widely distributed in the tissues with the exception of the central nervous system. Just under 80% of individuals also have the determinants (corresponding to their blood group) in tissue fluids and secretions (except CSF). Chemical studies on these antigens recovered in quantity from ovarian cyst fluid show that the difference between A and B determinants is determined by the nature of a single saccharide attached as the terminal sugar of an oligosaccharide chain. Group O individuals synthesize the oligosaccharide backbone which is known as H-substance. Group A individuals have a enzyme which adds D-N-acetylgalactosamine to the end of the H-substance to produce the A determinant. In Group B individuals D-galactose is added to H-substance to produce the B epitope. The oligosaccharide moiety is usually attached to lipids in the case of the cell-associated blood group antigens and to proteins in the secreted form.

Blood transfusion in relation to ABO groups

Transfusion of an individual with red cells from an individual of a different group results in exposure of the transfused cells to an isoagglutinin — anti-A or anti-B — and except in the case of O cells, which carry neither the A nor the B antigen, the cells will be destroyed with resulting haemoglobinaemia and haemoglobinuria. Although it is clearly best to administer blood only of the same group as the recipient, in an emergency group O cells can be given. Although the plasma of a group O individual (sometimes called a **universal donor**) contains anti-A and anti-B isoagglutinins, these are so diluted by the recipient's plasma (a pint of blood would be diluted about 1 in 12) to have only a negligible effect except when large quantities of blood have to be administered. Group O individuals whose serum contains anti-A and anti-B isoagglutinins cannot accept blood of any group except O. Since an individual of group AB has neither anti-A nor anti-B isoantibodies he can accept blood of any of the four groups and has therefore been called a **universal recipient**.

This relatively straightforward scheme is unfortunately slightly complicated by the existence of a number of subgroups of A (probably five in all). However, only A_1 and A_2 are of importance as far as transfusion is concerned. The frequency of occurrence in Caucasians of the six different ABO groups is shown in Table 6.1.

Transfusion reactions

Transfusion of large amounts of ABO incompatible blood can be fatal whilst incompatible transfusion involving other blood groups is usually less severe. Clinical symptoms include fever, chills, pain at the site of injection with later dyspnoea, hypotension and joint pains. Renal failure may accompany severe reactions.

Haemolytic transfusion reactions are brought about by antigen/antibody complexes on the erythrocyte membrane with activation of complement and kinins. Bradykinin leads to hypotension whilst erythrocytes coated with C3b are cleared by phagocytes, resulting in

Table 6.1 **Blood group distribution in Caucasians**

Blood group	Frequency	Isoantibodies
O	43.5%	Anti-A (+ anti-A$_1$), anti-B
A$_1$	34.8%	Anti-B
A$_2$	9.6%	Anti-B (occasionally anti-A$_1$)
B	8.5%	Anti-A (+ anti-A$_1$)
A$_1$B	2.5%	None
A$_2$B	0.8%	None (occasionally anti-A$_1$)

extravascular haemolysis. Clotting mechanisms are also activated, leading to intravascular coagulation.

Transmission of infection by blood transfusion has become of increasing importance, particularly with the worldwide spread of infections such as those caused by HIV and hepatitis viruses. Cytomegalovirus may also be transferred and this is particularly dangerous in immunocompromised patients. Other infections are relevant to certain areas such as those where malaria, Chagas' disease, brucellosis or leishmaniasis are prevalent. Careful selection of blood donors and screening procedures are important considerations to avoid transmission of these infections.

The Rhesus blood group system

This system is the next most important system to the ABO groups. The Rhesus (Rh) blood group antigens are present in the red cells of 85% of Caucasians and 94% of Afrocaribbeans. The most common of the Rhesus antigens are C, c, D, d, E and e, and Table 6.2 shows some of the various combinations which can exist and their frequency in Caucasians.

The Rhesus group of an individual must be taken into account for transfusion purposes. Of these antigens D is the most potent although immunization by D and at the same time by the C or E antigens can occur. A variant of D named D^u has been described and cells carrying this antigen are not agglutinated by routine anti-D sera. For transfusion purposes recipients carrying the D^u antigen are considered to be Rh-negative, whilst donors in this category are regarded as Rh-positive.

Rhesus incompatibility

The clinical importance of the Rhesus groups lies in the ability of the red cells of a Rhesus-positive fetus to immunize its Rhesus-negative

Table 6.2 Combinations of Rh antigens and frequency in Caucasians

Genotype	Frequency	
CDe/cde	31.7%	
CDe/CDe	16.6%	Rh-positive
CDe/cDe	11.5%	
cDE/cde	10.9%	Rh-negative
cde/cde	15.1%	

mother. Immunization usually takes place following the trauma of parturition with the result that the maternal immune response does not develop until a **second** pregnancy. The maternal anti-Rh antibody is passed to the subsequent fetus via the placenta and causes haemolytic destruction of its erythrocytes. This condition is known as **haemolytic disease of the newborn** or erythroblastosis fetalis. Since the original description of the disease it has been found that blood group antigen systems other than the Rh system can be responsible for the condition. For example, a group O mother can occasionally be immunized by fetal antigens if the father is A_1, A_1B or B.

The serious nature of haemolytic disease of the newborn, necessitating complete exchange of the infant's blood (exchange transfusion) to remove the maternal antibody, has now been alleviated by a rather ingenious immunological manoeuvre. This is based on the observation that attempted immunization by an antigen in the presence of its specific antibody tends to inhibit synthesis of the antibody to the injected antigen. It is known, for example, that immunization of infants is best delayed for a few months after birth to allow the levels of maternal antibody to fall.

Rh-immunization can be suppressed almost entirely if high titre anti-Rh immunoglobulin is given within 72 hours after maternal exposure to Rh positive cells. In the case of a recognized Rhesus incompatibility it is now the practice to give a small dose of potent anti-Rh antibody to Rh-negative mothers within 3 days after delivery of a Rh-positive infant. The antibody appears to inhibit the response to the Rhesus antigen, possibly by diverting the cells carrying the antigen from the antibody-forming tissues or perhaps by a direct 'feedback inhibition' effect on the antibody-forming cells (Fig. 6.1).

The detection of anti-Rh antibodies

After the recognition of the association between haemolytic disease of the newborn and Rhesus immunization, it soon became apparent that the standard method of demonstrating anti-Rh antibody — by direct

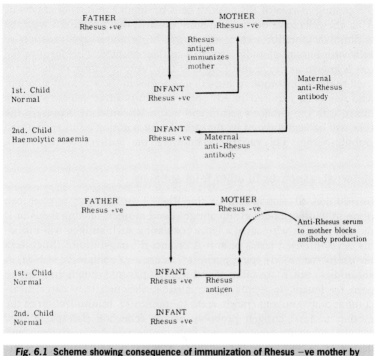

Fig. 6.1 Scheme showing consequence of immunization of Rhesus −ve mother by Rhesus antigen of Rhesus +ve child.
Prevention obtained by injection of anti-Rhesus serum after delivery of first child.

agglutination of a saline suspension of Rh-positive cells by serum — was not able to show up the presence of antibody in one-half to two-thirds of sera tested. A solution to the problem was found by the substitution of a dilute protein solution, e.g. bovine albumen, for the normal saline diluent. Visible agglutination could then be readily demonstrated in the majority of cases. The form of serum antibody responsible for agglutination, demonstrable only in protein diluent, became known as **incomplete** antibody in contrast to the saline active **complete** antibody.

Another very important method for demonstrating incomplete antibodies is the Coombs' **antiglobulin test**. An antiserum is prepared in rabbits against human immunoglobulins and this is used to react with Rh-positive cells previously coated with human incomplete antibody. The second antibody brings about agglutination simply by linking together the molecules of human globulin attached to the red cells (p. 323 and Fig. 10.9).

One of the advantages of this method is that it can be used to detect the coating in vivo of Rh-positive cells by small amounts of antibody. After the cells have been thoroughly washed, they are mixed with the antihuman globulin serum which will bring about agglutination of cells with human globulin attached to their surface. This form of the test is known as the 'direct Coombs' test'. Another form of the test is used to detect incomplete anti-Rh antibodies in the serum of a patient who has been exposed to Rh antigens. Rh-positive cells are simply mixed with the patient's serum and if anti-Rh antibody is present the cells will be agglutinated by the subsequent addition of an antihuman globulin serum. This variation is known as the 'indirect Coombs' test'.

Maternal responses to other fetal antigens

In addition to responding to the Rhesus antigen the mother can respond to other blood group antigens and mothers lacking the A or B red cell antigen who carry a fetus possessing such antigen will probably develop raised levels of anti-A or anti-B isoagglutinins. Such sera are useful for blood-typing purposes, as are sera containing anti-HLA antibodies, which are often found in multiparous women and can be used for leucocyte typing. Spermatozoa, although they carry histocompatibility antigens, rarely seem to immunize. Immunization of the mother to fetal antigen probably occurs following passage of fetal blood (by small haemorrhages) into the maternal bloodstream and occurs more frequently as pregnancy progresses. The fetus represents an allograft containing potentially immunogenic antigens derived from paternal antigens of the major histocompatibility complex (MHC). The mother makes both humoral and cell-mediated responses to these antigens but the fetus survives because the placenta appears to be an immunologically privileged site and does not allow effector cells or antibodies to affect fetal development. The placenta seems to be able to absorb out antifetal antibodies from the maternal blood and H-2K and H-2D antigens of paternal type have been found on mouse placenta. There is evidence that MHC disparity is associated with fetal survival. Women who have chronic abortions share more HLA antigens with their husbands than predicted by chance. The placenta is believed to be responsible for balancing the tendency for rejection of the fetus with 'facilitation' that allows the fetus to survive to term. Immunochemical studies have identified two sub-populations of trophoblast on the basis of HLA class I expression. Extravillous trophoblast is MHC class I positive whilst villous trophoblast is MHC class I negative. Maternal antibodies to fetal antigens, where the parents are genetically dissimilar, appear to offer protection to the fetus. This finding has been used with some success to prevent recurrent abortion, where no other obvious abnormality is present, by immunizing mothers with paternal lymphocytes.

A complement-regulating protein called membrane cofactor protein is found on the trophoblast. Its role appears to be to regulate complement activation via the alternative pathway by preventing amplification of C3 deposition. A number of pregnancy-associated substances, such as alphafetoprotein, 17β-oestradiol, prostaglandin synthetase inhibitor and β1-microglobulin, may play a role in regulating the immune response in pregnancy. It has also been found that natural killer cells are absent in neonates. It is becoming increasingly apparent that a certain degree of foreignness may actually assist human reproduction and viviparity. An IgG 'blocking factor' has been found in maternal serum that inhibits production of lymphokines by maternal lymphocytes sensitized to antigens on the trophoblast and paternal lymphocytes. Women who undergo recurrent abortions of unknown aetiology lack the blocking factor. Preliminary trials in which 'blocking factor' is induced by immunization with pooled leucocyte infusions have given encouraging results.

Recent evidence in animals indicates that locally produced colony-stimulating factor (CSF-1) is required for a successful pregnancy and probably acts by regulating trophoblast function and haemopoietic cells in the uterus.

Other blood group systems

In 1927 Landsteiner described two human antigens, M and N. The use of antisera against these antigens can divide individuals into three types, half having the MN genotype and 28% and 22% respectively having MM and NN genotypes. A further antigen was later found, the S antigen, and the group is known as the MNS blood group system. This group is of limited clinical importance although a few instances of haemolytic disease of the newborn have been reported due to incompatibility of these antigens.

Landsteiner's P antigen is noteworthy because a naturally occurring anti-P cold agglutinin is found in a large proportion of the 20% of individuals who are P-negative. Amongst a number of blood group systems described, including those of Lutheran, Kell, Lewis, Kidd, Duffy and Diego, special mention should be made of the Lewis system because naturally occurring antibodies to Lewis antigens are frequently found in human serum. They sometimes act as cold agglutinins and have been found occasionally to be the cause of haemolytic transfusion reactions. These antigens are unique in that they are not part of the red cell structure but are soluble antigens found in body fluids, which adsorb on to the red cell surface.

Antigens of blood leucocytes and platelets

As will be discussed in the section on transplantation antigens, blood leucocytes in humans carry major histocompatibility antigens (HLA molecules). The appearance of antibodies against donor leucocytes and also platelet antigens is a common finding after blood transfusion. This results in rapid destruction of the transfused cells and although immunization occurs more frequently than anti-red cell immunization the consequences are less dangerous.

Leucocyte and platelet groups fall into two types: those with antigens which they share in common with red cells and those with antigens which are restricted to leucocytes, platelets and other tissue cells. The blood group antigens A and B are the main antigens shared with erythrocytes. The important antigenic group limited to leucocytes, platelets and other tissue cells is the HLA system.

A reaction between antileucocyte isoantibodies and transfused leucocytes often gives rise to febrile transfusion reactions and their incidence can be correlated with the number of transfusions given. Although these reactions are not usually severe they can be a disadvantage to patients for whom repeated transfusions are necessary.

The transfusion of fresh platelets is of value in patients suffering from haemorrhagic disorders due to thrombocytopenia and although, theoretically, selection of compatible platelets is desirable, in practice platelets are usually obtained from a small number of donors, if possible related to the recipient.

ABO blood groups, secretor state and susceptibility to infection

As noted above, ABO incompatibility between mother and fetus predisposes to haemolytic disease of the newborn and also to spontaneous abortion. Associations have also been reported between blood group and a wide variety of infective agents. In particular, blood group B is associated with infections of the mucous membranes of the urinary tract, gastrointestinal tract and respiratory tract. ABO blood group substances are secreted in about 75% of individuals into the tissue fluids and other secretions, under control of a dominant gene independent of the genes determining the ABO blood groups. Some populations have a higher proportion of non-secretors, for example Iceland with nearly 50% of non-secretors. Studies in the author's laboratory have shown that non-secretors appear to be immunocompromised. There is a higher incidence of non-secretors among women with recurrent urinary tract infections than in the general population. The same is true for individuals with oral or vaginal infections caused by *Candida albicans* and *Neisseria meningitidis* infections in Scotland, Iceland and northern Nigeria. The reasons for this increased susceptibility of non-secretors to such infections of the mucous membranes have not yet been established.

Recent evidence indicates that some common respiratory viruses are more likely to cause disease in secretors of ABO blood group antigens and heterosexual transfer of HIV appears to occur more frequently in secretors and less frequently in non-secretors. Another recent finding indicates that the HIV envelope may be glycosylated by the blood group A glycosyl transferase and that this interferes with the ability of the virus to infect individuals of other blood groups, possibly due to the presence of anti-A antibodies. The ability of viruses to activate genes for cellular enzymes such as glycosyl transferases seems likely to underlie these phenomena.

FURTHER READING

Bowman J M 1988 The prevention of Rh immunization. Transfusion Medical Reviews 2: 129

Huestis D W et al 1988 Practical blood transfusion. 4th edn. Little Brown, Boston

Mowbray J F et al 1985 Controlled trial of treatment of recurrent abortion by immunization with paternal cells. Lancet 1: 941

Race R R, Sanger R 1975 Blood groups in man, 6th edn. Blackwell, Oxford

Stites D P, Terr A I (eds) 1994 Basic and clinical immunology. 8th edn. Appleton and Lange, Norwalk, Conn.

The immunology of tissue transplantation

The tissue cells of animals contain molecular structures that are specific for the species of origin of the cell and which if implanted into an animal of another species will induce an immune response. This response rapidly destroys the implanted cells and has the characteristics of the primary and secondary immune response as already described for antigens in general. In addition to species-specific antigens, differences also exist between individual members of the same species so that transfer of tissue cells between members induces a similar immune reaction. The closer the relationship between two individuals of the same species, the more likely are implanted cells to survive. In the case of identical twins survival is assured. Inbred strains of animals, particularly mice, have been developed which are genetically identical and these are widely used in experimental work on tissue transplantation immunology. Table 7.1 summarizes the terminology used in transplantation studies.

In humans, surgical techniques are available to enable transplantation of many organs and tissues but unfortunately a high proportion of organ transplants fail because of rejection by the immune response or because of the side-effects of attempts to suppress the immune response, due to toxicity of the drugs or their depressive effect on resistance to infection.

Transplantation antigen systems

The first systematic studies on the antigens carried by cells which determine whether a graft will be rejected or not were carried out in inbred strains of mice of known genetic make-up.

It was found that there were very many antigenic differences between tissues of different strains of mice, the number of separate antigens involved being estimated at between 15 and 500 in different

Table 7.1 Transplantation terminology (older terminology in brackets)

Relationship between donor and recipient	Term applied to relationship	Prefix applied to graft, antigen or antibody
Of different species	Xenogeneic (heterogeneic)	Xeno- (hetero-)
Of same species but different genetic constitution	Allogeneic (homologous)	Allo- (homo-)
Of same inbred strain (genetically identical)	Syngeneic (isogeneic) (isologous)	(iso-)
Same individual	Autologous	Auto-

experiments. However, it was found that, just as in the red cell antigenic system, some antigens were very 'strong' and others very weak. The strong transplantation or 'histocompatibility' antigens of the mouse are controlled by the H-2 genetic locus and in humans are controlled by the HLA locus (see Ch. 3).

MHC-encoded molecules are identified and characterized by tissue typing. This is done with a panel of various monospecific HLA antisera, often obtained from women who had multiple pregnancies or, increasingly, with monoclonal antibodies prepared against HLA antigens.

The test is carried out with lymphocytes from the individual to be typed incubated with the various antisera and complement. Other types of assays using fluorescent or enzyme-linked antibodies are also used.

Grafts between HLA identical siblings are the most successful and have a greater chance of survival than HLA-A and HLA-B matched grafts that are not necessarily identical at other loci.

Leucocyte grouping

The strong antigens of the HLA system are widely distributed in the tissues but absent from the red blood cells which contain only the ABH antigens.

Fortunately blood leucocytes carry all the known HLA antigens and it is therefore possible to test for the presence or absence of antigens of the system using leucocyte agglutination and cytotoxicity tests (p. 329). In principle the leuco-agglutination test is performed with leucocytes separated from the erythrocytes of anticoagulant-treated blood. Specific antisera for HLA antigens are then used to agglutinate the leucocytes and the tests are read under the microscope. The cytotoxic test is carried out with a purified suspension of blood lymphocytes which are mixed with antisera to HLA antigens in the presence of complement. If the lymphocytes carry the appropriate antigens the antiserum will combine and in the presence of complement will damage the cell membrane. The resulting increased cell membrane permeability is usually detected by dye uptake into the cell. Matching donor and recipient for HLA antigens, including the MHC class II molecules, is normally carried out prior to grafting.

Despite the very great diversity among HLA alleles of unrelated subjects, it is encouraging to find that about a third of kidneys from unrelated donors survive for a year or longer although only a third of them show normal kidney function. Although this partial success must be dependent to an extent on the use of immunosuppressive agents, differences in the 'strength' of individual HLA antigens is probably partly responsible.

Mechanisms of graft rejection (Fig. 7.1)

Passenger antigen-presenting cells in the graft are believed to provide the main stimulus for graft rejection and include dendritic cells and monocytes expressing MHC class II molecules. These cells present graft antigens to $CD4^+$ T-cells along with interleukin-1 (IL-1) and initiate an immune response with the production of effector T-cells and plasma cells. Effector cells that destroy the graft develop from both $CD8^+$ and $CD4^+$ subsets of T-lymphocytes. In addition to cytotoxic effects, interferon-gamma is produced that increases expression of MHC-encoded molecules on graft tissue and makes the graft more vulnerable to destruction by effector cells.

There are two main types of graft rejection process: (1) the so-called 'first set' response which occurs about 10 days after a first graft from an unrelated donor and (2) the 'second set' response occurring in about 7 days in an animal which had previously received a graft from the same unrelated donor. This phenomenon of first and second set rejection can be compared to primary and secondary immunization — the accelerated secondary response being brought about by stimulation of an already sensitized or 'primed' immune system.

The role of lymphoid cells

It can be shown histologically that grafts undergoing rejection are heavily infiltrated with lymphocytes and that there is extensive vascular damage. Other types of cells of the immune system, such as plasma cells and macrophages, are also frequently found in association with

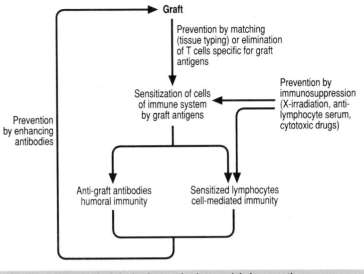

Fig. 7.1 Schematic view of rejection mechanisms and their prevention.

graft rejection. The ability to reject grafts can readily be transferred from one animal to another by a process known as **adoptive transfer** of lymphoid cells from an immune animal (i.e. one capable of a second set graft rejection) to a non-immune recipient of the same inbred strain. Lymphoid cells appear to be able to transfer this ability most effectively when taken before the circulating antibody level reaches its peak. Contrary to expectation, it is possible to show, using isotope-labelled cells, that it is not the transferred cells which migrate to the graft but those of the recipient. The donated cells, in the main, home to the lymphoid organs, as no more are found in the graft than at control sites.

From what is known about the recirculating lymphocyte pool (p. 97), it seems likely that there is a good chance of cells with a specific ability to react to an antigen coming in contact with such material in a graft during the process of lymphocyte recirculation. Donor lymphocytes carried over as 'passengers' in the vascular bed of the graft are a source of transplantation antigens that can sensitize the host. Removal of APC from the graft can be shown to promote graft survival when only minor antigen incompatibility is present. Strong incompatibility is associated with responses induced by host APC, therefore MHC class II molecules are involved.

The role of circulating antibody

The ability to reject grafts cannot be transferred from one animal to another by means of passively injected antibody. This does not rule out the possibility that antibody can play a part in graft rejection because when the serum, containing at best about 1% specific antibody, is injected into a recipient the diluting effect of the blood and tissue fluids considerably reduces the possibility of the antibody reaching the graft site in an adequate concentration to influence the viability of the graft. The same antibody-containing serum can readily be shown in vitro to be cytotoxic, in the presence of complement, for cells containing antigens to which the antibody was produced. However, this is an artificial situation and does not take into account the dilution effects discussed above. Kidney grafts which have survived for some time, perhaps months or years, can, it seems, be rejected by serum antibody alone without any evidence of invasion of the graft by lymphoid cells. Deposits of immunoglobulin and complement can be detected particularly in the walls of blood vessels. Although at this stage no antibodies may be detected in the serum, if the rejected kidney is removed they soon appear, suggesting that the antibodies were rapidly removed by combination with kidney antigens. The kidney is rejected by the development of a progressive vasculitis affecting glomerular and other vessels. Attempts have been made to recover antibody by elution from rejected kidneys removed from 27 patients. Seven of the kidneys contained recoverable antibody and this often differed from that found in the patient's serum, supporting the view that grafted incompatible kidneys filter out antibody from the circulation.

Locally produced antibody and non-antibody lymphocyte factors

The possibility is quite strong that antibody made locally in a graft by the infiltrating lymphoid cells is present in a sufficiently high concentration in the area immediately surrounding the antibody-producing cell to damage incompatible cells of the graft. This situation can be compared to the observation made in vitro with the Jerne plaque technique in which lymphocytes can be shown to be producing antibody to sheep red blood cells which produces a surrounding halo of lysis of the red cells in the presence of complement. Indeed, lymphocytes and plasma cells invading grafts can be shown to contain immunoglobulin. Evidence that immunoglobulin is combining with antigen during graft rejection is provided by a detectable fall in the serum complement level The role of complement in xenotransplantation is discussed later (p. 250).

There are a number of other possible direct ways in which the infiltrating lymphocytes can influence survival of the graft: (1) the antibody which they produce may activate the various pharmacological mediators of immediate hypersensitivity reactions such as histamine (p. 272) and these will bring about changes in the vessels of the graft, (2) the lymphocytes on contact with antigen may release lymphokines that will cause accumulation of macrophages in the graft and (3) lymphokines produced by sensitized lymphocytes can influence non-immune lymphocytes to behave aggressively towards cells in their vicinity and induce cytotoxic effects.

Experimental evidence has shown that only a low percentage of the lymphocytes infiltrating a graft are specifically reactive to graft alloantigens. Lymphokines secreted by helper T-lymphocytes may be responsible for the migration and proliferation of the majority of the infiltrating inflammatory cells. Graft rejection can be inhibited by in vivo administration of antisera against lymphokines. Adoptive transfer experiments in T-lymphocyte-depleted mice indicate that CD4$^+$ T-cells are critical to skin-graft rejection in mice. Furthermore, injections of interleukin-2 can greatly enhance heart graft rejection in rats.

Other cell types may influence graft rejection and it has been found that monocytes and macrophages accumulate in large numbers early in human renal graft rejection.

It can thus be seen that the reaction against a graft depends upon a complex series of interrelated phenomena, some of which are specifically induced by the foreign nature of graft antigens. Other phenomena are non-specific in the immunological sense and occur as part of an inflammatory process.

Clinical transplantation

The first successful kidney transplant was carried out in 1954. Improvements in techniques, including the use of immunosuppressive drugs, have reduced the incidence of complications. The use of cyclosporin and monoclonal antibody therapy have greatly improved the success rate. Transplant therapy is now also available with the likelihood of success for heart, liver and pancreatic grafts and has transformed the outlook for patients with chronic and debilitating disease of these organs. The most successful transplants are those given at an early stage of the disease.

Donor selection normally depends on ABO and HLA compatibility and testing by cross-matching of patient's serum and donor tissue. Improved immunosuppression and preoperative conditioning procedures have enabled donor tissue to be used that shares two, one or no haplotypes with the recipient. Preoperative random blood transfusion is correlated with improved allograft survival believed to be due to development of suppressor T-cells or anti-idiotype antibodies.

Advances in histocompatibility typing, prevention of graft-versus-host (GVH) disease and supportive care have resulted in successful transplantation of bone marrow for several previously fatal diseases. It is the treatment of choice for severe combined immune deficiency (SCID) and is used with varying degrees of success in aplastic anaemia, acute and chronic myelogenous leukaemia and acute lymphoblastic leukaemia.

Efforts to use marrow from partially matched family donors or phenotypically matched unrelated donors show increasing success. 'Purging' techniques with monoclonal antibodies against leukaemic neoplastic cells are in the process of development.

Liver transplant rejection appears to be due to different mechanisms than kidney rejection. Donor selection depends more on ABO matching rather than HLA. Liver seems to be able to resist acute rejection but the mechanisms are not understood. Cyclosporin therapy has had a major effect on the results of transplantation.

In heart transplantation evaluation of donor tissue and recipient depends on HLA typing and detection of any preformed anti-HLA antibodies. A mononuclear cell infiltration of the tissue is found if rejection is taking place along with electrocardiographic abnormalities. There is a 70% survival rate at 5 years.

In bone transplantation autografts, or autografts in conjunction with allografts, are the most commonly transplanted tissue. Allografted cells induce antibody production and cell-mediated immunity with resulting bone destruction. Slow revascularization usually occurs and new cartilage and bone is laid down. About 10% of grafts fail. Conventional immunosuppression is rarely used in bone transplantation. A new technique is under development in which donor bone is coated with a biodegradable cement that covers HLA antigens for sufficient time for them to lose their antigenicity.

Immunosuppression

Graft rejection, as has been noted, involves a sequence of separate phenomena developing from initial contact of the foreign antigens with the host immunological system through to rejection itself. The steps include establishment of lymphatic drainage, antigen release, its contact with cells of the immune system, proliferation of antibody-forming cells of the lymphoid tissues, the inflammatory response and release of pharmacological mediators and cytotoxic effects of lymphoid cells and/or antibody on the graft tissues.

Prevention of sensitization: tolerance to graft antigens

Interference with any of these stages would be likely to interfere with the rejection process. One of the most interesting approaches, which is as yet unfortunately only at the experimental stage, is interference with what might be termed the afferent arc of the process of rejection, namely the initial sensitization of the lymphoid cells. If it were possible to induce immune tolerance to the strong histocompatibility antigens of tissue grafts, then immunological rejection would not take place.

The tolerant animal, although unable to react against the antigen to which it is tolerant, can still respond to other antigens such as potentially infective agents like bacteria, fungi or viruses; this obviates one of the greatest difficulties associated with immunosuppressive procedures.

Mitchison (using serum protein antigens) has shown that there are two types of tolerance (p. 142), so-called 'high-dose' tolerance, where the immune system is overloaded with excess antigen, and 'low dose' tolerance, where only minute quantities of antigen are administered. Although the molecular processes underlying these phenomena are not as yet understood, the 'low dose' tolerance phenomena has great potential application to transplantation problems. When it becomes possible to extract purified transplantation antigens from tissue, it should then be possible to prepare an individual for graft acceptance by inducing low dose tolerance to the appropriate antigens.

Some progress has been made recently in the induction of specific tolerance against transplantation antigens in rats by eliminating the T-lymphocytes which normally respond to graft antigens. It has been done by preparing antibodies against the T-cell antigen receptors. Another approach that involves T-cell receptors is the induction of tolerance by means of anti-idiotypic antibodies against the receptor so that recognition of graft MHC antigens is blocked.

Another approach to inducing transplantation tolerance is the repeated injection of massive doses of serum into neonatal rats. The serum contains small amounts of histocompatibility antigen and this is sufficient in neonatal rats to induce a lasting tolerance to certain skin grafts showing strong histocompatibility differences between donor and recipient. The practical value of this approach is clearly limited by the requirement that tolerance be induced in neonatal animals. Recipients of grafts who have received previous blood transfusions have shown improved graft survival. The mechanism is not understood but the most significant improvement occurs when the donors and recipients are well matched for MHC antigens.

Another approach that may have important implications for transplantation, so far limited to studies in adult mice, indicates that it is possible to induce tolerance to an antigen without permanently suppressing the total ability of the immune system. This is done by injecting the mice with a monoclonal antibody directed at the T-helper cells (anti-CD4) at the same time as an antigen is injected. After a short period of almost complete immunosuppression the T-cell population recovers and the animal is found to be tolerant to both the anti-CD4 and the antigen that was injected along with it. If this technique can be extended to humans it could provide a way of inducing transplantation tolerance without the loss of other immune functions. Recent experimental attempts have been made in mice to induce graft tolerance by intrathymic injection. These and other approaches involving interruption of cytokine pathways offer possible future strategies for the control of rejection.

Immunological enhancement

Another phenomenon relevant to the maintenance of incompatible grafts is 'immunological enhancement'. This is brought about by antibody produced against graft antigens that can under certain circumstances protect the graft from attack by cells of the immune system. This system has been used successfully in rats with incompatible kidney grafts, the animals being previously immunized with tissue from the prospective donor. The grafts exhibit normal renal function for a year or more afterwards. The method has been applied in a few instances to human kidney grafts and the results suggest that the method may be of considerable future value. The mechanism may involve coating of the cells of the graft by non-complement-fixing antibody and/or direct inhibition of antibody production by removal of T-helper cells coated by immune complexes of antibody and graft antigen. Another suggestion is that enhancing antibody binds to passenger leucocytes in the graft that express alloantigens so that they are removed and fail to stimulate a response against the alloantigens. The danger of the antibody damaging the graft will require the use of antisera (directed against the histocompatibility antigens) that has been treated so as to eliminate any cytotoxic effects. This could be achieved by making use of antibody fragments (Fab) that do not bind complement.

Practical approaches

Complement in xenotransplantation

Shortage of donor organs has led to studies into the possibility of using pig organs for transplantation. A critical barrier is complement-mediated hyperacute rejection brought about by natural IgM antibodies to the endothelium of the donor organ. Complement is activated and results in damage and rejection of the donated organ. A variety of approaches are available including removal of the IgM antibody and decomplementation. More recently, advancing knowledge of complement regulatory proteins (p. 25) has led to trials involving the inhibition of complement activity using, in particular, complement receptor 1 (CR1) in which the region encoding the transmembrane and cytoplasmic portions of the molecule are deleted. The resulting molecule has been shown in vitro to be a powerful inhibitor of complement from several species and in experimental cross-species transplantation has proved to be valuable in graft survival. Much effort is being directed at studying complement regulatory molecules and it is likely that in the near future inhibition of complement will become an accepted clinical procedure in transplantation and probably also in situations where blood is exposed to foreign surfaces.

In practice there are at the moment three main approaches to the problem of immunosuppression: (1) X-irradiation to knock out the lymphoid tissues and abolish the immune response, (2) immuno-suppressive drugs — antimetabolites and anti-inflammatory agents to prevent proliferation of antibody-forming cells and (3) immunological methods — antilymphocyte serum (ALS) produced, for example, in the horse to attack the lymphocytes directly and destroy them before they attack the graft.

Pancreas transplantation

Transplantation of the pancreas is a well-established procedure and dramatic advances have been made in graft survival in the last few years. New immunosuppressive drugs for both pancreas and kidney transplantation are becoming available for clinical trials and donor-specific bone marrow infusions are under investigation to enhance chimerism in the hope of reducing allospecific immune responses of recipients. Much research is targeted at transplanting the purified endocrine components of the pancreas (e.g. islets of Langerhans). In rodents tolerance induction has been achieved by intrathymic implanta-tion of islet cells or cell extracts and the use of fetal placenta has been shown to be effective in immunodeficient animals. Proliferation of human beta cells in vitro has been achieved after stimulation with hepa-tocyte growth factor. It is hoped that these procedures will lead to major progress in clinical islet cell transplantation in the next few years.

Immunosuppressive therapy

Most immunosuppressive drugs in current use are capable of inhibit-ing the immune response non-specifically. The aim is to develop agents (drugs, monoclonal antibodies, cytokines) with the ability to act on specific components of the immune system.

Amongst the most commonly used drugs are the corticosteroids that are effective in suppressing inflammatory processes and immune responses. Corticosteroids transiently (4–6 hours after injection) reduce the numbers of circulating leucocytes, increasing neutrophils and reducing lymphocytes, monocytes and eosinophils. The counts return to normal by 24 hours. The release of phagocyte proteolytic enzymes (collagenase, plasminogen activator) is decreased and in vitro lymphoproliferative responses are impaired along with reduced IL-2 secretion. Delayed hypersensitivity skin tests are inhibited by pro-longed treatment. Reduced expression of Fc and complement recep-tors also occurs, contributing to impaired phagocytic activity.

Table 7.2 Cyclosporin

Uses	Action on T-helper cells Inhibits IL-2 production Possible reduction of IL-2 receptors
Toxic effects	Liver and kidney damage Hypertension Neurotoxicity Haemolytic uraemic syndrome

Four cytotoxic drugs are in clinical use for immunosuppression: cyclophosphamide, azathioprine, methotrexate and chlorambucil. They are not selectively toxic for lymphocytes and to varying degrees affect all the cells of the immune system (and non-lymphoid proliferating cells), resulting in increased susceptibility to opportunistic infections. Side-effects include pancytopenia, gastrointestinal disturbances and reduced fertility. These drugs are used to treat autoimmune diseases including rheumatic disorders.

Cyclosporin (CsA) (Table 7.2) is a more selectively immunosuppressive agent and is able to act on T-helper cells without affecting other T-cell functions, B-lymphocytes, granulocytes or macrophages. This drug has been used for the prevention of transplant rejection. Its major activity appears to be inhibition of IL-2 synthesis and secretion and it may impair T-helper cell responses to IL-2. Corticosteroids and cyclosporin act synergistically. Cyclosporin like other cytotoxic drugs has been associated with B-cell lymphomas and can have effects on the CNS, and can cause liver and kidney disease. A more recent immunosuppressive drug (tacrolimus) FK506 has a similar action to CsA, binding to cytosolic-binding proteins. The resulting complex inactivates the calcium-dependent phosphatase calcineurin, resulting in inhibition of the interleukin-2 gene. FK506 was incidentally found to be useful in a variety of inflammatory skin diseases such as psoriasis and atopic dermatitis. Monoclonal antilymphocyte antibodies have been used to reverse transplant rejection and to treat graft-versus-host reactions following marrow transplants. Polyclonal antilymphocyte antibodies are not selective for T-lymphocytes and heterologous antibodies are recognized as foreign protein. They have been used mainly to prevent transplant rejection and graft-versus-host disease.

Antilymphocyte serum has the advantage of primarily affecting the thymus-dependent lymphocytes of the spleen and lymph nodes, and lymphocytes circulating in the blood. This results in a suppression of the cell-mediated immune response with only a slight effect on the circulating antibody response. Thus, whilst suppressing the graft rejection mechanisms, ALS leaves the animal able to produce circulating antibody against infecting microorganisms and their products. However, infections caused by intracellular agents, such as viruses in which protection depends on cell-mediated immunity (Ch. 5), still remain a possible complication in this form of immunosuppression and different preparations of ALS may vary in their effect on the antibody response. Furthermore, ALS can destroy platelets because of shared platelet and leucocyte antigen and may require prior absorption with platelet suspensions. Anaphylactic reactions may occur because of the foreign nature of the protein and severe pain frequently occurs at the injection site. The combination of ALS with donor-specific bone marrow cells has given promising results in a mouse model of kidney transplantation.

Interference with the activity of IL-2 by blocking its receptors on T-lymphocytes with anti-receptor antibodies is under trial and indicates that consideration needs to be given to interruption of cytokine pathways as possible strategies for immunosuppression. Another approach to controlling the interaction of cells of the immune system with allografts involves interference with the cell-adhesion molecules (p. 98) by antibodies.

FURTHER READING

Brent L (ed) 1991 Transplantation. Current Opinion in Immunology 3: 707–757

Inverardi L, Ricordi C 1996 Transplantation of pancreas and islets of Langerhans: a review of progress. Immunology Today 17: 7

Mason D W, Morris P J 1986 Effector mechanisms in allograft rejection. Annual Review of Immunology 4: 119

Michel G, Kemeny L, Homey B, Ruzicka T 1996 FK506 in the treatment of inflammatory skin disease: promises and perspectives. Immunology Today 17: 106

Stites D P, Terr A I (eds) 1994 8th edn. Basic and clinical immunology. Appleton and Lange, Norwalk, Conn.

8 Malignant disease

The ability of normal cells to proliferate in response to cell loss is rigidly controlled within an organ or tissue. In some pathological states the stimulus for cell proliferation exceeds that required for replacement, leading to polyclonal expansion and hypertrophy of tissue. In most circumstances the expansion and hypertrophy of tissue comes under control with reduction of the growth stimulus. For cells to proliferate out of control requires a transforming event so that the daughter cells continue to proliferate independent of external growth control. Humans have 100 or so specialized genes that control the growth of cells. If they mutate, a single DNA base may change or whole sections of the message are lost. Certain virus oncogenes are inserted into the DNA and these may be responsible for harmful mutations. Most mutations occur in parts of the DNA that do not contain meaningful instructions, or mutations may affect critical areas of the DNA essential for survival of the cell.

In discussing the general biological significance of immune reactions in maintaining the integrity of the cellular systems of the body, Burnet points out that in humans, in whom more than 10^{14} cells are constantly reproducing, there is sufficient evidence to make it likely that at any given genetic locus an error occurs with a frequency in the range of 10^{-5} to 10^{-7} per replication. This means that in the cell population there must be many millions of errors or mutations occurring every day of life. It seems inconceivable that complex and long-lived multicellular animals could have evolved unless some means of dealing with this eventuality had been developed. Recently, however, doubt has been expressed on this view and it has been suggested that 'this daily development of malignant cells is not supported by the experimental evidence, and that spontaneous malignant transformation in vitro appears to be dependent more on cell-to-cell interactions than to be an intrinsic property of single cells.'

The role of immunological mechanisms in the suppression of malignant cells has been appreciated since the work of Paul Ehrlich at the beginning of the century but it is only in the last 10 years or so that immunologists have begun to unravel the details of the immunological processes underlying the control of tumours, the antigenic changes in tumour cells themselves, and the extent and activities of the immune response arising as a result of these changes. Tumour immunology involves knowledge of the antigenic properties of transformed cells and the ability of the host to mount an immune response to such antigens. Tumour growth itself can have effects on the immune system and these have to be taken into account in designing immunotherapeutic measures to control tumour growth.

EVIDENCE FOR THE ROLE OF IMMUNE MECHANISMS

Mention is made in Chapter 5 of the increased incidence in thymectomized mice of tumours induced by chemical carcinogens and viruses. This seems likely to be due to a deficiency of the cell-mediated immune mechanisms which are under the control of the thymus (p. 89). Thus neonatally **thymectomized** animals are unable to reject incompatible tissue grafts and do not give delayed hypersensitivity reactions of the tuberculin type. These activities depend on intact cell-mediated, thymus-dependent immune reactivity and it is the absence of this reactivity which allows tumour cells to grow unhindered.

The experimental evidence in support of this view is conflicting. Thymectomy of mice does appear to increase the incidence of skin tumours to certain chemical carcinogens (polycyclic hydrocarbons) and of tumours induced by DNA viruses. However, early thymectomy seems to have no significant effect on development of spontaneous tumours in mice and there are reports of a decreased incidence of tumours, such as mouse mammary carcinoma, following thymectomy. It thus appears that the effects of thymectomy are variable and depend to some extent on other factors, such as the agent responsible for tumour development.

Another example where deficiency of the cell-mediated immune mechanisms is associated with tumour formation is in a condition known as **graft-versus-host** disease. This condition is produced in mice by injecting spleen cells into an unrelated recipient, the reaction of the spleen cells against the host resulting in destruction of its lymphoid tissues. This can be demonstrated by using two inbred strains of mice, e.g. CBA and C57 Black, and injecting the spleen cells of one of the parents into the offspring of such a mating. CBA cells injected into a CBA/C57B recipient will recognize the C57B component of the host lymphoid cells as foreign but will not be themselves rejected because the recipient itself carries the CBA antigens.

The destruction of the recipient's lymphoid tissues, and thus its cell-mediated immune response, produces a defect in the control of neoplastic cell proliferation. These mice frequently develop tumours of the lymphoid tissues having many of the features of Hodgkin's disease of humans.

A herpes virus (Epstein–Barr) has been isolated from the human lymphoid tumour known as **Burkitt's lymphoma** and it has been proposed that the tumour is of virus aetiology. Evidence in patients with Burkitt's lymphoma has added considerable support to the significance of cell-mediated immune mechanisms in the control of the tumour. Only 1 of 12 patients, on skin testing with extracts of their own tumour cells, had positive delayed hypersensitivity reactions. However, when the tumour growth was suppressed with cyclophosphamide, skin tests became positive in 7 of the 12 indicating a recovery of the cell-mediated immune mechanisms which is associated with remission of the tumour.

Serological studies have demonstrated a strong association between the presence of high titres of antibody to EB virus in both Burkitt's lymphoma and postnasal carcinoma. However, antibody to the virus is widespread throughout the world and association can be found with a number of diverse disease states. The virus can be found not only in leucocytes of patients with Burkitt's lymphoma but also in leucocytes of patients with infectious mononucleosis and even in some normal individuals. The virus appears to be able in vitro to **transform** leucocytes into virus-containing cells capable of continuous growth. The virus appears to have a predilection for cells of the lymphoid organs and it cannot yet be excluded that the virus is a 'passenger' trapped within lymphoid cells present in the tumour rather than the prime cause of the tumour. Recent evidence suggests the possibility that the herpes viruses may act indirectly on cells by activating a latent RNA tumour virus. Ultraviolet light irradiated herpes simplex virus, whilst unable to destroy mouse cells, resulted in the activation of an endogenous virus similar to the RNA tumour viruses.

The possible involvement of a transmissible viral agent in human sarcomas has been proposed in the last few years. A common surface antigen has been found on sarcoma cells derived from bone, cartilage, fat and muscle and induces a detectable antibody response in patients' serum. This antigen can be transferred to normal human fibroblasts by exposing them to the filtered culture medium from sarcoma cells. That the antigen is transmissible to other individuals is suggested by the finding that cohabitants of sarcoma patients have the anti-sarcoma antibody in their serum. Papillomaviruses have been recently implicated as the cause of neoplastic changes along with herpes viruses in cervical tumours.

Retroviruses, oncogenes and tumours

The Rous sarcoma virus (RSV) that induces sarcomas in chickens was the first of the retroviruses to be implicated in tumour formation. It consists of two genetic subunits, one being required for viral replication in the host cell and the other determining its capacity to induce sarcomas. This latter subunit is termed an oncogene — in this case src — and is not required for normal viral growth. Using radioactive DNA probes synthesized from RSV using reverse transcriptase, the src oncogene could be demonstrated in normal chicken cells. Since then oncologists have shown that the src oncogene is present in a wide variety of species. The gene appears to be a normal cellular gene that was in some way picked up by the virus. Its finding has led to the identification of some 20 retroviral oncogenes that can be subdivided into families that share sequences. The way the cellular oncogene is activated so that a virus-infected cell becomes transformed to a tumour cell appears to be by the insertion of proviral DNA that carries sequences that function as control centres for gene expression. The sequences activate the oncogene and lead to overproduction of its protein product and transformation of the cell. Several of the proteins encoded by oncogenes are likely to be abnormal versions of cell surface receptors for growth factors and at least one encodes a portion of a growth factor itself. Several of the proteins are found on the inner surface of the plasma membrane so that they may serve to transduce signals received from growth factors acting outside the cell. Such activation phenomena are likely to happen only rarely in virus-infected cells, as viral DNA seems to enter the chromosome of the host cell in a random way. It appears that every human cell contains sets of genes (at least 20 and less than 100) that may become oncogenes when incorporated into retroviruses.

These findings emphasize the need for an understanding of growth factors and their controlling mechanisms so that tumour cell formation can be elucidated. The experimental systems are unfortunately very complex and are ill-understood. Growth factors for various cell types, for example T-cell growth factor, interleukin-2 (p. 126), colony-stimulating factors and epidermal growth factor, have the common features of stimulating DNA synthesis in their target cells. It is significant that transforming retroviruses can substitute for growth factors that are normally essential for maintenance of cell lines in culture. The M-CSF receptor may be identical or closely related to the c-fms proto-oncogene.

One of the cellular oncogenes, c-myc, is joined directly to immunoglobulin genes during chromosomal translocation in B-cell tumours and activation of both T-lymphocytes and fibroblast proliferation is associated with increased production of c-myc. This area of research is clearly crucial to the detailed understanding of transformation of cells to tumours.

Further understanding of the role of retroviruses in the transformation of cells has been achieved by the recent discovery of a gene in one of the retroviruses HTLV-1 (the transacting or tat gene) acting at a distance, which appears to be responsible for inducing T-lymphocytes to produce various cytokines including both IL-2 and IL-2 receptors thus inducing abnormal growth. The virus has also been shown to affect the integrity of the T-cell receptors by inhibiting the expression of the CD3 gene. The HTLV-1 virus has been associated with a form of adult T-cell leukaemia found mainly but not exclusively in south western islands of Japan and in the Caribbean basin. The origin of the virus is believed to be Africa where a closely related virus has been found in certain species of monkeys. Spread of the virus to other parts of the world may have been due to trading activities. The lymphocytes from patients with adult T-cell leukaemia can be shown in the laboratory to transform T-cells from normal infants into cells showing immortal precancerous characteristics and the virus itself can transform $CD4^+$ cells in culture over a period of 5 to 7 weeks. Such transformed cells when put into hamsters cause malignant tumours. Disease caused by the HTLV-1 virus is rare except in the endemic areas although it is suggested that the virus may be spreading in populations who are at increased risk of infection, such as intravenous drug users. The HTLV-2 virus is associated with a less aggressive form of leukaemia known as hairy-cell leukaemia and, like the HTLV-1 virus, can transform cells in culture and shares the same transacting mechanism having been shown to contain a tat gene (tat 2).

In summary, the leukaemia-causing retroviruses can be divided into three groups according to their genetic structure and pathogenic mechanism. The chronic leukaemia viruses, such as the mouse leukaemia viruses, contain only the basic viral genome coding for core proteins, reverse transcriptase and the envelope proteins. The acute leukaemia, or sarcoma viruses, have another DNA sequence known as the one gene that regulates cell growth. The third group, including the HTLV-1 and 2 viruses, contain the tat genes with their ability to induce IL-2 production in lymphocytes as described above.

HIV is not a transforming virus and is thus not directly responsible for the lymphomas and skin tumours found in AIDS patients. The crucial factor in AIDS is the associated immunodeficiency that interferes with normal immune surveillance mechanisms. These tumours can thus be compared to the opportunistic infections characteristic of AIDS.

Papillomas resulting from human papillomavirus are commonly associated with immunodeficiency states (p. 285) as are EBV-induced tumours (Burkitt's lymphoma).

Immunity to tumours

Carcinomas of the gastrointestinal tract can be shown to contain an antigen absent from normal adult gut cells but present in those of embryos. The antigen termed **carcinoembryonic antigen** (CEA) has been found in the blood of patients with such tumours and their lymphocytes appear to be able to act in vitro against their cultured tumour cells in contrast to control lymphocytes that have no effect. Based on animal models using anti-CEA monoclonal antibodies, it has become possible to detect tumours and metastases with radiolabelled anti-CEA or fragments and this may lead to useful immunotherapeutic procedures.

The incidence of cancer in humans is highest at the two extremes of life and it is just at these times that the immune system is least efficient. All these observations point to the probable important role played by the intact mechanisms in keeping the body free of undesirable mutant neoplastic cells.

There is considerable discussion amongst immunologists concerning the particular cells of the immune system that may be responsible for **surveillance** mechanisms to deal with neoplastic cells or host cells altered in other ways. Cytolytic T-cells (CD8$^+$ cells) are known to be the key effector cells in the immune attack against experimental tumours. Recent evidence in humans indicates the existence of tumour antigens that induce cytolytic T-cells. Tumours are often heavily infiltrated with macrophages and transfer of such cells in an activated state to mice with experimental tumours has been shown to lead to tumour suppression. Macrophages undoubtedly have the ability to recognize and bind to surfaces (with and without antibody) of various foreign materials such as bacteria and altered cells (e.g. red cells), and it is not unreasonable to suppose that this ability might extend to recognition of neoplastic cells.

A view has recently been expressed by some tumour immunologists that offers an alternative approach to the idea of immune surveillance. This is based on a failure of growth and differentiation control rather than escape from immune surveillance. The regulatory mechanisms that determine the self-renewing proliferative capacity of cell populations and their differentiation to mature cells are not fully understood. The control of cell apoptosis by p53 gene products and deficient p53 gene activity in some tumour cells is under current study. There is growing evidence that there is reciprocal communication between the immune system and several other cell systems (e.g. the neuroendocrine system). Disturbance (destabilization) in these regulatory systems could conceivably disturb normal homeostasis so that the self-renewing proliferative capacity of a particular cell type becomes predominant and differentiation to the mature form is depressed. The consequences of such a series of events could thus lead to uncontrolled proliferation — tumour growth.

TUMOUR ANTIGENS

It can be deduced from the foregoing discussion that for the immunological system to react against tumour cells these cells must be changed in some way so that they are no longer recognized as self. That this is indeed so is substantiated by many examples of tumours which have been found to develop **new antigens** as part of their cell structure.

Tumour antigens can be divided into two major categories: those that are unique to a particular tumour, i.e. tumour-specific, and those that whilst found on normal cells are qualitatively or quantitatively different on tumour cells; these are termed tumour-associated antigens. The first category are much more likely to be good targets for the immune response. The latter category is best characterized by the oncofetal antigens. These antigens may be expressed on some normal cells at a particular stage of differentiation. A well-known example is carcinoembryonic antigen (CEA) found in tumours of the gastrointestinal tract. This glycoprotein is not normally found on adult colon but only in fetal gut. CEA can be found in the serum but is unfortunately not a reliable marker for the presence of a tumour as inflammatory lesions such as pancreatitis and colitis can also lead to the expression of the antigen. Monitoring of the level of CEA is, however, useful in predicting the response to therapy of colonic tumours. Another oncofetal antigen, alphafetoprotein, normally secreted by fetal liver, is found in the serum of patients with liver and germinal cell tumours. Other antigens found in normal cells may be produced in excess by tumour cells and include T-cell antigens such as CD5 in chronic lymphatic leukaemia and CD10 in acute lymphatic leukaemia.

There are numerous examples of tumour formation which seem to be associated with these changes. The SV40 virus induces tumours in monkeys, the Rous sarcoma virus in chickens and the polyoma virus in mice. The tumours induced in mice by the polyoma virus have recently been shown to consist of two sorts of cells, cells that are malignant on introduction into another mouse and cells that do not survive transplantation. It seems possible that the latter cells are destroyed by the immune system because they carry recognizable foreign antigens on their surface. When cells of the non-transplantable variety are cultured in vitro variants appear which have lost their antigenicity and can thus transfer the tumour. This raises the possibility that attempts to eliminate malignant cells by increasing the immune reaction against them may result in the 'selection' of 'non-antigenic' variants which would allow the tumour to spread.

The tumour-specific antigens are comparable to the weak histocompatibility antigens (Ch. 7) and their strength has been found to vary for different aetiological groups. Methylcholanthrene-induced sarcomas in mice have been found to be more strongly antigenic than similar sarcomas induced by dibenzanthracene. Among the virus tumours, Moloney virus-induced lymphomas of the mouse are quite strongly antigenic, whereas the Gross agent induces a similar tumour with very weak tumour-specific antigens. Consistent with the finding that the specificity of tumour antigens varies even with one chemical carcinogen is the finding that the strength of these antigens varies also. These antigens have been identified as cell surface glycoproteins and intracellular antigens that belong to the family of stress-induced or heat shock proteins. Similar antigens have also been found in tumours induced by oncogenes in fibroblasts. A recent view is that these heat shock proteins may act as carriers of immunogenic peptides that may be involved in presentation of the peptides by MHC class I molecules, thus leading to recognition by cytolytic T-lymphocytes.

Most tumour cells carry MHC class I antigens on their surface that should induce tumour-specific cytotoxic T-lymphocytes (CTLs), particularly if associated with immunogenic molecules. As already indicated, many tumour antigens are only weakly immunogenic and this has led to attempts to enhance the generation of CTLs by supplying the appropriate co-stimulatory signals. Transfection of MHC class I B7 molecules into tumour cells in animal experiments has resulted in the development of effective CTL-mediated responses against tumours that would otherwise have grown progressively. In another experimental system tumour immunity is mediated by $CD4^+$ T-cells but as most tumours do not express class II MHC antigens attempts have been made to transfect the cells with both class I and class II MHC antigens. The resulting tumour cells can thus act as an antigen-presenting cell via MHC class II and at the same time induce CTLs via the class I MHC molecules.

Recent work with a human melanoma cell line expressing MHC class II antigen showed that it was able to induce clonal anergy in a specific, MHC-restricted $CD4^+$ T-cell clone. The conjugates formed between the melanoma cell line and the T-cells failed to induce IL-2 production or proliferation of the T-cells. It was concluded that whilst the melanoma cell line was able to deliver antigen-specific signals to the T-cell clone it was incapable of producing the necessary co-stimulatory signals, e.g. a B7/CD28 interaction. Transfection of the melanoma cells with an expression vector containing a B7 cDNA resulted in a fully competent antigen presenting cell, IL-2 synthesis and T-cell proliferation. If these findings are applicable to other tumour cell T-cell interactions the procedure may lead to new strategies in tumour immunotherapy.

Dendritic cells (p. 106) are particularly effective as antigen-presenting cells and are believed to play an important role in generation and regulation of tumour immunity. The antigen-presenting epidermal cells of the skin lose their ability to induce tumour-specific immune responses after UV-B irradiation.

Immune mechanisms

Having established that antigenic changes occur in neoplastic cells and that immunological processes are apparently involved in the body's reaction to tumours, the question is, how in fact does any tumour grow and spread throughout the body in the face of the body's immune reaction? Some of the factors which tip the balance in favour of tumour growth have already been discussed in relation to central defects of the immune response.

As noted above, some tumour-specific antigens are not strongly antigenic and the degree of immunity developed is insufficient to cause the rejection of a rapidly growing tumour. In experiments in mice with primary tumours induced by chemical carcinogens, it has been shown that if a mouse is pre-immunized with tumour cells (inactivated by X-irradiation) the animal can then develop a state of immunity on transfer of living tumour cells, provided that the number of transferred cells is not too large to overcome the induced immunity.

The abnormal social behaviour of tumour cells is well known in that they generally fail to form stable intercellular adhesions. It would not be surprising if the interaction between tumour cells and cells of the lymphoid system would likewise be abnormal, leading to escape of the tumour cell from the potentially cytotoxic effects of lymphocytes.

Tumour formation within existing structures is accompanied by profound changes of the stroma that include altered matrix production and intense angiogenesis and eventually invasion of the surrounding connective tissue. To metastasize a tumour must detach from the original group of tumour cells and pass through the stroma to enter the lymph system or blood capillaries and then attach to and pass through the endothelium and underlying basement membrane of the target organ. The molecules that are mainly responsible for cell–cell contacts are called cadherins. These are a superfamily of transmembrane glycoproteins that mediate calcium-dependent homophilic cell–cell adhesion. Integrins (transmembrane receptors that recognize cellular matrix proteins such as collagens, laminins, fibronectin, vitronectin and fibrinogen) play a crucial role in cell adhesion to matrices.

Cadherins and integrins maintain the integrity of normal tissues and are involved in the processes controlling cellular growth and differentiation. Adhesion molecules are believed to prevent tumour progression by anchoring cells in the extracellular matrix. In transformed cells destructive changes in the adhesion system lead to abnormal relationships between cells and their extracellular matrix. Recent descriptions of mutations in the gene for E-cadherin in human carcinomas and the association of the adenomatous polyposis coli tumour–suppressor–gene product with beta-catenin (a receptor for E-cadherin) suggest that cadherins and catenins play an important role in the cellular growth-control system or participate in the function of tumour–suppressor–gene products. Further understanding of the functions and expression patterns of cadherins and integrins may lead to the development of new anticancer therapy strategies.

Another way in which tumours could escape the attention of lymphocytes sensitized to the tumour antigens is by the **shedding** from the tumour of excess antigen. Such antigen present in the serum of patients with malignant disease is believed to account for the inhibitory effect of such serum on lymphocyte cytotoxicity for the tumour. Free tumour antigen or antigen/antibody complexes could conceivably 'blindfold' sensitized lymphocytes, thus preventing them from identifying and attaching to tumour cells themselves.

Experiments in vitro have shown that complexes of tumour antigen and antibody can interfere with the potentially cytotoxic effects of lymphocytes, presumably by preventing access of the lymphocytes to the tumour cell surface. Recent evidence based on studies of murine tumour cell lines has provided strong support for masking of antigenic epitopes in tumours by antibody so that even a strongly antigenic tumour continues to grow despite the presence of cell-mediated cytotoxic immunity.

Antibody interacting with the surface antigens of tumour cells can induce modulation of expression of the antigen. This leads to shedding of the antigen and redistribution of the antigen in the tumour cell membrane so that it is not available to interact with antibody. Tumour antigens that are carried to a local lymph node may be present in sufficiently large amounts to induce tolerance and also to trap sensitized lymphocytes within the infiltrated node.

The possibility arises that tumour products other than antigens could interfere with immunity, for example prostaglandins are known to reduce the expression of MHC class II molecules on antigen-presenting cells and can also suppress NK cell activity.

Tumours that are potentially immunogenic can develop in the presence of an intact immune system. This has been ascribed to induction of low-zone tolerance by repeated stimulation of small amounts of antigen. This has been termed 'sneaking through' in which the immune system adapts through a process of selection to tumour growth.

In the last few years attention has been directed to the role of T-lymphocyte sub-populations (including helper and suppressor activities) in the generation of specific cytotoxic cells and antibodies against tumours. The development of T-lymphocytes with suppressor activity can be shown in mice when the tumour burden becomes great. Suppression of immune responses in both mice and humans has also been attributed to the activities of B-lymphocytes and macrophages.

The immune response against tumour antigens is thus likely to be modified in a variety of ways (Table 8.1) with consequences that are very difficult to predict. It is likely that a precise understanding of the role of the immune system in tumour immunity will only be gained when the local response at the site of the tumour is analyzed. Thus, for example, in the estimation of the role of T-cell suppression, it may be

Table 8.1 Restrictions on tumour immunity
Immune suppression by tumour cell components
Excessive tumour size
Enhancing or blocking factors
Antigenic modulation of tumour antigens
Development of T-cell suppression
Tumour cells situated in site inaccessible to immune system

necessary to take into account only those cells in the local tumour environment.

Glioblastoma tumour cells and the cells of acute T-cell leukaemia have been found to produce TGF-beta, which has the ability to suppress T-cell and B-cell growth, IgM and IgG production, and virus-specific cytotoxic T-cells. This phenomenon may be important in reducing immune responses against tumours, allowing them to escape immune surveillance.

In tumours of mice associated with vertically transmitted viruses such as the Gross virus, there is no evidence of a specific immune response to virus or tumour and it is assumed that the presence of the virus from the early development of the animal leads to immunological tolerance to the virus. The search for a similar situation in human tumours has not been fruitful and histological examination of tumours and associated lymph nodes all point to absence of tolerance.

Non-specific immunodeficiency is often found associated with rapidly growing tumours in humans but it is not clear if this is cause or effect. It appears that patients with early tumours do not usually show lack of immunological competence and that this only appears after fairly extensive tumour growth. This is believed to be due to the appearance of suppressor T-lymphocytes and is interpreted to be a consequence of tumour growth rather than a failure of the initial immune surveillance mechanism. Recent understanding of the molecular basis for T-cell dysfunction against tumours indicates that there may be abnormalities in signal transduction in T-cells (e.g. altered patterns of protein tyrosine phosphorylation by protein kinases) taken from mice with progressively growing tumours. Similar abnormalities have been found in B-cell lymphomas from humans that showed decreased protein tyrosine phosphorylation compared with control peripheral blood lymphocytes. These results are interpreted as suggesting that signals regulating mRNAs or nuclear factors required for gene transcription might be defective in tumour-bearing hosts.

Much recent research has concentrated on the role of cytokines in regulating tumour immunity and, for example, cytokines such as GM-CSF appear to play an important role in enhancing tumour antigen presentation and in some experiments transfection of tumour cells with cytokine genes leads to tumour rejection. Since many cytokines show this effect it is difficult to evaluate the specificity and biological relevance of such studies. T-cells stimulated by solid tumours often fail to secrete cytokines without which proliferation and differentiation of effector T-cells is deficient, thus justifying transfection with cytokine genes using disabled viruses or liposomes containing cDNA. The most recent approaches have established that rejection of established tumours could be induced by immunization with tumour cells that secreted IL-2, IFN-gamma, IL-4 and GM-CSF. As a result of this work Phase I trials have been initiated in cancer patients (Table 8.2). Many other cytokine genes have been shown in experimental systems to reduce tumorigenicity when present in high levels within the tumour microenvironment. These include IL-3, IL-6, IL-7, IL-10, IL-12 and TNF-alpha.

Other research has identified that over-expression of T-cell receptor (TCR) beta-chain variable gene segments is a common feature of T-cells infiltrating tumours and in a study of melanoma patients the dominant sequences were expressed in T-cells that mediated antitumour effector functions in vitro. It is suggested that, if this is confirmed, TCR expression could provide a molecular marker to select and expand specific T-cell populations for use in adoptive transfer and immunotherapy.

Summary of immune effector mechanisms

The T-cell response to tumour antigens with the help of antigen-presenting cells is responsible for the activation of the immune system. $CD4^+$ and $CD8^+$ T-cell responses are of major importance in tumour immunity and can mediate eradication of the tumour. Table 8.3 summarizes the roles of various cells of the immune system. Antitumour

---

Table 8.2 Approaches to cytokine therapy and targeted gene delivery

1. Bispecific monoclonal antibodies capable of carrying cytokine and recognizing tumour antigen
2. Fusion of gene coding cytokine to C-terminus of immunoglobulin heavy chain whose Fab recognizes tumour antigens.
3. Delivery of cytokines in haemopoietic stem cells, irradiated tumour cells or T-cells
4. Use of viral vectors to introduce genes into proliferating target cell (e.g. gene for *Herpes simplex*, thymidine kinase, which when metabolized administers ganciclovir to toxic compound that destroys target cell). Mutant adenovirus that only infects p53 gene deficient tumour cells.

Table 8.3 **Summary of immunity to tumour cells**

Natural immunity	Natural killer cells, neutrophil polymorphs, activated macrophages
Acquired immunity Positive effects	Natural killer cells amplified by gamma-interferon from T-cells activated by tumour antigen
	Macrophages acted on by lymphokines MIF, MAF and chemotactic factor from T-cells activated by tumour antigen
	Macrophages and K-cells that recognize antibody on tumour cells by their Fc receptors (ADCC)
	Complement components produced in inflammatory response that are chemotactic for neutrophils and cause enzyme release from macrophages
Negative effects	PGE$_2$ from macrophages and tumour cells suppress NK cell activity

Cytolysins for tumour cells include: natural killer cell cytotoxic factor, perforins, cytolysins, lymphotoxins and tumour necrosis factor. Their mechanisms of action are not understood; perforin in mice, which shows a 27% amino acid homology with C9, has a similar molecular mass and shares antigenic determinants.

antibody is sometimes found in patient serum and can act by complement-mediated lysis or by antibody-dependent cell-mediated cytotoxicity (ADCC). ADCC may be a more important mechanism than complement lysis. Natural killer cells, particularly if activated by cytokines such as IL-2 and IFN-γ, are cytotoxic for tumour cells and are believed to be a first line of defence against tumours as well as being recruited later after T-cell stimulation.

CANCER IMMUNOTHERAPY

There are four main approaches that are under investigation for the immunotherapy of tumours.

1. Non-specific immunotherapy has a long history starting with the use of microbial products and more recently synthetic agents and cytokines.

2. The use of tumour-specific antibodies (passive immunotherapy) to mediate the effector functions of antibodies or as carriers of radio-chemicals, chemotherapeutic agents or toxins.

3. Transfer of T-cells from a donor who has been immunized with tumour antigens (adoptive immunotherapy).

4. Active immunization to induce protective immunity against emergent or existing cancer cells.

Non-specific immunotherapy

Passive immunotherapy and immunostimulants

The most hopeful approach in this form of therapy is the use of tumour-specific monoclonal antibodies linked either to toxins, such as diphtheria toxin or ricin, or to agents that suppress cell proliferation such as ^{131}I or cytotoxic drugs. Another possibility with promising preliminary results is the use of anti-idiotypic monoclonal antibodies against B-cell lymphomas — the immunoglobulin expressed on the lymphoma being the target.

Agents known to stimulate the cells of the lymphoid tissues in a non-specific manner have come into vogue in the last few years as a form of cancer immunotherapy. This interest derives from the work in France of Mathe who has employed BCG treatment as part of the therapy of acute lymphoblastic leukaemia in children. The length of the remissions in such cases appeared to be prolonged. The possible value of **non-specific stimulation** of the immune system is thought to be work with such an agent, *Corynebacterium parvum*. Mice injected with C parvum and given vigorous antitumour chemotherapy showed complete remission in up to 70% of mice with a chemically induced sarcoma. The effect was found only when the two treatments were combined. Other experiments in mice showed that BCG was most effective if given a week or more before the injection of tumour cells. This indicated that the treatment is not likely to be effective in the presence of an established tumour unless some steps are taken to reduce the tumour mass by drug or X-ray therapy. Recent evidence indicates that these microbial agents are inducers of cytokines and that these are at least in part responsible for the antitumour effects. It is not at present clear what factors determine whether or not a tumour will respond to these agents and the unpredictability of responses in individual patients.

Corynebacterium parvum and BCG injected directly into mouse tumours can be shown to suppress tumour growth dramatically. The effect appears to be largely due to a cell-mediated immune response to the antigens of the microorganisms in which lymphoid cells are attracted to the injection site in large numbers and appear to act not only on the bacterial antigens but also on the surrounding tumour cells.

Another effect of these organisms is to **activate** the macrophages of the injected animal in such a way that they can be shown in vitro to become cytotoxic for cultured tumour cells. It is difficult to be sure that this effect operates in vivo but it is possible, at least where tumour cells are circulating in the bloodstream or free in a body cavity, that activated macrophages could capture and destroy them.

Alpha-interferon

This interferon is now commercially available in both genetically engineered form and from lymphoblastoid cell lines and is licensed by the Committee on Safety of Medicines for the treatment of a rare form of leukaemia — hairy cell leukaemia. It is under trial for a variety of other tumours, including leukaemias and lymphomas, and preliminary evidence suggests that it may be valuable for the treatment of non-Hodgkin's lymphomas. It is also being injected into localized tumour sites such as the bladder and peritoneal cavity and it is hoped that trials may establish its value for the treatment of bladder and ovarian tumours. Alpha-interferon is also under consideration for use in multiple myeloma and Kaposi's sarcoma. A form of alpha-interferon prepared from human leucocytes is extensively used in Cuba for treatment of some viral diseases, including dengue fever, and for some forms of throat cancer.

Alpha-interferon has a general cytostatic effect and inhibits tumour growth as well as modulating the actions of cells of the immune system. The antiviral effect is believed to be due to interferon-induced changes in intracellular enzymes that block viral replication. In order to reduce the side-effects of large doses of interferon, tests are being carried out using conjugates of interferon and monoclonal antibody targeted at colonic tumour cells. A similar procedure proved effective in vitro in preventing proliferation of Epstein–Barr virus infected cells. Conjugation of interferon with a cytotoxic drug (cisplatinum) has been shown to be effective against cultured tumour cells from lung cancer.

Other forms of immunotherapy

Human and mouse lymphocytes cultured in the presence of interleukin-2 have been shown to develop cytotoxic activity against a large variety of tumour cells. These cells are called lymphokine activated killer (LAK) cells (see p. 121). A study in humans showed 50% reduction in tumour mass in 11 of 25 patients with various types of tumour. Another approach that has been proposed (based on experiments in mice) involves the injection of small amounts of IL-2 or gamma-interferon that are likely to activate cytotoxic T-cells and natural killer cells. The NK cell activity does not depend on the expression of antigens by tumour cells and the T_c-cells should provide immunological memory to tumours that do express antigens.

Adoptive transfer of tumour-specific T-cells has been used successfully in a number of animal models and with the recognition of specific tumour antigens and may lead to effective therapy in human malignancies, possibly in combination with cytokines to promote T-cell activity and antigen presentation.

In conclusion, it seems possible that immunotherapy may have an important role in the future treatment of malignant disease. It seems likely to be most effective when the tumour mass is small or can be reduced by chemotherapy. The spontaneous disappearance of tumours and complete recovery of patients with widespread cancer does, on rare occasions, happen and is usually explained as divine intervention. A more readily acceptable explanation of such phenomena is that for some other reason the balance between tumour growth and the immune reaction against it has been tipped in favour of the immune response.

Chemotherapy is widely used to control tumour growth but tumour cells can develop multidrug resistance. This appears to be due to the 'pumping out' of the anticancer drug from the cell and is brought about by p glycoprotein. This glycoprotein is found on cells of the biliary system and elsewhere in the gut and is involved in the removal of toxins. The p glycoprotein can be blocked by cyclosporin so that the anticancer drugs are not so rapidly eliminated. In trials of cyclosporin treatment combined with chemotherapy the cyclosporin is given at 3-weekly intervals so as to minimize its effects on the immune system (see p. 252).

The major difficulty confronting the oncologist in the use of immunotherapy is that there is at present such an incomplete understanding of the relationship of tumours with the immune system that it is not possible to make rational decisions on whether immunotherapy will be of value in any particular situation. Present efforts are initiated largely on an empirical basis that in theory might work but the background knowledge is inadequate to provide a proper scientific basis for treatment. In this situation available resources should clearly be allocated to this end and the attractive option of trying out yet another form of immunotherapy should be resisted. The history of medical progress, however, is full of examples where empirical observations were found to have real therapeutic value. Nevertheless, it is probably true to say that in most instances they occurred before the recent enormous advances in scientific progress in the cell biological and molecular biological sciences, and that it is no longer justifiable to turn aside from a systematic scientific investigation of a disease state.

FURTHER READING

Becker J C, Brabletz T, Czerny C, Termeer C, Brocker E B 1993 Tumour escape mechanisms from immunosurveillance: induction of unresponsiveness in a specific MHC-restricted CD4[+] human T-cell clone by the autologous MHC class II[+] melanoma. International Immunology 5: 1501

Bischoff J R, Kim D H, Williams A et al 1996 An adenovirus mutant that replicates selectively in p53-deficient human tumor cells. Science 274: 373–376

Burnet F M 1962 The integrity of the body. Oxford University Press, London

Burnet F M 1970 Immunological surveillance. Pergamon Press, London

Grabbe S, Beissert S, Schwarz T, Gramstein R D 1995 Dendritic cells as initiators of tumor immune responses: a possible strategy for tumor immunotherapy? Immunology Today 16: 117

Glukhova M, Deugnier M-A, and Thiery J P 1995 Tumour progression: the role of cadherins and integrins. Molecular Medicine Today 1: 84

Klingeman H-G, Dougherty G J 1996 Site-specific delivery of cytokines in cancer. Molecular Medicine Today 2: 137

Manson L A 1991 Does antibody-dependent epitope masking permit progressive tumour growth in the face of cell-mediated cytotoxicity. Immunology Today 12: 352–355

Odd L J (ed) 1991 Cancer. Current Opinion in Immunology 3: 643–705

Sensi M, Parmiani G 1995 Immunology Today 16: 588

Stites D P, Terr A I (eds) 1994 Basic and clinical immunology. 8th edn. Appleton and Lange, Norwalk, Conn.

Zier K, Gansbacher B, Salvadori S 1996 Preventing abnormalities in signal transduction of T-cells in cancer: the promise of cytokine gene therapy. Immunology Today 17: 39

9 Immunopathology

In the earlier chapters of this section, the immune system has been considered in relation to its role in protection from infection or tumour development and in graft rejection or reaction to transfused blood cells. Such responses can be considered as advantageous to the host in terms of removal of foreign material. As has been noted in Chapter 5, protection is sometimes associated with disadvantageous consequences to the host, as is illustrated by the finding of immune complexes with their effects in the kidneys and elsewhere. In other situations the functioning of the immune system is affected by its exposure to infective agents and in rare instances by inherited defects. In Chapter 4 it was pointed out that in normal individuals self-tolerance and the ability to discriminate between self and non-self was an essential feature in the development of the immune system. This ability of the cells of the immune system is not absolute and conditions (largely ill-defined) can arise where self-reactivity, or autoimmunity, occurs. In this chapter an outline is given of these disadvantageous immune responses under the three headings hypersensitivity, immunodeficiency and autoimmunity.

HYPERSENSITIVITY

Immunity was first recognized as a resistant state that followed infection. The immune system protects the host not only from infectious agents but reacts against foreign material such as tissue grafts, blood products and various bland chemical substances none of which bear any relationship to infectious agents. However, some forms of immune reaction, rather than providing exemption or safety, can produce severe and occasionally fatal results. These are known as **hypersensitivity reactions** and result from an excessive or inappropriate response to an antigenic stimulus. The mechanisms underlying these deleterious reactions are those that normally eradicate foreign material but for various reasons the response leads to a disease state. When considering each of the four hypersensitivity states it is important to remember this fact and consider the underlying defence mechanism and how it has given rise to the observed immunopathology.

Various classifications of hypersensitivity reactions have been proposed and probably the most widely accepted is that of Coombs and Gell. This recognizes four types of hypersensitivity, which will be considered in turn here.

Type I: anaphylactic

If a guinea-pig is injected with a small dose of an antigen such as egg albumin no adverse effects are noted. If a second injection of the same antigen is given intravenously after an interval of about 2 weeks a condition known as **anaphylactic shock** is likely to develop. The animal becomes restless, starts chewing and rubbing its nose, begins to wheeze and may develop convulsions and die. The initial injection of antigen is termed the sensitizing dose and the second injection the shocking dose. Post-mortem examination shows contraction of smooth muscle, especially of the bronchioles and bronchi, and dilation of capillaries. Similar reactions are seen in humans especially after a bee sting or injection of penicillin in sensitized individuals. Localized reactions are seen in patients with hay fever and asthma. In all these situations the host responds to the first injection by producing IgE and it is the level of IgE produced to a particular antigen that will determine whether an anaphylactic reaction will occur on re-exposure to the same antigen.

Mechanism

When first exposed to an antigen the immune system will respond by setting in motion the interaction that gives rise to host defence mechanisms that will effectively combat the foreign material. The processes involved and some of the control mechanisms have been outlined earlier. The types of response that are generated depend on a number of factors including the type of antigen, its route of entry, the dose and also the genetic make-up of the host. The humoral response to an antigen will start with the production of IgM and with time other isotypes will be produced. In normal individuals extremely low levels of IgE will be produced. However, atopic individuals, those with a genetic predisposition to allergy, respond to certain antigenic stimuli by synthesizing larger amounts of IgE. This is believed to be determined by the cytokine milieu during the initial phase of the immune response that results in the predominance of either T_H1 or T_H2 T-cells (see p. 125). The T_H2 subset of T-cells plays a prominent role in immediate hypersensitivity by producing IL-4, which is the critical stimulus for the switch to IgE antibody production.

The IgE produced becomes associated with two types of cell, mast cells and basophils. Two types of mast cells have been described both of which bind IgE but differ in their anatomical distribution (mucosal or connective tissue), granular contents and response to growth factors. Basophils are leucocytes normally present at very low levels only in the blood. All these cell types possess a high affinity receptor for the Fc portion of IgE. In the normal situation an individual will have produced extremely low levels of IgE against many epitopes. This spectrum of antibodies will be reflected on the cell surface, i.e. there will be many IgE molecules present but most will have different specificities (Fig. 9.1A). An allergic individual will produce the same extremely low amounts of IgE against most antigens but will synthesize relatively large amounts of IgE against certain antigens, i.e. allergens. In this individual the mast cells and basophils will again mirror the picture in serum and this time a high proportion of the surface-bound IgE will be directed against a specific epitope (Fig. 9.1B). As well as in type I hypersensitivity, IgE levels are raised in a number of other situations (Table 9.1). The biologically active molecules that are responsible for the manifestations of type I hypersensitivity are stored within mast cells and basophil granules or are synthesized after cell triggering. The

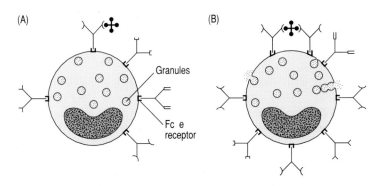

Fig. 9.1 Type I hypersensitivity.
Release of mediators from a mast cell or basophil is triggered by the crosslinking of surface-bound IgE. (A) A normal individual produces low levels of IgE directed against many different epitopes. These IgE molecules bind specifically to Fcε receptors on the surface of mast cells and basophils. (B) An atopic individual produces high levels of IgE against a particular stimulus (+). As in (A) the IgE binds to the Fc receptors on the surface of mast cells and basophils but since a greater amount is present that recognizes a particular epitope it is possible to get crosslinking of the bound IgE when the antigen is encountered. This causes degranulation with the release of preformed mediators.

Table 9.1 Causes of raised total IgE

Allergic	
Rhinitis	
Asthma	Allergy to environmental allergens
Dermatitis	
Aspergillosis	Allergy following bronchopulmonary exposure
Non-allergic	
Parasitic infections	Protective immunity against parasite
IgE myeloma	Plasma cell neoplasm
Ataxia-telangiectasia	Possible T-suppressor cell defect
Wiskott–Aldrich syndrome	Origin unknown

signal for the release or production of these molecules is the crosslinking of surface-bound IgE by antigen. For this to happen the antigen must be at least divalent with respect to the epitopes recognized and the spatial arrangement of the IgE on the responding cell must be such that this can happen. In the normal individual the likelihood of this occurring to any extent is remote due to the spatial distribution of the specific IgE molecules. However, in an allergic individual, crosslinking is more likely to occur since IgE molecules that recognize the same antigen are more likely to be close to each other on the cell surface.

In both situations the bridging of IgE on the surface of the cell will lead to the release of mediators by the activation of a biochemical cascade involving phosphatidyl inositol turnover, Ca^{2+} ions and various enzymes. This process leads to the secretion of granule contents into the surrounding tissue and to the release from membrane lipids of arachidonic acid, which is the substrate for the production of the newly synthesized mediators (Table 9.2).

The preformed mediators include histamine, heparin, a number of chemotactic factors and platelet activating factor (PAF). In some species 5-hydroxytryptamine (serotonin) is produced in place of, or as well as, histamine. Histamine is the most abundant and fast-acting of these substances. It induces smooth muscle contraction, vasodilation and increases vascular permeability; all of which are responsible for the symptoms of anaphylaxis described above. The other preformed molecules attract cells to the site or have actions similar to histamine. The metabolites of arachidonic acid — the leukotrienes, prostaglandins and thromboxanes — cause the same effects as histamine but more slowly and over a longer time course. It must be emphasized that this is the normal inflammatory process and these molecules play a key role in normal host defence. It is only when the situation gets out of hand and there is a massive release of these substances, often to an inappropriate signal, that the hypersensitivity state develops.

Table 9.2 **Mediators from mast cells — triggered by crosslinking of IgE by antigen or anaphylatoxins (C3a or C5a)**

Constitutive	
(preformed in granules)	
Histamine	Initial inflammatory response by increased capillary permeability and vasodilation
Heparin	Acts as anticoagulant
Eosinophil and neutrophil chemotactic factors	Chemotaxis of eosinophils and neutrophils
Platelet activating factor	Formation of microthrombi
Tryptase	Proteolysis
Induced	
(via arachidonic acid metabolic pathways)	
Leukotrienes (LT) LTC4 and LTD4	Early inflammatory response by vasoactive bronchoconstrictive and chemotactic effects
Prostaglandins, thromboxanes	Late inflammatory response Bronchoconstrictive and vasodilatory with oedema and mucous secretion

Since mast cells are found in the mucosa and connective tissue, exposure to allergens can lead to a wide spectrum of symptoms. The systemic form of anaphylaxis is likely to develop if an allergen is injected parenterally, as in the case of a drug such as penicillin or by the bite or sting of an insect. The symptoms of dyspnoea with bronchospasm and laryngeal oedema, a fall in blood pressure and occasionally death are caused by the release of mediators into the circulation. If, on the other hand, the antigen comes in contact with the respiratory mucous membrane, e.g. grass pollen or animal dander or faeces of the house dust mite, then in a sensitized individual the local forms of anaphylaxis will develop, i.e. hay fever or asthma. If the intestinal mucous membranes of a susceptible individual come in contact with the appropriate antigen, e.g. nuts, fish or strawberries, then a mixed form of reaction can develop with intestinal symptoms, skin rashes (urticaria) and sometimes the symptoms of asthma.

The IgE levels of normal individuals are low and it has been shown that the higher the level the greater the chance of allergic predisposition. There is a strong familial association with the development of atopic allergy. If neither parent has a history of allergy then there is about a 15% chance of the offspring developing allergic reactions. This rises to 30% if one parent is affected and almost 50% if both parents are sufferers. There is a link to particular HLA haplotypes within families but no association with a specific HLA type has been identified. Other factors that are involved include the degree of exposure to allergens, the nutritional state of the individual and the presence of chronic infections or acute viral infections.

Clinical tests

The possible cause of an individual's allergic reactions can be determined by a simple skin test. Small amounts of highly purified extracts of common allergens are introduced under the skin. Since the injection site is small many different substances can be tested, at the same time, on a person's back. In less than 30 minutes a wheal and flare reaction, caused by the release of mediators, will be seen at the injection site of the guilty substance(s). There are also specific laboratory tests available to measure total and specific IgE levels.

Therapy

On consideration of the mechanism of anaphylaxis it would seem likely that there are many ways to interfere with the allergic reaction. The simplest is to avoid contact with known allergens. In families with a known disposition to allergy it is advisable to avoid cow's milk in the very young since this can be a potent allergen. Once sensitized, avoidance of the allergen would be a sensible precaution. This will be easier if the allergen is, for example, animal dander than if it happens to be grass pollen.

Preventing the antigen from reaching the tissue-fixed IgE would also have the desired effect. This was the theory behind desensitization therapy. Extremely small doses of the allergen are injected over a long period of time with a gradual increase in the amount. This therapy is successful for a proportion of patients but some individuals never respond and in others the benefits are short-term. The precise mechanism underlying this immunotherapy is still unknown. In some patients the serum IgG to the antigen rises and it is thought that this blocking antibody will mop up the antigen before it reaches the IgE on the mast cells. As might be expected this method is much more effective in preventing systemic anaphylaxis than the local forms where antigen never enters the blood. However, since the production of IgE is T-cell dependent the benefits of injecting small amounts of antigen may be related to the induction of tolerance or even suppressor T-cell effects.

Symptomatic treatment of allergies commonly involves the use of antihistamines and corticosteroids to block the effects of the released mediators. Theophylline increases the level of cyclic-AMP thereby inhibiting mediator release while sodium cromoglycate and isoprenaline bind to other receptors on mast cells making them resistant to triggering.

Role of IgE

As pointed out above, the mediators present in mast cells play a central role in inflammation. The controlled release by physical damage of products of an immune reaction, such as the anaphylatoxins or IgE, will be of considerable benefit to the infected host. IgE has also been implicated in the control of parasitic worms, a health problem that afflicts one-third of the world's population. Antigens from parasitic worms enter the body through the gut mucosa and enter the draining lymph node. The type of antigen, its site and probably other factors result in the production of specific IgE. This worm-specific antibody will bind to maturing mucosal mast cells in the lymph node. These cells will leave the lymph node and migrate via the lymphatics, thoracic duct and blood back to the mucosa. If worm antigens bridge the membrane-bound IgE then mediators will be released. This leads to increased vascular permeability and the attraction of eosinophils and neutrophils to the area. The increased vascular permeability will also allow the influx of complement and IgG. All these mechanisms help in the elimination of the parasite.

Type II: cytotoxic

If antibody interacts with an epitope on a cell then the cell can be destroyed by a number of mechanisms (Fig. 9.2). The cell can be engulfed by a phagocytic cell by a reduction in the surface charge caused by the interaction with antibody, by direct opsonization and uptake by Fc receptors, or by complement receptor uptake after activation of complement by antigen/antibody complexes. Cell death can be mediated by the activation of complement and the action of the membrane attack complex. The cell can also be attacked by a distinct cytolytic mechanism that requires the presence of specific target cell-bound antibody. Phagocytes cannot phagocytose large targets so granule and lysosomal contents are released in apposition to the sensitized target causing its destruction. The Fc portion of this bound antibody is recognized by the effector cells which destroy the target through an extracellular release of toxic molecules. This antibody-dependent cell-mediated cytotoxicity (ADCC) is performed by both phagocytic and non-phagocytic myeloid cells (neutrophils, eosinophils and monocytes) and by large granular lymphocytes that have been called 'killer cells'. These killer cells are almost certainly natural killer cells that recognize an unknown target cell structure in the absence of antibody but can use antibody if it is present.

Type II reactions can be initiated by the binding of an antibody to an antigenic component of a cell and include the cytolytic effects seen in mismatched blood transfusions and in Rhesus incompatibility. The production of antibodies to a patient's own cells will give rise to

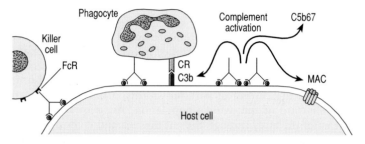

Fig. 9.2 Type II hypersensitivity.
The defect is the production of antibody that binds to a host cell surface. The antibody is directed against an epitope (●) that can be a self molecule, in autoimmune disease, or a molecule such as a drug or microbial product passively adsorbed onto a cell surface. The bound antibody can stimulate cell damage by a number of effector mechanisms. Antibody alone or in conjunction with complement components can opsonize the cell so that phagocytes can recognize and engulf the cell using Fc receptors (FcR) or complement receptors (CR). Antigen/antibody complexes will produce C3b that can act as an opsonin but the membrane attack complex (MAC) can also be generated to give direct lysis. Bystander lysis, mediated by C5b67, can affect adjacent cells adding to the area of tissue affected. Crosslinking of Fc receptors can result in the production of oxygen radicals and other molecules by phagocytes that are unable to engulf large particles. Antibody-dependent cell-mediated cytotoxicity, by killer cells, can also be generated. All these mechanisms will lead to the destruction of the host cell and the stimulation of an inflammatory response.

autoimmune diseases. Autoantibodies to an individual's own red blood cells are present in autoimmune haemolytic anaemia. Patients with Hashimoto's thyroiditis have antibodies which, in the presence of complement, destroy human thyroid cells. Activation of the complement cascade by autoantibodies to the glomerular basement gives rise to kidney damage in patients with Goodpasture's syndrome. Myasthenia gravis is caused by the stripping of acetylcholine receptors from muscle end-plates by autoantibodies. The possible mechanisms that give rise to these autoimmune diseases will be discussed later.

There are many examples of these cytotoxic or cytolytic reactions which are brought about by an immune reaction to foreign substances attached to the cell membranes of erythrocytes, leucocytes or platelets. One of the best-known examples of this phenomenon is Sedormid (apronal) purpura. The complexing of the drug Sedormid with platelets results in the induction of an antibody response directed against the platelet-absorbed drug. This antibody then binds to platelets that have the drug attached and causes destruction of the platelets, and purpura. As a result of the elucidation of the mechanism of this disease by Ackroyd in London, Sedormid was withdrawn from use. This type of reaction may be more widespread than generally recognized. A variety of infectious diseases due to salmonella organisms and mycobacteria are associated with haemolytic anaemia. There is evidence, particularly in studies in salmonella infections, that the haemolysis is due to an immune reaction against a lipopolysaccharide bacterial endotoxin that becomes coated onto the patient's erythrocytes.

The proper functioning of many cells and processes is controlled by chemical messengers, such as hormones and neurotransmitters, that act by binding to a receptor on the surface of the responding cell. This interaction on the surface of the cell is then transmitted to the interior of the cell and signals the cell to perform the required activity. For example, thyroid-stimulating hormone (TSH) produced by the pituitary gland binds to a specific receptor on thyroid cells. This leads to the activation of a membrane adenylate cyclase and the production of the second messenger cyclic-AMP that stimulates the activity of the thyroid cell. Certain individuals produce an antibody against their TSH receptor that does not lead to the destruction of the cell but mimics the effect of TSH. Therefore, there is stimulation of the cells and an overproduction of thyroid hormones.

In type II hypersensitivity, the production of an antibody against a self molecule or to a foreign antigen bound to a cell surface, an infectious agent or inert material gives rise to damaging reactions. The damage is caused by the activation of host defence mechanisms in an inappropriate setting.

Type III: immune complex

As discussed previously, when a soluble antigen combines with antibody the size and physical form of the immune complex formed will depend on the relative proportions of the participating molecules (Fig. 3.22). The amount of antigen and antibody needed to form a large aggregate will depend among other things on the class of antibody and the valency of the antigen. Under appropriate conditions the complexes formed can precipitate out of solution. This precipitation reaction is maximal at what is known as equivalence and large complexes will form. Monocytes and macrophages, using Fc receptors, are very efficient at binding and removing large complexes. These same cell types can also eliminate the smaller complexes made in antibody excess but are relatively inefficient at removing those formed in antigen excess. The large complexes are also removed by neutrophils but they are inefficient at clearing the smaller, soluble ones. If a situation arises that mimics antigen excess, then the complexes formed are not cleared and their persistence can trigger an acute inflammatory response. This is part of the normal host response to infection; however, if the complex persists or becomes trapped in tissues then immunopathological reactions ensue. Type III hypersensitivity reactions appear if there is a defect in the system, involving phagocytes and complement, that remove immune complexes or if the system is over-loaded and the complexes are given a chance to become deposited in tissues. This latter situation occurs when antigens are never complete-ly eliminated, as with persistent infection with a microbial organism, autoimmunity and repeated contact with an environmental factor.

The tissue damage that results from the deposition of immune complexes is caused by the activation of complement, platelets and phagocytes, in essence an acute inflammatory response (Fig. 9.3). Complement activation will result in the production of the anaphyla-toxins, C3a and C5a, that trigger mast cells to release their granule contents. The increased vascular permeability and chemotactic factors produced lead to an influx of neutrophils that begin to remove the immune complexes. During this process some of the neutrophils release their granule contents of proteolytic enzymes. This leads to more tissue damage and intensifies the inflammatory response. The terminal components of the complement pathway can become attached to the surface of adjacent cells leading to their lysis.

Platelets can be activated to release vasoactive amines by the bind-ing of immune complexes to their surface or through the action of platelet-activating factor produced by the degranulating mast cells. The aggregation of platelets by the complexes also results in the for-mation of microthrombi that lead to local ischaemia and further cell damage.

In general, the degree and site of damage depends on the ratio of antigen to antibody. At equivalence or slight excess of either compo-nent the complexes precipitate at the site of antigen injection and a mild local type III hypersensitivity reaction occurs, e.g. Arthus' reac-tion. In contrast, the complexes formed in large antigen excess become soluble and circulate causing more serious systemic reactions, i.e. serum sickness, or eventually deposit in organs, such as skin, kid-neys and joints. The type of disease and its time course will depend on the immune status of the individual.

If a soluble antigen is injected intradermally into an individual who has pre-existing precipitating antibody then redness and swelling with associated heat and pain appear within a few hours and resolve after 24 hours. This Arthus' reaction is the result of immune complex depo-sition at the site of injection often within the walls of small blood ves-sels. Complement is activated and an inflammatory response is initiated. These reactions occurred in diabetics who had received many injections of insulin and have developed high levels of IgG to the insulin preparation (usually of bovine or porcine origin). With the introduction of recombinant human insulin this is no longer a prob-lem.

Arthus' reactions in the bronchial or alveolar wall may explain the late asthmatic reactions that occur 7 to 8 hours after inhalation of anti-gen. A number of employment/pastime-related conditions are caused

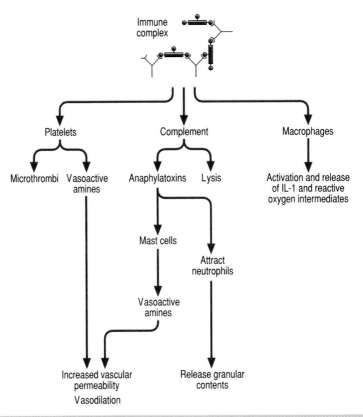

Fig. 9.3 Type III hypersensitivity.
Immune complexes will activate a number of defence mechanisms. They act on the complement cascade to produce C3a and C5a, the anaphylatoxins, that in turn cause mast cell and basophil degranulation. Complement can also cause cell lysis when the complex is deposited in tissues. Vasoactive amines produced from mast cells and platelets will lead to vasodilation and increased vascular permeability due to retraction of endothelial cells. Neutrophils will be attracted to the site and try to remove the complexes. If these are trapped in tissues some of the neutrophils will find it difficult to engulf the complex and release their granule contents. This will lead to more tissue damage. Platelet aggregation, through Fc receptors, will produce microthrombi which can lead to tissue damage by causing local ischaemia, i.e. lack of oxygen. Macrophages that take up the complexes may find them difficult to destroy and the continual stimulation of these cells leads to the release of various monokines and also macrophage activation.

by type III hypersensitivity reactions. Sufferers develop severe respiratory difficulties 6 to 8 hours after exposure to the antigen. Inhalation of antigens present in mouldy hay gives rise to the condition known as farmer's lung. Similar conditions, generally referred to as extrinsic allergic alveolitis are found in the brewing industry where maltworkers are sensitized to *Aspergillus clavatus* from contaminated barley, and even in the dairy industry where cheese washer's disease is caused by spores of *Penicillium casei*. Dust from the dried faeces of pigeons causes pigeon fancier's lung and rat serum proteins excreted in the urine can cause unpleasant effects for rat handlers.

The local release of antigens from an infectious organism can cause a type III reaction. A number of parasitic worms, although undesirable, cause little or no damage. However, if the worm is killed it can get lodged in the lymphatics and the inflammatory response initiated by antigen/antibody complexes causes a blockage of lymph flow. This leads to the condition of elephantiasis in which enormous swellings can occur. In some cases of tuberculosis, sarcoidosis, leprosy and streptococcal infections, vascular inflammatory lesions are seen mainly in the legs. These are variously referred to as erythema nodosum, nodular vasculitis and erythema induratum and may be due to the deposition of immune complexes and the development of an Arthus' reaction.

Serum sickness develops, as the name suggests, in individuals injected with a foreign serum and was described soon after the introduction by parenteral administration, for therapeutic purposes, of diphtheria antitoxin prepared in horses. Foreign serum protein, or other antigenic material, is eliminated from the circulation over a period of a few weeks but there may still be large amounts present at the time an immune response against the foreign material is developing (Fig. 9.4). This results in the formation of antigen/antibody complexes that become deposited in tissues and give rise to the symptoms of a general urticarial rash and painful swollen joints. To cause major problems the complexes must be of the right size. Large complexes are removed by macrophages of the reticuloendothelial system and very small complexes fail to induce an inflammatory response. The first thing that happens is that there is an increase in vascular permeability, due to immune-complex-mediated release of vasoactive amines from platelets or through an IgE or complement-mediated degranulation of mast cells. This leads to changes in the capillaries with a separation of the endothelial cells, allowing the complexes to attach to the exposed basement membrane. The clinical manifestations depend upon where the immune complexes form or lodge. Skin, joints, kidney and heart are particularly affected.

The site of deposition depends on a number of factors such as the production of vasoactive amines, the presence of antigen-binding sites, size of complexes, immunoglobulin class and haemodynamic processes. In the kidney, small complexes are able to pass through the glomerular basement membrane while large complexes cannot and accumulate between the endothelium and the basement membrane or in the mesangium. Deposition is most likely where there is high blood pressure, e.g. in the glomerular capillaries, and where turbulence

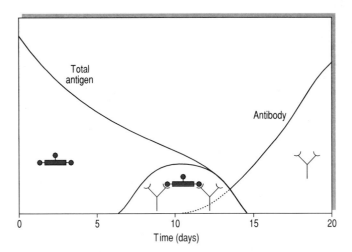

***Fig. 9.4* Time course of serum sickness.**
After exposure to a foreign material such as xenogenic serum or a drug there is a period where free antigen is present. This is the period necessary for the induction of immune response to the antigen. When antibody is produced immune complexes will form in the serum. While these complexes are present symptoms such as nephritis, arthritis or urticaria may occur if the complexes become deposited in tissues. Free antibody will not be detected until the antigen is saturated with antibody. When the antigen is finally removed, the free antibody level will rise, the complexes are cleared and the symptoms resolve.

occurs, such as at vessel bifurcations or at filters such as the choroid plexus or ciliary body of the eye. As antibody continues to be synthesized the antigen is cleared and the tissue is finally repaired.

Antigens other than serum proteins cause serum sickness. Nowadays the most likely cause is drugs such as penicillin and sulphonamides. The most susceptible patients will develop rashes (urticarial, morbilliform or scarletinoform), pyrexia, arthralgia, lymphadenopathy and perhaps nephritis some 8 to 12 days after being given the drug. It is likely that many bacterial and viral infections include development of similar symptoms — rashes, joint pains and sometimes haematuria — that resolve quickly and are probably a sign that the body is destroying the pathogen. In other situations the response to the pathogen may have more serious consequences. In post-streptococcal glomerulonephritis streptococcal antigens have been detected in the glomeruli. In viral hepatitis circulating immune complexes have been found associated with periarteritis nodosa. Many of the clinical features of the autoimmune disease systemic lupus erythematosus appear to result from arteritis, and deposits of immunoglobulin (probably complexed with DNA) and complement have been found in the skin lesions and glomeruli of patients with the disease.

Type IV: cell-mediated or delayed

This form of hypersensitivity can be defined as a specifically provoked, slowly evolving (24 to 48 hours), mixed cellular reaction involving lymphocytes and macrophages. The reaction is not brought about by circulating antibody but by sensitized lymphoid cells and can be transferred in experimental animals by means of such cells but not by serum. This type of response is seen in a number of allergic reactions to bacteria, viruses and fungi, in contact dermatitis and in graft rejection. The classical example of this type of reaction is the tuberculin response that is seen following an intradermal injection of a purified protein derivative (PPD) from tubercle bacilli in immune individuals. An indurated inflammatory reaction in the skin appears about 24 hours later and persists for a few weeks. In the human the injection site is infiltrated with large numbers of mononuclear cells, mainly lymphocytes, with about 10–20% macrophages. Most of these cells are in or around small blood vessels.

A normal cell-mediated immune response develops when first exposure to the antigen gives rise to a population of antigen-specific memory T-lymphocytes. These cells continuously circulate around the body until they come across the antigen expressed on the surface of an antigen-presenting cell in association with MHC class II. They are stimulated by this interaction to proliferate and to release lymphokines. The lymphokines are responsible for the cell-mediated host defence mechanisms that involve not only the attraction and activation of macrophages but also the stimulation of precursor cytotoxic T-cells into effector cells. These events lead to the elimination of the foreign material. The type IV hypersensitivity state arises when an inappropriate or exaggerated cell-mediated response occurs.

Cell-mediated hypersensitivity reactions are seen in a number of chronic infectious diseases due to mycobacteria, protozoa and fungi. Because the host is unable to eradicate the microorganism the antigens persist and give rise to a chronic antigenic stimulus. Thus continual release of lymphokines from sensitized T-cells results in the accumulation of large numbers of activated macrophages that can become epitheloid cells. These cells can fuse together to form giant cells. Macrophages will express antigen fragments on their surface in association with MHC class I and II and will therefore be the targets of cytotoxic T-cells and stimulate more lymphokine production. This whole process leads to tissue damage with the formation of a chronic granuloma and resultant cell death. Granuloma formation is the body's attempt to isolate a site of persistent infection. Granulomas can also form following exposure to indigestible inorganic materials such as silica and talc. The skin rash in measles and some of the lesions in herpes simplex infections may be due to cell-mediated allergic reactions where the damage is caused by cytotoxic T-cells. Therefore, the cell-mediated immune reactions, in a situation where they do not eliminate the pathogen, can lead to tissue destruction.

Type IV hypersensitivity reactions sometimes develop following sensitization to metals such as nickel and chromium, to simple chemical substances such as dyestuffs, potassium dichromate (affecting cement workers), primulin from primula plants, poison ivy and chemicals such as picryl chloride, dinitrochlorobenzene and paraphenylene diamine (from hair dyes). Penicillin sensitization is a common clinical complication following the topical application of the antibiotic in ointments or creams. These substances are not themselves antigenic and only become so on combination with proteins in the skin. The Langerhans cells of the epidermis are efficient antigen-presenting cells favouring the development of a T-cell response. These cells pick up the newly formed antigens in the skin and transport them to the draining lymph node where a T-cell response is stimulated. Substances that cause cell-mediated hypersensitivity often become directly attached to the surface proteins of Langerhans cells and are transported to the lymph node. Here the specific T-cells will be stimulated to mature and will then return to the site of entry of the offending material and release their lymphokines. In a normal situation these would help eliminate a pathogen but in this case the continual or subsequent exposure to the foreign material leads to an inappropriate response. The reaction site is characterized by a mononuclear cell infiltrate peaking at 48 hours. The clinical symptoms in these contact dermatitis lesions include redness, swelling, vesicles, scaling and exudation of fluid, i.e. eczema.

IMMUNODEFICIENCY STATES AND THE IMMUNOCOMPROMISED HOST

Primary and secondary immune deficiency

The immunologically competent cells of the lymphoid tissues derived from, renewed and influenced by the activity of the thymus, bone marrow and probably gut-associated lymphoid tissues, can be the subject of disease processes due either to defects in one of the components of the complex itself, or secondarily to some other disease process affecting the normal functioning of some part of the lymphoid tissues. In 1953 Bruton first described hypogammaglobulinaemia in an 8-year-old boy who developed septic arthritis of the knee at 4 years of age followed by numerous attacks of otitis media, pneumococcal sepsis and pneumonia. Electrophoretic analysis of the serum proteins showed almost complete absence of the gamma-globulin fraction. The child appeared unable to give an immune response to typhoid and diphtheria immunization. It is now recognized that this form of deficiency is only one of a group of specific deficiencies affecting the lymphoid tissues which can affect both sexes, manifest themselves at any age and be genetically determined or arise secondarily to some other condition.

Before considering specific defects in the acquired immune response there are a small number of defects that need to be considered in the innate immune mechanisms that possibly involve defects in phagocyte function.

Defective innate immune mechanisms

Defects in phagocytic function take two forms: (1) where there is a **quantitative** deficiency of blood leucocytes which may be **congenital** (e.g. infantile agranulocytosis) or **acquired** as a result of replacement of bone marrow by tumour tissue or the toxic effects of chemicals and (2) where there is a **qualitative** deficiency in the functioning of neutrophil leucocytes which, whilst ingesting bacteria normally, fail because of an enzymic defect to digest them. The clinical form of this defect is known as **chronic granulomatous disease** and is a sex-linked recessive condition characterized by increased susceptibility to infection in early life by microorganisms of low virulence to the normal individual. In this condition the monocytes and polymorphs fail to produce H_2O_2 due to a defect in the hexose monophosphate shunt nicotinamide adenine dinucleotide phosphate (NADPH) pathway that is normally activated by phagocytosis (see p. 32). Phagocyte enzyme defects can be detected by the NBT test (p. 340). The ability of the patient's phagocytes to kill bacteria to which they are not normally susceptible is much reduced and organisms can survive for 2 hours or more within the phagocyte.

Other enzyme defects include deficiency of white blood cell glucose-6-phosphate dehydrogenase. In such patients the NBT test may be normal but the intracellular activity of the phagocytes is reduced. Myeloperoxidase deficiency has also been described. This enzyme is necessary for normal intracellular killing but the phagocytes from patients with this defect also show normal NBT tests, superoxide and H_2O_2 production.

Defects in the ability of phagocytes to respond to chemotactic stimuli have been described. Such defects include the lazy leucocyte syndrome and Chediak–Higashi syndrome, the latter condition being a multisystem disorder characterized by giant cytoplasmic inclusions in white blood cells and platelets. In this condition the lysosomal granules are structurally and functionally abnormal, and there is an associated reduction in intracellular killing of microorganisms.

The complement system (p. 340) can also suffer from certain defects in function leading to increased susceptibility to infection. The defects that have been described include: C1q deficiency, C1r and

C1s deficiency, C2, C3, C6, C7, C8 deficiency, and dysfunction of the C5 component. Many of these disorders, which are very rare, are associated with an increased incidence of autoimmune disease (p. 295). The most severe abnormalities of host defences occur, as would be expected, if there is a defect in the functioning of C3. Severe deficiency or absence of C3 is associated with increased susceptibility to infection, particularly pneumonia, meningitis, otitis, and pharyngitis. Individuals with inherited C3 deficiency can be shown to have normal C1, C4 and C2 activation. Activation of the alternative pathway or components C5–C9 does not occur. Thus normal chemotactic (C5a) and leucocytosis promoting factors (C3e) are absent.

Individuals with C1, C4 and C2 deficiencies tend not to be particularly susceptible to infections due to their intact alternative pathway mechanisms. C5 dysfunction may lead to deficient phagocyte activity with associated recurrent infections and C6, C7 and C8 deficiency with ability to lyse susceptible bacteria such as *Neisseria*, Salmonella and *Haemophilus* organisms.

Diseases in which defects in complement components occur include sickle cell disease and systemic lupus erythematosus (SLE). In sickle cell disease (red cells contain abnormal haemoglobin) there appears to be a defect involving the alternative pathway and in SLE there is a reduction in levels of the C4 component, sometimes in the C2 component. In addition, persons with SLE appear to have a specific inhibitor of C5-derived chemotactic activity, with the associated susceptibility to infection.

Summary

Defects in the innate immune mechanism may be summarized as follows:

1. Congenital agranulocytosis.
2. Chronic granulomatous disease — due to defect in NADPH pathway of neutrophils or glucose-6-phosphate dehydrogenase deficiency.
3. Defective phagocyte responses to chemotactic stimuli.
4. Deficiencies of complement components (rare) — most common and severe is C3 deficiency. Sometimes associated with autoimmune diseases.

Primary defects

In the first category are the congenital defects affecting immunoglobulin synthetic mechanisms, cell-mediated immune mechanisms or sometimes both. Deficiency of immunoglobulin synthesis is complete in Bruton-type agammaglobulinaemia, an X-linked recessive character found in boys and in which the IgG level is reduced by about a tenth and the IgA and IgM by about a hundredth of normal values. Cell-mediated immune mechanisms function normally in these patients, who can reject grafts and develop normal delayed hypersensitivity to tuberculosis. However, they do not give the normal circulating antibody response to bacterial vaccines and are thus very susceptible to pyogenic infections. The lymphoid tissue in the appendix and Peyer's patches is somewhat reduced and patients do not develop plasma cells and germinal centres in lymph nodes.

Partial defects in immunoglobulin synthesis have been described affecting one or more of the main immunoglobulin classes. For example: (a) the IgG or IgA levels may be reduced and the IgM level raised, (b) the IgA and IgM may be reduced and the IgG level be normal or (c) the IgA level may be reduced and the others normal.

Electrophoresis of serum as shown in Figure 9.5 cannot distinguish between the various immunoglobulin deficiencies and will only show gross changes in total immunoglobulins. Gel diffusion and immunoelectrophoretic techniques (p. 319) using anti-immunoglobulin antisera are required for the detailed analysis of these deficiencies.

In (a), which is inherited as an X-linked recessive character, the lymphoid tissues appear normal histologically although the plasma cells appear to be making predominantly IgM. Patients are susceptible to pyogenic infections and the condition is often associated with anaemia, thrombocytopenia and neutropenia. In (b), even the IgG which is produced in normal quantity is thought to be abnormal in some way and unable to combine with antigen. Defect (c) occurs in 80% of patients with a condition known as hereditary ataxia telangiectasia who have increased susceptibility to infections of the upper and lower respiratory tract. There is a deficiency in plasma cells in the mucous membranes of the intestinal tract, where IgA is known to be produced in normal individuals, and the disease seems likely to be due to lack of protection at the level of the respiratory mucous membranes normally brought about by IgA secretion.

Both **cell-mediated** immune mechanisms and **immunoglobulin synthesis** are deficient in an X-linked disease of male children known as 'Swiss-type agammaglobulinaemia' or severe combined immunodeficiency (SCID). There is almost complete absence of lymphoid tissue in the body, the thymus is very small and the lymphoid tissues of the appendix and Peyer's patches are absent. Children with this condition cannot make antibodies or develop cell-mediated immune reactions, and they suffer from progressive bacterial and/or viral infection and die within 2 years of birth.

In another type of deficiency state only the cell-mediated immune mechanisms are affected and there is thymic dysplasia and deficiency

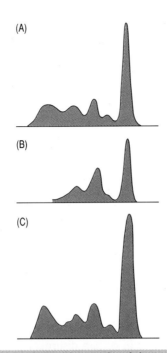

Fig. 9.5 Tracings obtained by ultraviolet scanning of electrophoretic patterns of human sera.
(A) normal serum, (B) reduced gamma-globulin (antibody deficiency syndrome possible B-cell defect) and (C) raised gamma-globulin (possible myeloma). Peaks right to left: albumin, alpha-, beta- and gamma-globulins (see Fig. 3.5).

of lymphoid cells from those areas of the spleen and lymph nodes which are under thymic control. Although children with this rare type of deficiency can produce circulating antibody, their inability to develop cell-mediated immunity renders them highly susceptible to virus infection. One form of this condition associated with thymic dysplasia and absence of parathyroid glands is known as Di George's syndrome.

The World Health Organization classification for antibody deficiencies is as follows:

1. Transient hypogammaglobulinaemia of infancy — as maternal IgG levels fall
2. Congenital hypogammaglobulinaemia — X-linked or autosomal recessive, i.e. male infants only
3. Common variable immunodeficiency — heterogeneous group of infants or adults
4. Immunodeficiency with raised IgM
5. Immunodeficiency with thymoma
6. Selective IgA deficiency

7. Selective IgM deficiency
8. Selective IgG subclass deficiency.

Table 9.3 summarizes the main primary immune deficiency states.

Secondary defects

Acquired deficiencies of the immunological mechanisms can occur secondarily to a number of disease states affecting the lymphoid tissues, such as Hodgkin's disease, multiple myeloma, leukaemia and lymphosarcoma. Deficiency of immunoglobulins can also be brought about by excessive loss of protein through diseased kidneys or via the intestines in protein-losing enteropathy. Malnutrition and iron deficiency can lead to depressed immune responsiveness, particularly in cell-mediated immunity. Viral infections can be immunosuppressive. For example, HIV, measles and other viruses infect cells of the immune system (p. 189). Medical and surgical treatment such as X-rays, cytotoxic drugs, steroids and catheterization can lead to the state referred to as the 'compromised host' in which there is interference with the effectiveness of the innate and acquired immune mechanisms (Table 5.1, p. 153).

In contrast to the deficiency states just described, raised immunoglobulin levels are found in certain disorders of plasma cell function, which amount to malignant proliferation of a particular clone or family of plasma cells. In this condition, known as multiple myeloma, a malignant clone is found to produce one particular class of immunoglobulin, usually IgG or more rarely one of the other classes. The frequency of occurrence among myeloma of particular immunoglobulin classes reflects their relative levels in serum. There is usually a decreased synthesis of normal immunoglobulins associated with a deficient immune response to infective agents. On electrophoresis of serum a distinct band can be seen in the immunoglobulin area and Figure 9.5 shows an example of the type of pattern found on simple paper electrophoresis. This abnormal band is produced by the raised levels of the myeloma immunoglobulin which is termed an M-type protein. In about 20–30% of patients with multiple myeloma immunoglobulin light chains are found in the urine. These occur as dimers and are known as Bence-Jones proteins. The condition is also associated with excess numbers of plasma cells in the bone marrow and X-ray evidence of myeloma cell deposits in bone. Table 9.4 gives a summary of secondary deficiencies and the types of microorganisms that can infect such patients.

Clinical aspects

Increased susceptibility to many types of infection is the outstanding

Table 9.3 A summary of the main primary immune deficiency states affecting T- and B-lymphocytes

Stem cell defects	Expression	Infections
Haemopoietic stem cell (autosomal recessive)	Severe combined immune deficiency affecting T-cells, B-cells and phagocytes	Early onset of infections in all systems, e.g. respiratory, alimentary, skin
Lymphocyte stem cell (autosomal recessive, some X-linked)	Diminished numbers of T- and B-cells	
Adenosine deaminase deficiency		
T-cell defects in development Thymus defects	1. Di George's syndrome (congenital but not usually familial) (thymic hypoplasia) with diminished numbers of T-cells 2. Ataxia telangiectasia (autosomal recessive) affecting T-cells and plasma cells — both reduced	Recurrent viral bacterial, fungal infections, including viral respiratory infections
Defects in T-cell sub-populations	Variable immunodeficiencies affecting Ts or T_H cells	Viral and bacterial infections
B-cell defects in development Arrested development at pre-B-cell level (X-linked)	Infantile agammaglobulinaemia with diminished numbers of B-cells	Mainly bacterial infections (occasional viral infections)
Defective terminal differentiation of B-cells	Selective deficiency of immunoglobulin classes with reduced numbers of plasma cells, B-cells and sometimes T-cells	Infection with pyogenic bacteria, if selective IgM deficiency

feature of the immunological deficiency states. The age of onset of the congenital types is rarely earlier than 3 to 4 months of age due to the protective effects of maternal antibody. The most frequently affected

Table 9.4 Summary of secondary immune deficiencies

Defects affecting lymphoid tissues
1. Infections of lymphocytes or macrophages, e.g. severe immunodeficiency in infections with HIV or the lymphadenopathy associated virus of AIDS. Transient deficiencies in cytomegalovirus infections, infectious mononucleosis, measles, rubella and viral hepatitis. Bacterial infections such as leprosy, tuberculosis and syphilis can induce deficient function of immune system.
2. Malnutrition
3. Lymphoproliferative diseases or secondary tumour deposits
4. Drugs, such as cytotoxic or immunosuppressive agents
5. Drugs that attach to leucocytes and lead to hypersensitivity reaction and leucopenia, e.g. sulfonamides
6. Antibiotics can affect neutrophil and macrophage functions, e.g. chemotactic responses in neutrophils and sometimes the phagocytic function of macrophages

Loss of immunoglobulins
1. Nephritic syndrome with loss of proteins including antibodies in the urine
2. Protein-losing enteropathy — loss of immunoglobulin in the gut. This also occurs in chronic inflammatory bowel disease
3. Burns with severe loss of tissue fluids — sometimes with associated immunodepression

Types of microorganisms involved
1. Viruses, e.g. Herpes simplex virus, Varicella-zoster virus, cytomegalovirus
2. Bacteria, e.g. *Escherichia coli, Staphylococcus aureus, Streptococcus faecalis, Pseudomonas aeruginosa, Pneumocystis carinii* and others
3. Fungi, e.g. *Candida* spp. *Aspergillus fumigatus*
4. Protozoa, e.g. *Giardia lamblia*

site is the respiratory tract, which is attacked by pyogenic bacteria or fungi. Lack of IgA antibody leads to particular susceptibility to chronic infection of the respiratory tract. Other clinical features frequently associated with immune deficiency states are skin rashes, diarrhoea, growth failure, enlarged liver and spleen and recurrent abscesses or osteomyelitis.

When there is deficiency of the cell-mediated immune mechanisms, resistance to virus infections is diminished and may be recognized by the severe necrosis that will occur at the site of smallpox vaccination. BCG vaccination can lead to generalized tuberculosis infection in such cases.

Investigation of suspected immunological deficiency states should include family studies for any abnormalities of immune function. Lymphocyte function may be assessed by stimulation (a) with non-specific agents such as PHA or concanavalin A (p. 339) or (b) with a specific bacterial antigen in subjects previously sensitized to the bacterial antigen by natural infection or immunization (e.g. the tubercle bacillus). Quantitative determination of immunoglobulin levels can be made (p. 321) and estimation of the response to immunization with standard antigens. Peripheral blood counts and X-rays of the thymus region may also prove useful.

Treatment of deficiency states includes use of an appropriate antibiotic and regular administration of pooled human immunoglobulins. Closely matched sibling bone marrow has been used successfully in some cases and a graft of fetal thymus has been used in the case of thymic aplasia. Bone marrow grafts can be rejected in the same way as other grafts (Ch. 7) unless closely related to the recipient. An additional complication arises in that the graft may attack host cells — a graft-versus-host (GVH) reaction (p. 247). In immune deficiency states graft rejection is likely to be the lesser of the two problems. Total lymph node irradiation has been found to be preferable to whole-body irradiation in the control of GVH reactions.

Below is a summary of the management of immune deficiency states:

1. Immunoglobulin replacement therapy
2. Grafting of immunocompetent cells
3. Genetic counselling
4. Antibiotic therapy
5. Possible use of interferon and other mediators, such as interleukin-1 and 2, as they become available through recombinant DNA technology
6. Polyethylene glycol coupled with adenosine deaminase (PEG-ADA) for SCID.

Table 9.5 gives the indications for, and forms of, immunoglobulin replacement therapy.

GENE THERAPY

Somatic gene therapy has evoked considerable optimism for the treat-

---

Table 9.5 Immunoglobulin replacement therapy

Indications
X-linked agammaglobulinaemia
Common variable agammaglobulinaemia
Severe combined immunodeficiency
Wiskott–Aldrich syndrome

Forms
1. Alcohol-salt fractionated pooled human plasma (immune globulin) for intramuscular use
2. Normal human plasma. Advantages are fewer adverse reactions than immune globulin and less painful injections. Disadvantages are possible hepatitis B or HIV infection
3. Modified (enzyme-treated) immune globulin as in (1) for intravenous use. Advantage is that it can be given in large doses intramuscularly with rapid action and less painful than (1). Disadvantage is rapid clearance of enzyme-treated preparations from blood

ment of genetic diseases. The procedure involves inserting normal genes into affected cell populations so that a normal gene product is produced rather than an absent or deficient form. Severe combined immunodeficiency, in which about one-third of patients have the autosomal recessive form with adenosine deaminase deficiency, has been treated by insertion into T-lymphocytes of the adenosine deaminase gene using retroviral-derived vectors. Initial results indicate that, as peripheral T-lymphocytes have a limited capacity to proliferate, long-term therapy will require insertion of the gene into pluripotent human bone marrow stem cells. It is difficult to isolate these and efficiently insert the required gene so more work is required before these procedures become clinically applicable.

The immunocompromised host

The number of patients with immunocompromised lymphoid tissues and cells has increased substantially with the advent of solid organ transplantation, HIV infection and increased use of tumour chemotherapy and bone marrow transplantation (BMT) procedures. In transplant patients there is a high risk of infection soon after the transplant and the patient may remain in an immunocompromised state either because of the interaction between the graft and the host (graft-versus-host disease) or as a result of the immunosuppressive therapy administered to prevent graft rejection. HIV-infected patients become increasingly more immunocompromised with progression of the disease. Loss of protective immunity to infectious agents and their toxins, e.g. to tetanus toxoid or polio virus, is a predominant feature of immunocompromised patients so reimmunization is frequently used to ensure the necessary immunity. Care needs to be taken if live-attenuated vaccines are to be used in view of the possibility of the agent proliferating in the patient. Several studies have shown loss of immunity in bone marrow transplant patients to tetanus, polio virus and diphtheria that can be re-established by appropriate immunization, which is best carried out later than 6 months after transplantation. European policy is that such patients should be immunized with tetanus toxoid, diphtheria toxoid, inactivated polio virus and influenza. Hib should also be considered in allogeneic BMT patients.

The safety of live-attenuated vaccines has been a matter of concern in HIV-infected patients. In trials in children with symptomatic HIV infection immunized with live-attenuated measles, mumps and rubella vaccines the serological responses were poor but no vaccine-related symptoms occurred. Specific antibody preparations of hyperimmune immunoglobulin or monoclonal antibodies are used largely for treatment rather than as prophylaxis. A possible complication of such treatment is due to the ability of intravenous immunoglobulin to down-regulate specific immune responses to antigen. To overcome this problem adoptive transfer of immunity has been used by infusing circulating lymphocytes from immunized donors. To re-establish effective cell-mediated immunity patients have been infused with stem cells derived from the blood that in some trials have been stimulated with colony-stimulating growth factors. Epstein–Barr virus infection has been reversed by donor leucocyte infusions and cytomegalovirus infections by cytomegalovirus-specific T-cell infusions. Other viruses that complicate organ transplantation and are the subject of much current interest are hepatitis viruses B and C. Treatment at present available is the use of interferon-alpha but this has an uncertain outcome.

AUTOIMMUNITY

A fundamental characteristic of an animal's immune system is that it does not, under normal circumstances, react against its own body constituents. Mechanisms, as we have seen, exist that allow the immune system to tolerate self and destroy non-self. Occasionally these mechanisms break down and autoantibodies are produced. In many individuals autoantibodies are present but do not appear to cause any problems. However, in other situations autoimmune disease may be the sequela to the formation of autoantibodies.

There is a wide spectrum of autoimmune disorders. Some of the diseases where autoantibodies play a role are shown in Table 9.6 along with the antigens to which they bind. At one extreme there are the organ-specific diseases where the autoantibodies are directed against components specific to the organ involved. An example of this is autoimmune thyroid diseases which fall into three categories: (1) Graves' disease or hyperthyroidism, (2) Hashimoto's disease or hypothyroidism and (3) myxoedema with almost no thyroid function. In many individuals there is a progression through these three states. The thyroid is an endocrine gland that synthesizes hormones, such as thyroxin, that are essential for proper growth and metabolism.

In Graves' disease there is an autoantibody that binds to the thyroid-stimulating hormone (TSH) receptor and causes the release of thyroid products in the absence of TSH. This is a type II hypersensitivity reaction and gives rise to an over-reactive thyroid. In Hashimoto's thyroiditis an antibody specific for a thyroid protein, thyroglobulin, is present. The gland becomes infiltrated with lymphocytes and phagocytes, causing inflammation and goitre (enlargement of the thyroid). In addition to the cell-mediated destruction, the antibody against thyroglobulin is thought to add to the disease process by causing complement lysis of thyroid cells that are coated in thyroglobulin. The more progressive destruction seen in myxoedema involves a number of immune mechanisms, including autoantibodies, against a

Table 9.6 **Range of autoimmune diseases**

Disease	Antigen	HLA-link	Relative risk[*]
Hashimoto's thyroiditis	Thyroglobulin	DR5	3.2
Primary myxoedema	Cell surface	DR3	5.7
Graves' disease	TSH receptor	DR3	3.7
Pernicious anaemia	Intrinsic factor	DR5	5.4
Insulin-dependent diabetes	Islet cells	DR3, DR4 DR3/4	5.0, 6.8, 14.3
Goodpasture's syndrome	Glomerular and lung basement membrane	DR2	13.1
Primary biliary cirrhosis	Mitochondria	—	—
Ulcerative colitis	Colon lipopolysaccharide	—	—
Rheumatoid arthritis	IgG	DR4	4.2
Systemic lupus erythematosus	DNA, nucleoproteins	DR3	5.8

[*]Relative risk is a measure of the increased chance of developing the disease for individuals of particular HLA antigen type relative to those lacking the antigen.

number of organ-specific components. The destruction is mediated by macrophages and almost all function is lost.

At the other end of the autoimmune spectrum are the non-organ-specific diseases where both the lesion and antibodies are not confined to one organ. Systemic lupus erythematosus (SLE) is an example of such a disease. This condition is characterized by a butterfly-shaped facial rash resembling the colouring of a wolf (*lupus* being Latin for wolf). It is systemic, i.e. has multi-organ involvement, and erythematosus refers to the redness of the skin rash. Autoantibodies against DNA are present but others are found that react with a number of cellular constituents. Immune complexes are formed between these antibodies and products of damaged cells, e.g. DNA. These immune complexes can form or become deposited at a number of sites. Generalized inflammation will be stimulated by these complexes as will antibody-dependent cell-mediated cytoxicity and activation of phagocytes. The disease can go into remission when the source of the antigen is removed and the immune complexes are cleared away. It will, however, return if more cell damage occurs.

In between these two extremes are disorders where the lesion tends to be localized to a single organ but the antibodies are non-organ-specific. In primary biliary cirrhosis the small bile ductule is the main target of the inflammatory cells but the antibodies are directed against an organelle found in all cells — mitochondria.

A number of patients with autoimmune diseases tend to suffer from more than one condition. When this happens the diseases tend to come from the same region of the autoimmune spectrum. Thus patients with thyroiditis have a much higher incidence of pernicious anaemia than would be expected in a random population. The same situation is found at the non-organ-specific end where SLE is associated with rheumatoid arthritis and a number of other disorders.

Genetic factors appear to play a role in the development of autoimmune diseases. Autoimmune diseases are found to run in families. Close relatives of sufferers tend to have elevated levels of autoantibodies although these may not manifest themselves as an overt disease. There are also strong associations between several autoimmune diseases and particular HLA specificities (Table 9.6) suggesting that Ir gene effects may be involved.

Other genetic associations have been proposed including association with immunoglobulin allotypes and idiotypes. T-cell receptor (TCR) genes have been considered but so far no convincing evidence exists for a relationship between particular TCR haplotypes or polymorphisms and predisposition to autoimmune disease. More compelling are studies on defects in gene structure, transcription and function of cytokines and their receptors.

In animal models cytokines and their inhibitors have been shown to affect autoimmunity with both enhancing and suppressive effects depending on the strategies used. Interference with the cytokine network may eventually provide useful approaches for the therapy of human autoimmune diseases.

The question now arises of how autoantibody formation can be triggered. There are a number of ways in which the self-tolerance mechanisms could be overcome. The first involves the exposure of the immune system to molecules that are normally sequestered within organs. It is proposed that any mishap that caused release of these molecules would provide an opportunity for autoantibody formation. Hidden or sequestered antigens do appear to exist and the best examples of these are sperm and lens tissue. However, it appears that the injection of extracts of these tissues does not readily elicit an antibody response and that many of these sequestered molecules do indeed enter the circulation. Therefore, the accessibility of a molecule to the immune system does not appear to be of major importance in the generation of autoimmunity.

What may be more important for the generation of an immune response is whether the molecule is presented to the immune system in a form, and at a concentration, that can stimulate a response. For an immune response to be generated the antigen will have to be presented on the surface of a cell in association with MHC class II molecules and this complex must be recognized by a helper T-cell. Since autoreactive B-cells can be easily detected and it appears that self peptides can associate with MHC molecules, the key to the control of autoimmunity must be at the level of the T-cell. As discussed above, when considering tolerance in the normal situation, T-cells can be unresponsive because of clonal deletion, active suppression caused by other T-cells or macrophages, or failure of antigen presentation. There are a variety of ways in which this unresponsiveness could be altered and give rise to autoimmunity.

Experimental studies of tolerance evasion by altered antigens have been carried out with purified proteins, conjugates of haptens and proteins, and with cellular antigens. Some of the most definitive work is that carried out by Weigle who showed that rabbits made tolerant to bovine serum albumin (BSA) and then immunized with the cross-reacting antigen human serum albumin (HSA) eventually made antibodies which could react with BSA. The same result was obtained with chemically modified BSA in place of the HSA. In the tolerized state B-cells with the potential to make anti-BSA antibodies are present but they are unable to produce any antibody because of the lack of T-cell help (Fig. 9.6). The BSA specific T-cells that could provide this help have been made unresponsive by the induction of tolerance. When HSA, which contains some B-cell epitopes in common with BSA, is injected the rabbit will be exposed to a new set of T-cell epitopes, carrier determinants, that can stimulate the HSA specific T-cells to provide help for the B-cells. A closer approximation to autoimmune disease is provided by experiments using thyroglobulin in rabbits; not only are anti-thyroglobulin antibodies induced by injection of altered thyroglobulin but inflammatory lesions are also found in their thyroid glands.

When certain drugs bind to tissue proteins they can induce structural modifications. The resulting complex, drug and self molecule, can give rise to a type II hypersensitivity reaction as described above. However, it can also generate a new carrier determinant that will induce help for autoreactive B-cells. An example of this is the autoimmune haemolytic anaemia associated with the treatment of hypertension by α-methyl dopa. A metabolic breakdown product of α-methyl dopa is thought to modify proteins on the surface of the red blood cells in such a way as to generate a structure that can give rise to a T-cell epitope. The stimulated T-cells are then able to provide help for B-cells that are reactive to the Rhesus e antigen. The autoantibody produced will then bind to the patient's own normal red blood cells and cause their destruction through a complement-mediated mechanism. There are other examples of this type of reaction, including isoniazid which gives arthritis and procainamide which stimulates the production of antinuclear antibodies.

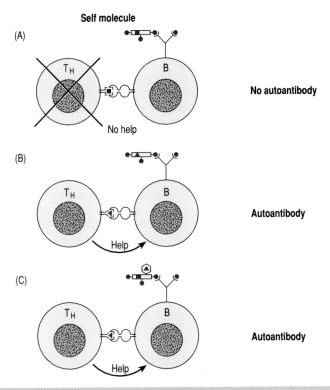

Fig. 9.6 Induction of autoimmunity by inducing T-help.
(A) In the normal situation B-cells are present that can bind self molecules. This molecule has a B-cell epitope (●) and will contain a sequence that a T-cell will recognize when associated with MHC molecules, a T-cell epitope (■). If a T-cell is produced, in the thymus, that reacts with this self antigen in the context of MHC then it will be functionally eliminated, i.e. deleted or suppressed. Therefore, the autoreactive B-cell does not receive help and no autoantibody is produced. If this B-cell is exposed to helper factors then autoantibodies will be produced. (B) The self molecule is altered so that a new T-cell epitope (▲) is produced or the individual is exposed to an antigen with the same B-cell epitope but different T-cell epitopes (as with Weigle's BSA). Then help can be supplied by T-cells responsive to this new epitope and autoimmunity develops. (C) A drug or component of a microbe binds to a self molecule and introduces a T-cell epitope (▲) that can then provide help for the production of autoantibodies. Although this illustration shows autoantibody production, the generation of effector T-cells also requires T-cell help and therefore similar mechanisms can occur for the generation of autoimmune cell-mediated responses. For simplicity B-cells are shown as the antigen-presenting cell but a similar mechanism can be envisaged using other types of antigen-presenting cell.

There are a number of examples where potential autoantigenic determinants are present in exogenous material. These preparations may provide a new carrier, i.e. T-cell stimulating, determinant that provokes autoantibody formation. The encephalitis sometimes seen after rabies vaccination is thought to result from a response directed against the brain that is stimulated by heterologous brain tissues present in the vaccine.

Microorganisms are a source of cross-reacting antigens sharing antigenic determinants with tissue components. These may provide an important way of inducing autoimmunity. There is an antigen in human colon, extractable even from sterile fetal colon, that cross-reacts antigenically with *Escherichia coli* 014. It is possible that the inflammatory condition known as ulcerative colitis, in which anticolon antibodies are found, is due to an immune response initiated by the cross-reacting bacterial antigen. Similarly the group A streptococci, which are closely associated with rheumatic fever, have an antigen in common with a human heart antigen. Heart lesions are a common finding in rheumatic fever and antiheart antibody is found in just over 50% of patients with this condition. Nephritogenic strains of type 12 group A streptococci carry surface antigens similar to those found in human glomeruli and infection by these organisms has been associated with the development of acute nephritis. Some of the immuno-pathology seen in Chagas' disease has been attributed to a cross-reaction between *Trypanosoma cruzi* and cardiac muscle (p. 204).

A new helper determinant may appear on a cell due to drug modification, as described above, or during viral infections. These new cell surface antigens (often known as neoantigens) then promote production of antibodies against other normal molecules. It has been shown that infection of a tumour cell with influenza virus produces a response towards uninfected tumour cells. Infection with *Mycoplasma pneumoniae*, which is responsible for a disease known as primary atypical pneumonia, is associated with the appearance of cold agglutinins. These IgM antibodies, often directed against blood group I, react with the patient's red cells in the periphery where the temperature is lowest.

Another way that autoimmunity may be triggered is by some breakdown in the immune network. This could occur at the level of cellular production or at a functional stage. At the level of production, defects could arise that allow self-reactive cells to survive. It is believed that suppressor cells play an essential role in maintaining non-reactivity to self antigens. Interference with suppressor cells may lead to autoimmune disease by allowing the immune system to interact positively with self antigens.

Autoimmunity can be induced by by-passing T-cells. Self-reactive cells can be directly stimulated by polyclonal activators that directly activate B-cells (Fig. 9.7). A number of microorganisms or their products are potent polyclonal activators; however, the response that is generated tends to be IgM and to wane when the pathogen is eliminated. Bacterial endotoxin, the lipopolysaccharide of Gram-negative bac-

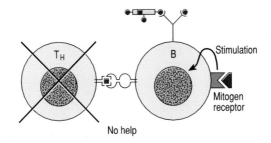

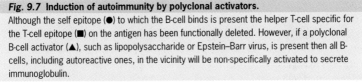

No help

Fig. 9.7 Induction of autoimmunity by polyclonal activators.
Although the self epitope (●) to which the B-cell binds is present the helper T-cell specific for the T-cell epitope (■) on the antigen has been functionally deleted. However, if a polyclonal B-cell activator (▲), such as lipopolysaccharide or Epstein–Barr virus, is present then all B-cells, including autoreactive ones, in the vicinity will be non-specifically activated to secrete immunoglobulin.

teria, provides a non-specific inductive signal to B-cells, by-passing the need for T-cell help. A variety of antibodies is present in infectious mononucleosis, including autoantibodies, that are caused by the polyclonal activation of B-cells by Epstein–Barr virus.

It has recently been proposed that self-reactive T-cells may form part of the normal immune repertoire and be responsible for maintaining peripheral tolerance. Peripheral tolerance requires the continued presence of antigen. Tolerance is not static but is flexible and reversible depending on differential signalling, regulation of co-stimulation and production of inflammatory cytokines. A proper understanding of these complex interactions may lead to development of new therapies for autoimmune diseases.

Breakdown in the idiotypic network is another way of activating self-reactive cells. Lymphocytes are linked in a network through interactions involving the variable regions of their surface receptors (discussed previously). Because T-cells have a receptor with a variable region they can also stimulate anti-idiotypic responses and their activities can be influenced through idiotypic interactions. In the normal, unstimulated situation these interactions keep the immune system in equilibrium but when antigen is introduced the network is initially tipped towards production of a response and then returns to the 'ground state' through the development of suppressor signals. It should be remembered that idiotypic interactions can act as either inhibitors or activators of the immune response, depending on the information received. There are a number of situations where signals could be generated that lead to an autoimmune response (Fig. 9.8).

The antibody produced in response to a microorganism could interact with the idiotope on a self-reactive cell to give a stimulatory signal and an autoreactive response (Fig. 9.8A). The foreign material might trigger the production of an antibody that has an idiotope that is found

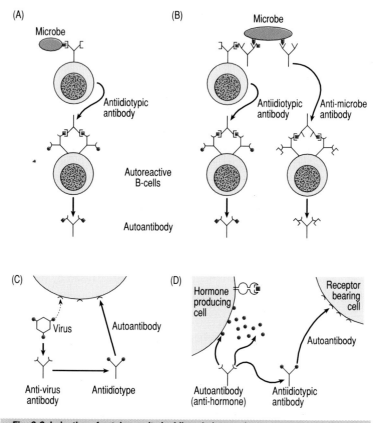

Fig. 9.8 Induction of autoimmunity by idiotypic interactions.
(A) Autoreactive B-cells carry an idiotope (■) that cross-reacts with microbial antigens. The antibody generated by exposure to the microbe can stimulate the production of autoantibody by idiotopic interactions. (B) Antibodies induced by microbe either share idiotopes with (left-hand side) or are anti-idiotypes to (right-hand side) autoreactive B-cells. (C) Antibody to attachment sites (●) on a virus will induce an anti-idiotype that can interact with the structure of the target cell (⌒) to which the virus attaches. This will be an autoantibody. (D) A T-cell epitope on a viral protein (■) stimulates the production of helper factors in the vicinity of a B-cell that can bind to the hormone (●) produced by the infected cell. This help stimulates the production of an antihormone antibody that could destroy the hormone-producing cell or mop up and inactivate the hormone. An anti-idiotypic antibody to this autoantibody will react with the hormone receptor (⌒) and could (i) destroy receptor bearing cells, (ii) stimulate them in the absence of hormone or (iii) inhibit hormone interaction.

on other immunoglobulins or T-cell receptors (a cross-reacting idiotope or public idiotope). This cross-reacting idiotope could stimulate autoreactive cells that share this idiotope or are linked through an anti-idiotypic interaction (Fig. 9.8B). Microorganisms use cell surface molecules as attachment sites, therefore if a response is generated against the microbial structure an anti-idiotypic antibody to this will be an autoantibody. The consequences for the host could be quite devastating since a number of microorganisms use important molecules as their site of attachment and entry (Fig. 9.8C). This can be extended to include the other mechanisms described above. In Figure 9.8D a viral infection has induced a neoantigen on the cell surface that is able to provide help for B-cells that produce antihormone antibody. This antibody will be capable of binding to the hormone-producing cells and instigating cell damage. In addition, anti-idiotypic antibodies generated against this antibody will have anti-receptor activity.

Since proper antigen presentation is essential for the initiation of an immune response it is possible that defects in antigen-presenting cells or aberrant expression of MHC class II antigens may lead to an autoimmune response. Undoubtedly, autoimmune diseases have a multifactorial aetiology and a number of the proposed mechanisms may contribute in different combinations to different disorders.

In the last few years the T_H1 subset of T-cells has been shown to be involved in the induction of experimental autoimmune diseases mainly based on the ability of adoptively transferred $CD4^+$ T-cells producing T_H1-type cytokines to transfer disease. This has been shown in models of experimental allergic encephalomyelitis (EAE) and insulin-dependent diabetes (IDDM). In human organ-specific autoimmune diseases, such as Hashimoto's thyroiditis and Graves' disease, T-cell clones isolated from lymphocyte infiltrates exhibit a clear-cut T_H1 phenotype. In addition T-cell clones derived from peripheral blood or cerebrospinal fluid of multiple sclerosis patients show a T_H1-type lymphokine profile. Cytokine expression in most samples of synovial material of rheumatoid arthritis patients show a T_H1-type pattern but the situation is less clear in other systemic autoimmune disorders such as systemic lupus erythematosus, Sjogren's syndrome and primary vasculitis.

In view of these findings interest is developing in the use of antagonists of IL-12 the critical product of T_H1 T-cells in the induction of autoimmunity. Anti-IL-12 antibodies have been shown to inhibit the development of experimental IDDM and EAE. The IL-12 receptor (IL-12R) subunit has recently been cloned and could be used as a possible antagonist.

Other diseases associated with autoimmune states

There is a large reservoir of diseases in which some form of autoantibody has been found but where neither the stimulus for autoantibody formation nor the role, if any, of immune reactions has been elucidated.

Rheumatoid arthritis

Rheumatoid arthritis (RA) is a condition in which an IgM antibody called rheumatoid factor is present in the serum. This antibody is detected in vitro by its ability to agglutinate red cells or latex particles which have been coated with IgG globulin (p. 337). The rheumatoid factor does not appear to be directly involved in the pathogenesis of the disease and no satisfactory explanation has been offered to account for its pathogenesis.

Rheumatoid factors react with the $C\gamma 2$ domain of the Fc fragment of IgG (rabbit or human) but not with the Fab fragment. Rheumatoid factors are sometimes found in patients with diseases other than rheumatoid arthritis. These include systemic lupus erythematosus, Sjogren's syndrome, scleroderma, lymphoproliferative disease and in certain persistent bacterial, protozoal and viral infections. Even healthy subjects sometimes have low titres of the factor in their serum, particularly in the older age groups.

Eighty to ninety percent of patients with RA express either the HLA-DR4 or DR1 products of the class II MHC genes with more severe forms of the disease associated with HLA-DR4. The proposal that susceptibility to RA is related to a shared epitope on the HLA molecule is supported by the finding of similar amino acid sequences between residues 70 to 74 in HLA-DR1 and HLA-DR4 subtypes Dw4, Dw14 and Dw15. The inheritance pattern of RA does not fit a single gene model and additional genetic factors appear to be involved.

In addition to the rheumatoid factor of the IgG class there are also IgA and IgM rheumatoid factors as well as antibodies against collagen types II, IX, XI and other matrix proteins. Other autoantibodies are found against chondrocytes, endothelial cells and granulocyte-specific antinuclear antibodies in addition to non-tissue specific antibodies to heat shock protein, antinuclear antibody and keratin antibodies. The IgG in patients with RA show reduced glycosylation in the Fc region associated with low levels of B-cell galactosyl transferase. This defect is not restricted to RA and its role, if any, in the disease has yet to be established.

Joint immunopathology in RA

Immune complexes containing IgG, IgM and complement components are found both in the circulation and in joints, and $CD4^+$ lymphocytes predominate over those with the $CD8^+$ marker in the synovium. Memory T-cells are also present expressing activation markers such as class II HLA and IL-2R. There are also abundant B-lymphocytes and other antigen-presenting cells. These synovial lymphocytes appear to be involved in the processes leading to autoantibody formation and development of immune complexes. Recruitment of these cells to the joints appears to be due to the effects of cytokines such as IL-1, TNF-alpha and IFN-gamma that augment the expression of adhesion molecules in the network of blood vessels in the synovial membrane. Chemotactic factors such as IL-8 and split complement products are present and contribute to cell migration into the joint. Immunochemical studies of mRNA in RA synovial membranes have confirmed the finding of proinflammatory cytokines in synovial fluid. The cytokine ligands TNF-alpha and IL-1 receptors are highly expressed by RA synovial cells. The cytokine TNF-alpha that has been identified in synovial fluid appears to be predominantly involved in the pathogenesis of the disease in view of its wide-ranging biological effects that include enhanced HLA class II expression and T- and B-cell activation along with induction of adhesion molecules on endothelial cells, bone and cartilage resorption. TNF-alpha also induces IL-1 and GM-CSF production and collagenase and prostaglandin E_2.

Developments in immunotherapy

The above findings, along with the success of experiments in a mouse model of arthritis in which TNF-alpha was neutralized by blocking antibodies, have led to controlled trials in RA patients of injected chimeric (human/mouse) monoclonal antibody to TNF-alpha. Significant clinical responses with reduction in acute phase protein, serum amyloid and IL-6 levels were found. Such approaches have suggested a variety of TNF-alpha blocking procedures such as blocking its cell receptor either with antibody or by soluble TNFR itself to mop up free TNF-alpha. This has been the most successful form of therapy to date although the relative roles of TNF-alpha and interleukin-1 are still unclear. It is believed that TNF-alpha is the lead cytokine responsible for the release of others although some workers consider that the two cytokines are responsible for different pathogenic processes. Results of trials in humans indicates that using anti-TNF monoclonal antibodies brings about suppression of active arthritis but the effect only lasts a matter of weeks. Another recent approach has been the use of anti-cytokine drugs such as tenidap, which appears in trials to be effective. It is to be hoped that procedures of this type will eventually revolutionize the therapy of this disabling disease.

An interesting new development based on animal models, oral tolerance, has been induced as a way of preventing and treating autoimmune diseases, for example using the autoantigen combined with recombinant cholera toxin B. This has been successful in treating autoimmune encephalitis, insulin-dependent diabetes and collagen-induced arthritis. Oral tolerance strategies for use in clinical trials have been developed in the USA for the treatment of multiple sclerosis, rheumatoid arthritis, uveitis and insulin-dependent diabetes. In rheumatoid arthritis, feeding with collagen type 2 reduced both the time to disease remission and disease severity at a statistically significant level. Induction of oral tolerance appears to be reflected in reduction of IgE and delayed hypersensitivity responses rather than IgG or IgA responses.

Possible initiating causes of RA

It is widely believed that rheumatoid arthritis is triggered by an unknown antigenic peptide presented to CD4$^+$ T-cells by a MHC class II molecule resulting in the triggering of an inflammatory cascade in the synovium involving infiltration by various cells of the immune system that produce cytokines and growth factors in the joint.

The possibility has been suggested that infective agents are involved, such as mycoplasma or chronic infective bacterial agents, and there are reports of the isolation of such agents from rheumatoid joints in humans and in arthritis in a number of other species. One suggestion is that the infective agent may modify the lymphoid tissues so that there is a failure of the normal tolerance control mechanisms (see above and p. 139). This might involve activation of pre-existing autoimmune T-cells inducing polyclonal B-cell activation, or the infective agent sharing epitopes with autoantigens on host cells. Experimental arthritis can be induced in rats by the injection of Freund's complete adjuvant containing killed tubercle bacilli. This is a polyarthritis with mononuclear cell infiltration similar to the arthritis found in a human illness known as Reiter's syndrome, the main features of which are urethritis and arthritis and which may occur in the presence of a mycoplasma infection. *Mycoplasma arthritidis* can also induce acute and chronic joint inflammation in rats and mice similar to that in rheumatoid arthritis. Uveitis, conjunctivitis and urethritis are also sometimes found. Mycoplasmas produce a mitogen (MAM) that is a potent inducer of gamma-interferon in both murine and human lymphocytes. MAM is a member of a group of microbial toxins known as **superantigens** that induce a polyclonal B-cell response through an action in mice carrying I-E molecules. MAM is believed to act as a bridge between T-helper cells and B-cells that express a receptor for MAM (I-E in mice).

The mechanism underlying the appearance of these rheumatoid (antiglobulin) factors is not clear. In chronic infections it is conceivable that the factor is a response to antigenic determinants on the IgG molecule that are exposed when IgG antibody complexes with the infective agent. In the healthy individual a low titre of rheumatoid factor may perhaps serve a physiological function as a way of clearing degraded immunoglobulin molecules arising during infective or inflammatory processes. HLA-B27 individuals who become infected with *Salmonella, Yersinia, Shigella* and gonococci often develop arthritis (ankylosing spondylitis), suggesting that HLA-B27 acts in conjunction with the bacterial infection to cause the development of autoantibodies. Transgenic rats expressing many copies of a B27 subtype gene (B*2705) and the human gene encoding β_2-microglobulin develop a form of arthritis that shares many features of ankylosing spondylitis. In the human disease no bacteria have been cultured so far from the synovial fluid of patients with this form of arthritis. The prevalence among B27$^+$ individuals of this form of arthritis is some fivefold higher than that in the general population in a Dutch study and increases another tenfold in B27 first-degree relatives of B27 patients indicating that genetic factors other than B27 must be involved in the pathogenesis.

Recent evidence has emerged indicating that patients with rheumatoid arthritis show enhanced responses to conserved bacterial products known as heat shock proteins and has stimulated considerable interest among immunologists and rheumatologists as a possible explanation for the pathogenesis of the disease. Heat shock proteins (HSPs) were first shown to be produced by cells in culture when their temperature was raised above 37°C. Their production has since been demonstrated in a wide range of eukaryotic and prokaryotic cells with extensive structural homology and cross-reactivity between foreign and self HSPs. HSPs are normally engaged in the stabilization of newly synthesized polypeptides in order to ensure correct protein folding and intracellular transport of proteins for secretion from cells. Since fever is a physiological stimulus to HSP production, it may exert beneficial effects on the repair of damaged proteins in inflammation. Because of the cross-reactivity between microbial and mammalian HSPs their generation within infected cells may lead to an autoimmune response. Raised levels of antibodies to the 65 kD HSP of mycobacteria have been found in the serum of patients with rheumatoid arthritis, their synovial T-lymphocytes proliferate in vitro to this HSP and epitopes of the HSP can be found in the synovial tissue. Additional evidence for the importance of HSPs in arthritis is the finding that Lewis rats that are susceptible to the development of adjuvant arthritis can be protected by vaccination with mycobacterial HSP. Furthermore, the sensitivity of individual animals to develop adjuvant arthritis seems to depend on the ability of their T-cells to respond to HSPs. It has recently been suggested that responses to HSPs may be related to a genetically inherited defect in the regulation of T-cell development so that a population of fetal type T-cells (with a $\gamma\delta$ T-cell receptor) and B-cells of B-1 (CD5$^+$) type are expanded in patients with rheumatoid arthritis. It is hoped that these various observations will lead to a clearer understanding of the mechanisms underlying the pathogenesis of rheumatic diseases.

Diabetes mellitus of the insulin-dependent type is believed to involve both an inherited susceptibility (Table 9.6) and environmental factors in the pathogenesis. The details of these interacting factors and their role are poorly understood. Susceptibility to the disease shows linkage to HLA haplotype inheritance within families, whatever the actual HLA phenotypes may be. A child that is of identical HLA phenotype to a diabetic sibling is likely to be susceptible. Peak incidence of the disease is between 10 and 14 years with a prevalence in white western populations of 0.25%, showing seasonal fluctuation and a slight predominance in males. More than 90% of patients have HLA-DR3, -DR4 or both and there is a negative association with HLA-DR2. A new susceptibility locus has recently been identified on the long arm of chromosome 11 and in some families linkage with loci on the long arm of chromosome 6, chromosome 18 and chromosome 8 has been noted.

Patients show evidence of lymphocytic infiltration (particularly CD8 T-cells) in the pancreatic islets even before glucose intolerance is found. Eventually destruction of beta cells occurs with atrophy and scarring. Autoantibody against pancreatic islet cells is found in 50–80% of these individuals and, when it is of the complement-fixing type, seems to lead to islet cell damage. The antibody appears early in the disease before clinically obvious diabetes and serves as a marker of islet cell damage before progression to insulin insufficiency. This suggests the possibility for development of measures to arrest islet cell destruction before diabetes occurs. More recently an insulin autoantibody has also been found in the prediabetic preinsulin treatment phase. In diabetes the pathological changes include the presence of inflammatory cells surrounding the islets (insulitis) and the presence of MHC class II molecules on islet cells. The latter finding led to the hypothesis that the MHC class II molecules might be responsible for presenting the islet cell antigens to T-helper cells but experimental studies on hyperexpression of MHC antigens on pancreatic islet cells have not so far supported this hypothesis. Local expression of interferon-gamma and other cytokines in the pancreas has been shown to lead to destruction of the islet cells and raises the possibility that a virus infection with a consequent host cytokine response could be responsible for the pathological changes. Although Coxsackie viruses are known to infect islet cells (as well as the myocardium) it has not been possible to implicate the virus in the pathogenesis of type 1 diabetes. Animal models of the disease suggest that there are defects in the immune regulation with depletion of a subset of T-cells (RT6$^+$ T-cells).

Multiple sclerosis (MS), another disease believed to have an autoimmune basis, is associated with a variety of HLA antigens (A3, B7, DR2) with DR2 showing the highest relative risk of 4.1 compared with approximately 2 for each of the other antigens. Subgroups of DR2 also appear to be involved. In a large survey of Canadian MS patients over half were DR2 compared to 28% in controls. Relative risk rates have been estimated as above 5% for siblings of patients and for their parents, aunts and uncles. In contrast, it is about 1% for children of patients compared with 0.1% for the population at large. The multifactorial basis of the disease is emphasized by the finding that Lapps and gypsies, over 50% of whom are DR2, have a very low incidence of MS. The increased prevalence of the disease at higher latitudes appears to be accounted for by the percentage of the population of Scandinavian ancestry. The DR2 association is a feature of northern European populations whilst in Japan the strongest association is with DR6. A large amount of contradictory data has been reported and it seems likely that different genetic backgrounds with various environmental factors may produce different susceptibility patterns. It is likely that loci in addition to HLA, along with environmental influences, are also involved. Recent evidence implicates particular haplotypes of the T-cell receptor (TCR).

Like rheumatoid arthritis the nature of the initiating event is unknown. A number of viruses produce demyelinating disease in animals, such as canine distemper virus, visna virus in sheep and goats and murine encephalitis viruses. This has led to the suggestion that molecular mimicry between viral antigens and host tissue antigens may exist and be responsible for autoimmunization. In a recent report, HTLV-like viral RNA has been found in cells cultured from the CSF of MS patients. The disease takes two main forms — relapsing–remitting or chronic progressing — and is characterized by perivascular cellular infiltrates and demyelination of the white matter of the central nervous system. The plaques that are formed show a depletion of oligodendroglial cells and proliferation of astrocytes. Evidence for a possible immune pathogenesis comes from the finding of macrophage-like cells with lipid inclusions and lymphoid cells in these lesions. Identification of the cell types has become possible using monoclonal antibodies to a variety of cell surface markers. Large numbers of cells bearing MHC class II molecules are present at the edges of the plaques decreasing towards the centre. $CD4^+$ and $CD8^+$ cells have also been found both around and within the plaques but no B-cells. The experimental disease in rats is believed to be mediated by $CD4^+$ T-cells that secrete IFN-gamma and TNF-beta. IFN-gamma up-regulates expression of MHC class II and adhesion molecules on cerebrovascular endothelial cells in the CNS which facilitate attachment and penetration of T-cells into the CNS parenchyma. Once past the blood–brain barrier inflammatory cytokines are released along with oedema due to permeability changes in the endothelium. There is extensive evidence from work with animal models of the disease in which demyelination can be induced by immunization with myelin basic protein and in which susceptibility can be transferred to normal animals by spleen cells of the immunized donors. More recently,

T-cell clones have been developed with specificity for myelin basic protein that produce typical disease in rats. Encephalitogenic epitopes have been identified in myelin basic protein and the immune response to these has been found to be dependent on the TCR repertoire and MHC class II restriction elements that are available to the responder animal strain. Some epitopes appear to be restricted by the rat homologue of I-A whilst others are restricted by the homologue of I-E.

Similar genetic associations have been reported in humans with strong associations with DR genes as noted above; these genes are also the human homologue of mouse I-E genes.

Therapeutic approaches

Work in the Lewis rat model of the disease has shown that rats could be protected by immunization with synthetic peptides corresponding to the CDR2 segment of $V_\beta 8$ TCR. This type of approach has led to clinical trials with TCR peptides and attempts to induce tolerance to MBP by oral feeding. No significant clinical improvement has so far been achieved by these approaches. More successful are trials in which patients are given subcutaneous injections of IFN-beta that have led to a significant reduction compared to placebo-treated controls in exacerbation rates and a marked decrease in active lesions as evaluated by magnetic resonance imaging. It is not clear if the effects are achieved by the antiviral activity of IFN-beta or its ability to down-regulate TNF and IFN-gamma.

Myasthenia gravis

The main feature of **myasthenia gravis** is muscle weakness due to a disorder of neuromuscular transmission. The prevalence is between 2 and 10 per 100 000 and can occur at all ages. There is sometimes an association with the presence of a thymoma, thymic hyperplasia and autoantibodies. Before the age of 40 and in the absence of a thymoma females appear to be more susceptible and there is an association with HLA-A1, -B8 and -DR3. In contrast, patients over 40 without a thymoma show an association with HLA-A3, -B7 and -DR2 with a preponderance of males. Patients with a thymoma over the age of 40 show no sex or HLA association. There is frequently an association with other autoimmune conditions (e.g. systemic lupus erythematosus).

Anti-acetylcholine receptor antibodies are found in 90% of patients. These antibodies and immune complexes induce complement-mediated destruction of the post-synaptic membrane with loss of receptor sites for acetylcholine. Anti-cholinesterase drugs and thymectomy are the mainstay of treatment as well as the use of immunosuppressive agents and/or plasmapheresis to remove the antibody. In experimental models of the disease in mice, monoclonal antibodies to $CD4^+$ T-lymphocytes suppressed established disease and prevented loss of acetylcholine receptors. Similar approaches have been applied to mouse models of systemic lupus, experimental autoimmune encephalomyelitis and collagen-induced arthritis. An interesting development is the use of monoclonal antibodies against a single T-cell clone specific for myelin basic protein that appears to protect rats from the development of experimental autoimmune encephalitis.

Although the possible side-effects of therapy that is directed at lymphocyte sub-populations (e.g. susceptibility to infection) are unknown it seems likely that this approach will be tested in patients with severe life-threatening forms of autoimmune disease in which other forms of therapy have proved ineffective.

Table 9.7 gives some examples of autoimmune diseases and the autoantibodies found.

Antibodies as a consequence of tissue damage

In considering the role of autoantibodies as a possible cause of autoimmune disease it should be remembered that antibodies of IgM type, directed at subcellular antigens, can be readily induced by various forms of tissue damage. These arise secondarily to the damage and appear to have no role in perpetuating it. Antibodies of this type have been shown in the author's laboratory and can readily be induced in rats by the injection of the hepatotoxic agent carbon tetrachloride. It was subsequently found that normal rats, mice and hamsters have some IgM antitissue antibody in their serum. A possible physiological

---

Table 9.7 Examples of autoantibodies in disease

Disease	Autoantibody specificity
Autoimmune haemolytic anaemia	Erythrocytes
Thrombocytopenic purpura	Platelets
Systemic lupus erythematosus	Nuclear antigens and antigens of various tissues and blood cells
Rheumatoid arthritis	Immunoglobulin G
Primary biliary cirrhosis	Mitochondria
Ulcerative colitis	Colon lipopolysaccharide
Hashimoto's thyroiditis	Thyroglobulin
Thyrotoxicosis	Cell surface thyroid-stimulating hormone (TSH) receptors
Pernicious anaemia	Intrinsic factor
Myasthenia gravis	Acetylcholine receptors (and certain muscle tissue)
Juvenile diabetes (type 1)	Islet cell surface

role for these antibodies is suggested by the finding in vitro of a chemotactic effect on rat polymorphs of a mixture of the antitissue antibody and its antigen. Thus the antibody might be responsible for initiating a phagocytic cell clearing process to deal with the breakdown products of normal cell turnover.

Recent evidence indicates that IgG antibody existing in the normal individual seems to be able to recognize glycoprotein determinants which appear on aged red blood cells. These determinants are exposed following the loss of sialic acid groups from the outside of the cells on ageing. Their exposure can be reproduced experimentally by treatment with neuraminidase. The IgG antibodies bind to the exposed glycoprotein and enable the attachment of the red cell to the Fc receptors on a macrophage. The aged red cell is then phagocytosed and destroyed by the lysosomal enzymes of the macrophage.

All autoantibodies are therefore not necessarily autoaggressive, although the history of immunity and protection inculcates the idea of antibodies acting solely as aggressive agents.

FURTHER READING

Hypersensitivity states
Coleman R M, Lombard M F, Sicard R E 1992 Hypersensitivity. Fundamental immunology, 2nd edn. Wm. C. Brown, Dubuque
Lawlor G J, Fischer T J, Adelmann D C (eds) 1994 Manual of allergy and immunology. 3rd edn. Little Brown, Boston
Middleton E et al (eds) 1993 Allergy principles and practice, 4th edn. C V Mosby, St Louis

Immune deficiency states
Ammann A J 1991 Antibody (B-cell) immunodeficiency disorders. In: Stites D P, Terr A I (eds) Basic and clinical immunology. Appleton and Lange, Norwalk, Conn., p. 322–361
Montagnier L, Gluckman J-C (eds) 1990 Immunodeficiency. Current Opinion in Immunology 2: 397–450
Seligmann M 1989 Primary immunodeficiencies: current findings and concepts. In: Melchers F et al (eds) Progress in immunology. Springer Verlag, Berlin

Autoimmunity
Burnet F M 1959 The clonal selection theory of acquired immunity. Cambridge University Press, Cambridge
Chapel H, Maeney M 1993 Essentials of clinical immunology. 3rd edn. Blackwell Scientific Publications, Oxford
Coleman R M, Lombard M F, Sicard R E 1992 Autoimmunity. Fundamental immunology, 2nd edn. Wm. C. Brown, Dubuque
Feltkamp T E W, Khan M A and de Castro J 1996 The pathogenetic role of HLA-B27. Immunology Today 17: 5
Gupta S, Talal N 1986 Immunology of rheumatic diseases. Plenum Publishing Corporation, New York
Kagnoff M F 1996 Mucosal Immunology: new frontiers. Immunology Today 17: 57

Kingseley G, Lanchbury J, Panayi G 1996 Immunotherapy in rheumatic disease: an idea whose time has come — or gone? Immunology Today 17: 9

Ottenhoff T H M 1996 Selective modulation of T-cell responses in autoimmunity and cancer. Immunology Today 17: 54

Schoenfeld Y, Isenberg D 1989 The mosaic of autoimmunity. Elsevier, Amsterdam

Schwartz R S (ed) 1990 Autoimmunity. Current Opinion in Immunology 2: 565

Taussig M J 1984 Processes in pathology and microbiology, 2nd edn. Blackwell Scientific Publications, Oxford

Taylor P C, Cope A P, Feldman M, Maini R N 1995 Autoimmunity and rheumatoid arthritis. Hospital Update 21: 462, 510

Theofilopoulos A N 1995 The basis of autoimunity: Part 11 Genetic predisposition. Immunology Today 16: 150

Trembleau S, Germann T, Gately M K, Adorini L 1995 The role of IL-12 in the induction of organ-specific autoimmune diseases. Immunology Today 16: 383

World Health Organization 1977 Immune complexes in disease. Report of a WHO scientific group. WHO, Technical report series no. 606

10 Interaction of antibody with antigen and applications in laboratory investigations

An antibody, as has been pointed out, is a molecule secreted into the tissue fluids from lymphoid cells which have been exposed to a foreign substance — and antigen. An antigen may be potentially harmful, such as bacterium or virus, or it may be a harmless bland substance such as foreign serum protein. The antibody can combine only with antigen which is identical or nearly identical with the inducing antigen and not with unrelated antigens. When antibody and antigen are brought together in solution, they interact with each other by the formation of a link between an antigen-binding site on the immunoglobulin molecule — part of the Fab portion known as the paratope — and the particular chemical groupings which make up what is termed the antigenic determinant or epitope of the antigen molecule. The molecules are held together by **non-covalent intermolecular forces** which are effective only when the antigen-binding site and the antigenic determinant group are able to make close contact. The better the fit, the closer the contact and the stronger the antigen–antibody bond. These factors determine what is often called the **affinity** of the antibody molecule. Antibodies of varying combining quality exist and the overall tendency to combine with antigen is the average ability of the antibodies to combine with antigen or the average intrinsic association constant. This can be calculated experimentally by application of the concepts of chemical equilibria to antigen–antibody interactions. Studies of this type have shown that the affinity of antibodies increases as immunization proceeds and that the dose of antigen can influence the quality of antibody (see p. 114).

The methods used for the detection of antigen–antibody reactions in the laboratory fall into two functional groups. The first group consists of procedures designed to elucidate the cytodynamics of antibody formation which involve the study of the behaviour of single cells or small populations of cells. The second group, which is the subject of the present discussion, concerns the detection and quantitation of **secreted antibody** circulating in the blood or present in the tissue fluids.

The methods used here range in their application from highly specialized studies of the physico-chemical aspects of antigen–antibody interaction to widely used procedures designed to aid in the diagnosis of disease.

PRIMARY INTERACTION AND SECONDARY EFFECTS

In practical terms, the union of antibody with antigen can be detected at two different levels. The first level is that following **primary union** of the two reactants and usually requires that one or other reactant is labelled with a suitable marker such as a fluorescent dye or a radioactive isotope. A simple example of this is the microscopic localization in a tissue of a particular microorganism utilizing an antiserum prepared against the microorganism and labelled with a dye that fluoresces under UV light. A widely used method in experimental immunology makes use of the fact that immunoglobulins are insoluble in 50% saturated ammonium sulphate. The test, developed by Farr, uses antigen labelled with ^{125}I that is mixed with antibody-containing serum and left to equilibrate. Ammonium sulphate solution is then added to the mixture, resulting in the precipitation of the antibody together with any labelled antigen bound to it. The unbound antigen remains in solution (only antigens that are themselves soluble in 50% ammonium sulphate can be used in this form of the test). The quantity of isotope-labelled antigen bound to the salt-precipitated antibody is then estimated by placing the washed precipitate in radioactive counting equipment. This sensitive and useful technique is a measure of the capacity of an antiserum to bind antigen.

The second level at which antigen–antibody combination can be detected depends on the development, after primary union, of certain changes in the physical state of the complex, resulting in precipitation or agglutination of the components or, alternatively, in the activation of non-antibody components such as serum complement or histamine from mast cells. Reactions of this type occurring subsequent to primary union are termed **secondary phenomena**. This discussion is concerned with the principles of a few of these secondary phenomena that are in common use.

Secondary effects: interpretation and applications

Before considering these reactions individually, it is important to be aware of the difficulties in interpreting the results of such tests. The initiation and development of the secondary phenomena constitute a complicated series of events involving many variables such as the type of antibody taking part, the relative proportions of antibody and antigen, characteristics of the antigen molecule, presence of electrolytes, inhibitory substances and unstable components.

Despite these formidable difficulties, the widely and long-used secondary phenomena, such as precipitation, agglutination and complement fixation, have an important role to play as aids in the diagnosis of disease and in the identification of microorganisms.

The secondary phenomena can bring about several readily observable changes when carried out in vitro. These are used in tests to demonstrate the presence of antibody in the sera of patients suffering from infectious disease or producing an antibody response to cell antigens as might, for example, occur after incompatible blood transfusion, tissue grafting or in autoimmune states.

Reactions of this type can also be used to identify antigens in the tissues or body fluids and, for example, would be utilized for blood grouping, tissue typing or the identification of microorganisms.

Among the most important of these reactions are **precipitation**, which occurs between antibody and antigen molecules in soluble form, **agglutination**, in which the antibodies directed against surface antigens of particulate materials such as microorganisms or erythrocytes link them together in large clumps or aggregates, and **complement fixation** in which antibody molecules, after reaction with antigen, activate the complex blood components that make up serum complement.

In addition to these widely used serological tests, a number of other effects of antigen–antibody interaction are of medical importance. These include **neutralization** tests used, for example, in virus identification, **immobilization** tests with bacteria and protozoa, and **skin tests** for the reaginic antibody characteristic of anaphylactic states.

Precipitation

Optimal proportions

As a result of the interaction of antibody and antigen molecules in solution, complexes of the two types of molecule will form and precipitation may occur depending on the relative concentration of the two reactants. If a series of tubes is set up (Fig. 10.1), each containing a constant amount of antiserum, and decreasing amounts of antigen are added to the tubes in the row, a haziness will start to appear in the tubes gradually increasing to clearly visible **aggregates** or **precipitates**. The amount of precipitation will be seen to increase along the row, reaching a maximum and then falling off with the lower antigen concentration. The tubes where most precipitate appears contain the

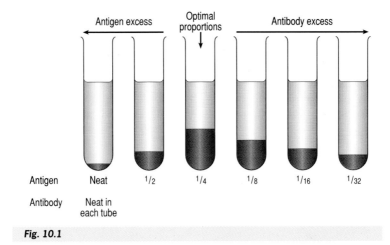

Fig. 10.1

optimal proportions of antigen and antibody for precipitation. The
composition of the precipitate varies with the original proportions of
the antibody and antigen; if antigen is in excess the precipitate will
contain relatively more of this component and similarly more antibody
if it is present in excess. As can be seen from Figure 10.2, on the antigen excess side of optimal proportions less precipitate appears. This is
due to the inability of the antigen–antibody complexes formed to link
up to other complexes and so a large aggregate or lattice is made,
which will appear as a visible precipitate (tube 1, Fig. 10.2). Large
aggregates of antibody and antigen can form best under conditions of
optimal proportions where the antibody and antigen proportions are
such that after initial combination of the molecules, free antigen-binding
sites and antigen determinant groups remain, enabling the complexes to
link up into a large lattice formation (as in tube 2 of Fig. 10.2). In antibody excess all the free determinants of the antigen molecule are soon
taken up with antibody, so that very little linking can take place
between the complexes (as in tube 3 of Fig. 10.2).

Applications

The precipitin test can be carried out in a quantitative manner by esti-
mating the protein content of the precipitate at optimal proportions.
The qualitative test is much more widely used and is of considerable
value in detecting and identifying antigens, having applications in the
typing of streptococci or pneumococci. This is done by layering an
extract of the organism over antiserum. After a short while, a ring of
precipitate forms at the interface (this is called the ring test). The technique is also used in forensic studies and in detecting adulteration of

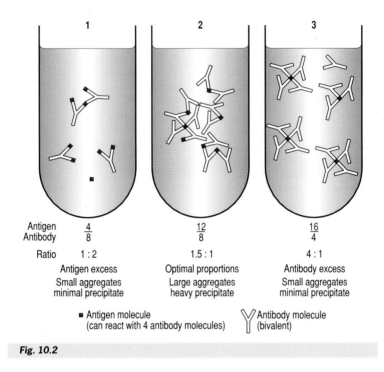

Antigen	$\frac{4}{8}$	$\frac{12}{8}$	$\frac{16}{4}$
Antibody			
Ratio	1 : 2	1.5 : 1	4 : 1
	Antigen excess	Optimal proportions	Antibody excess
	Small aggregates minimal precipitate	Large aggregates heavy precipitate	Small aggregates minimal precipitate

■ Antigen molecule (can react with 4 antibody molecules)   Y Antibody molecule (bivalent)

Fig. 10.2

foodstuffs. A modification of the test in which precipitation is allowed to occur in **agar gel** is very widely used for detecting the presence of antibody in serum or antigen in unknown preparations, and is valuable for showing the identity of different antigen preparations (Fig. 10.3). A concentration gradient forms in the gel, the concentration of a substance decreasing as the molecules diffuse away from the well in which they were placed. **Precipitin bands** form in the gel in the position where the antigen and antibody molecules reach optimal proportions after diffusion.

Applications

When a large number of different antigens are present in a solution, it is difficult to separate the precipitin bands for each of the antigen–antibody reactions by the simple gel-diffusion method just described. In such a situation, a variation of this method can be used to identify the individual components. This modification is particularly valuable in analysing a multicomponent system such as serum. The individual components of serum are first separated by electrophoresis in agar gel and an antiserum, prepared against the serum, is allowed to diffuse

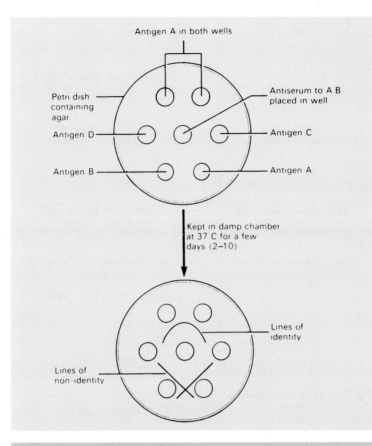

Fig. 10.3 Immunodiffusion or gel diffusion test.
Wells are cut in a layer of agar in a Petri dish. Antiserum and antigen solutions are placed opposite each other in the wells and after allowing a few days for diffusion to take place precipitin bands will form where antibody and antigen meet in suitable proportions (optimal proportions). No reactions take place with antigens C and D as the antiserum in the central well contains antibodies only for antigens A and B. Lines of identity as formed between the two A wells enable the technique to be used for identifying unknown antigens.

towards the separated components, resulting in the formation of precipitin bands (Fig. 10.4). This method, known as **immunoelectrophoresis**, is particularly valuable for showing the presence of abnormal globulin constituents in the serum of patients with myelomatosis and other serum protein abnormalities.

A microimmunodiffusion test with wells cut in a layer of agar on a microscope slide is a convenient modification of the Petri dish method. This procedure has been used for the detection in human

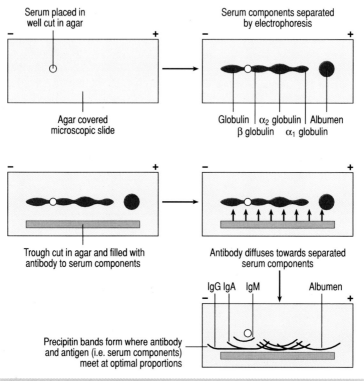

Serum placed in
well cut in agar

Serum components separated
by electrophoresis

Agar covered
microscopic slide

Globulin | α₂ globulin | Albumen
β globulin   α₁ globulin

Trough cut in agar and filled with
antibody to serum components

Antibody diffuses towards separated
serum components

IgG IgA   IgM   Albumen

Precipitin bands form where antibody
and antigen (i.e. serum components)
meet at optimal proportions

Fig. 10.4 Immunoelectrophoresis.
The antigen, for example serum, is placed in a small well cut in a layer of agar on a
microscope slide. A direct current is applied and differential migration of the serum
components takes place. (They are not normally visible in the agar and will show up only if
suitably stained.) After electrophoresis for an hour or so, a trough is cut longitudinally in the
agar and an antiserum against the electrophoresed antigen is placed in the trough. The two
components diffuse towards each other and precipitin bands form. These can be shown up
more clearly by staining with a protein stain. This is a very powerful analytic technique and
can show up about 30 different components in human serum compared with 4 or 5 by
electrophoresis.

serum of the **hepatitis B antigen** which is associated with serum
hepatitis although a radioimmunoassay (see p. 330) is now available.
The routine screening of blood products by this technique using
specific antisera prepared in animals is likely to become an important
laboratory test in the prevention of serum hepatitis outbreaks.

Instead of placing antibody and antigen in separate wells and allowing them to diffuse towards each other, the antibody can be incorporated in the agar and the antigen placed in wells. This technique is
known as **single radial immunodiffusion** and depends upon diffusion of antigen from the well until a point is reached where the con-

centration is optimal for precipitation to occur. Close to the antigen well the concentration of antigen will be high and although the antigen will combine with antibody in the agar, the complexes will be unable to form the large lattice structure necessary for precipitation to take place (Fig. 10.2) and will thus remain as soluble complexes. The precipitin band that forms at optimal proportions of antigen and antibody will show up as a ring around the antigen well. The distance the ring forms from the antigen well will be dependent on the concentration of the antigen in the well. In practice the **diameter** of the ring is measured around a well containing an unknown concentration of antigen and this is compared with the diameter of the rings formed with known concentrations of the antigen, thus enabling the estimation of the concentration of antigen in the unknown preparation.

This technique is widely used to estimate the quantity of the various immunoglobulin classes in human serum samples. An antiserum to a particular immunoglobulin class (e.g. IgG) is incorporated in the agar and the test serum sample is placed in a well. The diameter of the precipitation band that forms after incubation is then compared to the diameter obtained with standard IgG preparations of known concentration. The diameters of the rings with the **standard** IgG preparations (e.g. three or four dilutions of a known concentration) can be plotted graphically against the concentration of IgG and the diameter obtained with the unknown sample can be read off against concentration on this reference graph (Fig. 10.5).

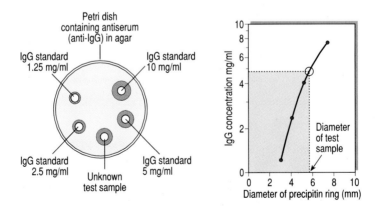

Fig. 10.5 **Diagram of single radial immunodiffusion plate with antiserum incorporated in agar and antigen dilutions and test sample in wells.**
Reference graph drawn using three concentrations of antigen standard showing the diameter of precipitin ring obtained with each concentration (●). Diameter of unknown sample (○) when plotted enables determination of its antigen concentration.

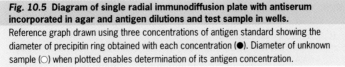

Agglutination

In this reaction the antigen is part of the surface of some particulate material such as a red cell, bacterium or perhaps an inorganic particle (e.g. polystyrene latex) which has been coated with antigen. Antibody added to a suspension of such particles combines with the surface antigens and links them together to form clearly visible aggregates or agglutinates (Fig. 10.6). In its simplest form an agglutination test is set up in round-bottomed test tubes or perspex plates with round-bottomed wells and doubling dilutions of the antiserum are made up in the tubes (neat, 1:2, 1:4, 1:8, etc.). The particulate antigen is then added and after incubation at 37°C agglutination is seen in the bottom of the tubes. The last tube showing clearly visible agglutination is the end point of the test. The reciprocal of the antiserum dilution at the end point is known as the **titre** of the antiserum and is a measure of the number of antibody units per unit volume of serum, e.g. if the end point occurs at a 1/256 dilution of the antiserum and if the test has been carried out in 1 ml volumes, the titre of the serum is 256 units per ml of serum.

One practical difficulty of importance in agglutination tests is the occasional inhibition of agglutination in the first tubes of an antiserum dilution series, agglutination occurring only in those tubes containing more dilute antiserum. This is known as the **prozone phenomenon** and is probably, in part, due to the stabilizing effects of high protein

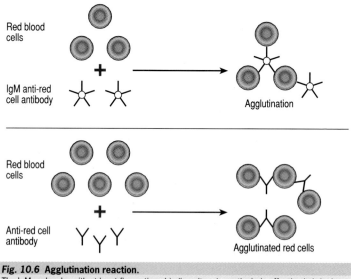

Fig. 10.6 Agglutination reaction.
The IgM molecule, with at least five antigen-binding sites, is particularly effective in bringing about agglutination.

concentration on the particles. The protein coats the particles, increases their net charge and so brings about increased electrostatic repulsion between individual particles, thus opposing the efforts of the antibody molecules to link the particles together. However, once the protein concentration is reduced by dilution the antibody molecules can then exert their aggregating effect and bring about agglutination. The agglutination reaction has been shown to require the presence of electrolytes in the suspending medium and is usually performed for this reason at physiological salt concentration.

Applications

One of the classical applications of the agglutination test in diagnostic bacteriology is the **Widal test** used for the demonstration of antibodies to salmonellae in serum specimens taken from suspected enteric fever cases. Agglutination is the basic technique used in blood grouping, the A, B, or O group of the red cells under test being determined by agglutination with a specific antiserum — an anti-A serum, for example, will agglutinate A cells but not B or O cells. Red cells and inert particles such as polystyrene latex can be coated with various antigens and suitably coated particles are used in a variety of diagnostic tests such thyroid antibody tests using thyroglobulin-coated cells or latex particles. Hormone-coated red cells or inert particles are used in many hormone assay procedures which are based on the inhibition of the antibody-induced agglutination of the hormone-coated particles by hormone added in the sample under test (Fig. 10.7). Tests of this type are in wide use in pregnancy diagnosis.

Certain viruses, e.g. the myxoviruses causing influenza and mumps, have the property of bringing about agglutination of red cells (haemagglutination). **Inhibition of haemagglutination** by antibody in patient's serum is a widely used diagnostic procedure. The presence of antibody in the patient's serum is thus detected by its ability to link with virus particles and prevent them from bringing about agglutination of the red cells (Fig. 10.8).

IgM antibodies capable of agglutinating human red cells (including those of the individual producing the antibody) between 0 and 4°C are sometimes found in certain human diseases including primary atypical pneumonia, malaria, trypanosomiasis and acquired haemolytic anaemia.

The presence of antibody globulin on a red cell may not result in direct agglutination of the cells, for example in some Rh-negative mothers with Rh-positive infants or in acquired haemolytic anaemia. It is, however, possible to show that the red cells are coated with antibody by using an **antiglobulin** serum (produced in the rabbit by injecting human globulin) which will bring about agglutination of the cells (Fig. 10.9). This is the basis of the Coombs' test which is a very

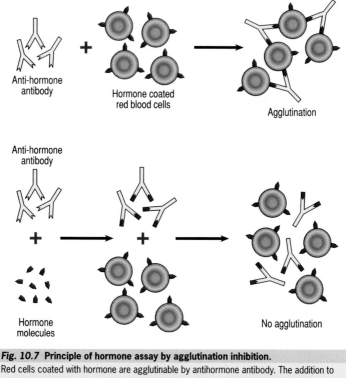

Fig. 10.7 Principle of hormone assay by agglutination inhibition.
Red cells coated with hormone are agglutinable by antihormone antibody. The addition to the antiserum of a test sample containing free hormone will block the antigen-binding sites and prevent agglutination. The test can be carried out quantitatively by comparing the activity of a known standard hormone preparation with the test sample.

widely used serological procedure. The coagulation test depends on the presence of protein A (p. 156) on *Staph. aureus* (Cowan strain 1) that binds to the Fc region of IgG leaving the Fab sites free. Staphylococci with specific antibody attached in this way can be used to detect bacteria in serum or urine or microbial antigens in such fluids. Clumping of the staphylococci indicates a positive test.

Complement fixation

The fact that antibody, once it combines with antigen, is able to activate the complement system is used as a way of showing the presence of a particular antibody in a serum, e.g. the **Wassermann** antibody in syphilis, or in identifying an antigen such as a virus.

The complement of most species will react with antibody derived

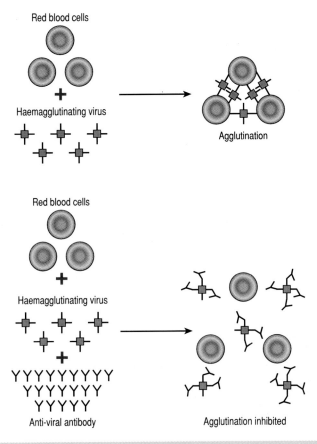

Fig. 10.8 Virus haemagglutination inhibition test.
Red cell agglutination is brought about by a variety of viruses (see text). This can be inhibited by mixing the virus with antiviral antibody as shown in the diagram. The test can be quantitated by comparison of serial dilutions of virus alone and virus-antibody mixture.

from other species and guinea-pig serum is a common laboratory source of complement.

For most antigens the reaction of the complement system with the antigen/antibody complex causes in itself no visible effect and it is necessary to use an indicator system consisting of sheep red cells coated with anti-sheep red cell antibody. In a test the antibody, complement and antigen are first mixed together and after a period of incubation the indicator system, antibody-coated sheep cells, is added. The complement will, however, have been used up during the incubation stage by the original antibody/antigen complex and will not be available to

Anti-red-cell antibody
combined with buried
surface antigen

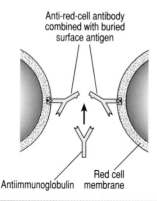

Antiimmunoglobulin   Red cell
membrane

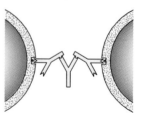

Antiimmunoglobulin combines with
attached anti-red-cell antibody and
link cells together for agglutination

Fig. 10.9 Coombs' antiglobulin test.
The red cell antibody, probably because it is directed against an antigen situated deep in the
cell wall, cannot link two red cells together for agglutination. The addition of an
antiimmunoglobulin (antiglobulin) serum brings about agglutination by linking two attached
immunoglobulins to one another.

lyse the red cells. Thus, a **positive** complement-fixation test is indicated by **absence of lysis** of the red cells whilst a negative test, with
unused complement, is shown by lysis of the red cells (Fig. 10.10).

Indicator system

    +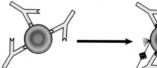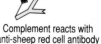

Complement   Sheep red cell coated
with anti-sheep red cell
antibody

Complement reacts with
anti-sheep red cell antibody
and lyses cell

Positive test

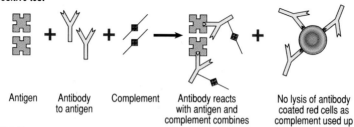

Antigen   Antibody   Complement   Antibody reacts   No lysis of antibody
to antigen   with antigen and   coated red cells as
complement combines   complement used up

Fig. 10.10 Complement fixation test.
The indicator system (sheep red cells coated with antibody to sheep red cells) is normally
lysed in the presence of complement (fresh guinea-pig serum) — top. If another
antibody–antigen system is first mixed with the complement it will no longer be available to
lyse the indicator system — bottom.

Applications

The classical complement fixation test is the Wassermann reaction used in the diagnosis of syphilis. The test system consists of Wassermann antigen mixed with dilutions of the patient's serum in the presence of guinea-pig complement. After the antigen and patient's serum have had time to react and take up the limited amount of complement available in the system, the indicator system is added to show whether or not there is free complement. Controls are included to ensure that none of the reagents are anticomplementary (able to take up complement non-specifically as might occur, for example, with contaminated serum) and positive and negative control sera are tested in parallel. Complement fixation tests are used routinely for detecting viruses in tissue cultures which have been inoculated with specimens of blood or tissue fluids from humans with probable virus infections.

Antigen–antibody reactions using fluorescent labels

The precise localization of tissue antigens or the antigens of infecting organisms in the body, of antitissue antibody and of antigen/antibody complexes was achieved by the introduction of the use of fluorochrome-labelled proteins by Coons and Kaplan in 1950. The adsorption of ultraviolet light between 290 and 495 nm by fluorescein and its emission of longer wavelength green light (525 nm) is used to visualize protein labelled with this dye. The technique is more sensitive than precipitation or complement fixation techniques and fluorescent protein tracers can be detected at a concentration of the order of μg protein per ml body fluid.

Applications

Some of the uses to which the technique has been put include the localization of the origin of a variety of serum protein components, for example immunoglobulin production by plasma cells and other lymphoid cells. The demonstration and localization in the tissues of antibody globulin in a variety of autoimmune conditions has been shown, including an antinuclear antibody in the serum of patients with systemic lupus erythematosus and thyroid autoantibodies in the sera of patients with Hashimoto's thyroiditis. In the diagnostic field most human pathogens can be demonstrated by immunofluorescence and a tentative diagnosis may be made much sooner than by cultivation. The fluorescent method at present can be used to supplement rather than replace conventional methods.

There are two main procedures in use, the direct and indirect methods (Fig. 10.11). The **direct method** consists of bringing fluorescein-tagged antibodies into contact with antigens fixed on a slide (e.g. in

Direct method

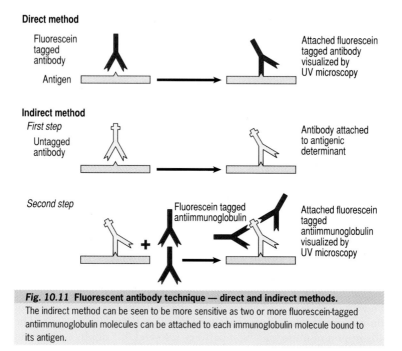

Fig. 10.11 Fluorescent antibody technique — direct and indirect methods.
The indirect method can be seen to be more sensitive as two or more fluorescein-tagged antiimmunoglobulin molecules can be attached to each immunoglobulin molecule bound to its antigen.

the form of a tissue section or a smear of an organism), allowing them to react, washing off excess antibody and examining under the UV light microscope. The site of union of the labelled antibody with its antigen can be seen by the apple-green fluorescent areas on the slide. The **indirect method** can be used both for detecting specific antibodies in sera or other body fluids and also for identifying antigens. This method differs from the direct method in the use of a non-labelled antiserum which is layered on first, in the same way as described above. Whether or not this antiserum has reacted with the material on the slide is shown by means of a fluorescein-tagged **antiglobulin serum** specific for the globulin of the serum applied first. Such an antiglobulin serum can be used to detect antibody globulin in sera to a variety of different antigens which gives it a considerable advantage over the direct test. It is also more sensitive.

Other types of labelled antibody test have been developed on the same principles as the fluorescent methods. Horseradish peroxidase and other enzymes can readily be linked to antibody leaving the antibody still able to combine with its antigen. After this has occurred (e.g. in a tissue section layered with the peroxidase-labelled antibody and then washed) the site of localization of the antibody can be visualized by using the enzymes to develop a coloured product. Ferritin (an electron-dense blood pigment) conjugated antibody has also been used in electron-microscope studies to show the localization of cell antigens.

Cytotoxic tests

Tests of this type are used in combination with red blood cell agglutination for studying histocompatibility antigen systems in tissue typing.

The cytotoxic test consists essentially of determining whether or not the **permeability** of cells changes after their incubation with antibody and complement (Fig. 10.12). Cytotoxic antibody, after combination with the target cell, will activate complement components and bring about changes in the permeability of the cell membrane. The permeability changes can affect the ability of the cell to exclude a dye such as trypan blue which will penetrate the cell and be visible by simple microscopic examination.

Although the test is applicable to a wide range of nucleated cells and

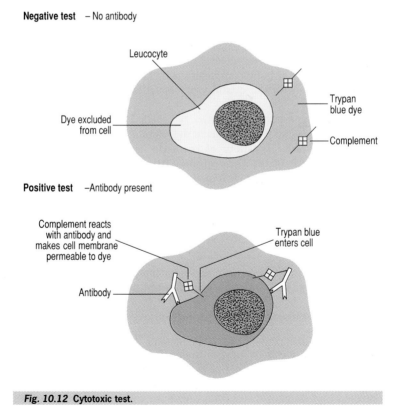

Negative test – No antibody

Leucocyte

Trypan blue dye

Dye excluded from cell

Complement

Positive test –Antibody present

Complement reacts with antibody and makes cell membrane permeable to dye

Trypan blue enters cell

Antibody

Fig. 10.12 Cytotoxic test.

is the test of choice with blood leucocytes, it is rather less sensitive than the red cell haemagglutination tests and more laborious to perform.

Radioimmunoassay methods

Increasing use has been made over the last few years of immunologically based assay methods for the accurate quantitative estimation of **polypeptide hormones**. These methods offer a unique combination of specificity, precision and simplicity and are already available for the assay of some 14 of the 20 or so polypeptide hormones in humans. Monoclonal antibodies are now used extensively in the tests.

The principle of the assay methods is that radio-iodine-labelled (purified) hormone competes with the non-labelled hormone of a sample under test for the antihormone antibody with which the labelled and non-labelled hormone are mixed. The more of the hormone there is in the test sample the less chance the labelled hormone has of combining with the limited number of antibody molecules that are available in the antihormone serum. Thus, by measuring the quantity of labelled hormone combined with antibody (using isotope counting equipment), a measure of the hormone in the test sample can be obtained. The more labelled hormone combined with antibody, the lower the hormone level in the test sample. The quantity of isotope labelled hormone complexing with the antihormone antibody varies inversely with the quantity of unlabelled hormone in the test sample.

In order to measure the amount of labelled hormone attached to antibody it is necessary to separate the hormone/antibody complexes from the mixture. A variety of methods have been developed to achieve this, perhaps the most common being attachment of antibody to inert particles that can be removed by centrifugation (Fig. 10.13). Figure 10.14 illustrates the principle of these assays.

An assay for IgE levels in serum has been developed using iodine-labelled IgE and anti-IgE linked to cellulose, and assays using these principles are being developed for the detection of hepatitis B antigen in human serum.

Immunoassays using enzyme-linked antibody or antigen

Enzyme-linked immunosorbent assay (ELISA)

Labels other than radioactive isotopes and fluorescent dyes can be linked on to antibody or antigen molecules. Enzymes such as horseradish peroxidase or alkaline phosphatase are linked to antibody or antigen molecules. The presence of the enzyme-linked molecule is detected by means of the enzyme substrate and can be measured by

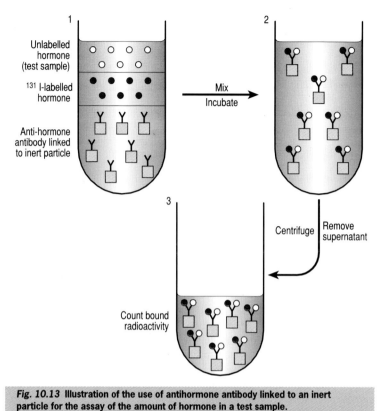

Fig. 10.13 Illustration of the use of antihormone antibody linked to an inert particle for the assay of the amount of hormone in a test sample.
The quantity of ^{131}I-labelled hormone complexing with the antihormone antibody varies inversely with the amount of unlabelled hormone in the test sample. A standard curve can be prepared using known concentrations of purified hormone in the same way as illustrated in Figure 10.5. This will enable the result obtained with the test sample to be plotted and its concentration obtained.

spectrophotometry. Either the labelled antigen or the antibody can be attached to an insoluble support, such as plastic beads or plastic agglutination plates. After the material has attached and the excess has been washed away, enzyme-linked antigen or antibody is added, together with the test substance. The antigen or antibody (whichever is being measured) in the test solution competes with the added labelled antigen or antibody reagent for the material attached to the plastic plates. The amount of enzyme-labelled reagent can then be estimated by the addition of enzyme substrate. The product of the reaction between enzyme and substrate is finally determined by spectrophotometry.

There are a number of variations of the technique similar to those used with fluorescent antibodies. These include a sandwich technique

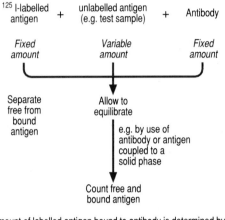

^{125} I-labelled antigen + unlabelled antigen (e.g. test sample) + Antibody

Fixed amount   Variable amount   Fixed amount

Separate free from bound antigen   Allow to equilibrate

e.g. by use of antibody or antigen coupled to a solid phase

Count free and bound antigen

(Amount of labelled antigen bound to antibody is determined by the amount of unlabelled antigen that competes in test sample)

Fig. 10.14 The principle of competitive binding radioimmunoassay.

with antigen bound to the plastic plate, the antibody to be assayed as the second layer and enzyme linked to immunoglobulin as the top layer. Enzyme substrate is finally added and the product determined in the spectrophotometer by colour change.

The technique has been applied widely in detection of bacterial and viral antigens and antibodies, particularly for rotavirus and cytomegalovirus. It has also been of use in the study of a variety of parasitic diseases due to helminths and protozoa.

These assays are increasingly used for qualitative and quantitative determinations of macromolecules. The development of monoclonal antibody technology and the subsequent availability of unlimited quantities of pure antibody has improved the selectivity of these assays. The drawback of the limited surface area of the wells of the microtitre plates used in the assay can be overcome by the use of macrobeads (e.g. polystyrene latex or Dynal copolymer beads). The beads are coated with the appropriate reagent and the detection stage involves the use of fluorescent or enzyme conjugates. The sensitivity of tests of this type tends to be lower than that of assays in ELISA plates.

Some common diagnostic applications of antigen–antibody reactions in medical microbiology

Agglutination tests

The agglutination test already referred to for the serodiagnosis of salmonella infections is known as the Widal test. It is usual to test dilutions of the patient's serum against standard suspensions of somatic (O) antigen and flagellar (H) antigen of each organism likely to be encountered in the patient's environment. The test usually becomes positive with both suspensions a week after the onset of the illness but may be weakly positive with one of the antigens even earlier. The titre in an acute infection rises to a maximum by the end of the third week. Complications in interpretation of the results may arise in patients who have been immunized with typhoid–paratyphoid vaccine (TAB). A **rising titre** may be of some help in diagnosing an infection; furthermore, some months after immunization, the titre of O agglutinins tends to fall off leaving only H agglutinins. Normal sera sometimes have low titres of agglutinins for *Salmonella* organisms and this varies in populations in different parts of the world. These difficulties make the test of questionable diagnostic value and its use is now limited.

Another widely used agglutination test is the **Paul-Bunnell** reaction. This is used for the diagnosis of infectious mononucleosis in which agglutinins develop for sheep erythrocytes. Normal serum may agglutinate sheep cells in low dilutions and a titre of 128 is taken as suggestive and 256 as positive for the test. In some individuals who have received horse serum as a therapeutic agent (e.g. antitetanus serum) agglutinins develop for sheep cells because of the presence in the horse serum of an antigen very widespread in nature, known as the **Forssman** antigen. This antigen is present in the red cells of sheep and the cells of a number of other species, including the guinea-pig. The usual way of differentiating the two types of antibody is to mix the serum with minced guinea-pig tissue (usually kidney). This treatment will absorb out the anti-Forssman antibody leaving the anti-sheep cell antibody unaffected. Ox red cells, which contain both the Forssman antigen and an antigen similar to that on sheep cells which reacts with the Paul-Bunnell antibody, will absorb out both types of antibody.

Complement fixation tests

These tests (described on p. 324) have wide applications in the diagnosis of bacterial and viral infections. One of the most commonly used methods is the Wassermann test used in the diagnosis of **syphilis**. This reaction depends upon the fixation of complement by the patient's antibody after it has reacted with cardiolipin, an alcoholic extract (a phosphatide lipoid) from normal animal tissues, usually ox heart. Why antibodies against this material develop in syphilis is not clear. Some workers suggest that it results from autoimmunization with host lipids made antigenic in some way by the spirochaete (*Trep. pallidum*) responsible for syphilis, whilst others believe that the spirochaete contains a cell wall antigen related to the tissue antigen.

Interpretation of the results of the Wassermann test is difficult and a final assessment depends on the results of both this and other serological tests and the clinical findings. **False-positive** reactions are sometimes found in leprosy, malaria, sleeping sickness, tuberculosis, infectious mononucleosis and other febrile diseases. Persistent false-positive reactions are sometimes found in autoimmune haemolytic anaemia, systemic lupus erythematosus and liver cirrhosis. A commonly performed test is a slide flocculation test using cardiolipin mixed with the patient's serum. This test is preferred by many laboratories because of its simplicity as an alternative to the Wassermann test. It is known as the VDRL (Venereal Diseases Research Laboratory) slide test. When there is doubt a more specific test may have to be employed, e.g. the treponemal immobilization test, in which motile treponemata can be seen to be immobilized when examined microscopically after exposure to patient's serum. This test is, however, technically complicated and has largely been replaced by an indirect fluorescent antibody (p. 328) test (fluorescent treponemal antibody absorbed, FTA-ABS, test). The test is highly specific and sensitive; it is able to detect antibody at all stages of syphilitic infection. The enzyme-linked immunosorbent assay (ELISA) described on page 330 has the potential for large-scale application in syphilis serology.

Complement fixation tests are used widely in the diagnosis of virus diseases. The source of the antigen is usually the infected tissues of animals, or eggs, or infected tissue cultures. The virus is usually extracted from the tissues or cells by differential centrifugation or sometimes by purifying the virus by adsorbing it on to red cells and then eluting it later.

Haemagglutination inhibition tests

Another useful procedure for the diagnosis of some types of virus disease is the **haemagglutination inhibition** test. This depends on the fact that certain viruses, e.g. those of influenza, mumps and parainfluenza, will agglutinate chicken, human and guinea-pig red cells (Fig. 10.8). Other viruses, e.g. the adenoviruses, agglutinate rat or monkey red cells, the reoviruses and many enteroviruses, agglutinate human red cells. The test is performed by mixing the virus with the appropriate red cells in the presence of patient's serum. If antibodies to the virus are present the virus will be unable to bring about haemagglutination. These tests are very valuable because of their extreme specificity and their ability to distinguish antibodies to various substrains and variants of viruses, e.g. the influenza virus. The complement fixation test on the other hand is less valuable for detecting these fine differences.

LABORATORY INVESTIGATIONS IN CLINICAL IMMUNOLOGY

Increasing attention is now being paid in the clinical laboratory to the investigation of the role of immune reactions in the **pathogenesis** of disease and to methods of assessing the **functional status** of the immune system in situations where apparent immune dysfunction exists.

Many of the disease states in which immune reactions are believed to be involved in disease pathogenesis have been considered briefly in preceding sections on hypersensitivity reactions and autoimmune states. Immune deficiency states are referred to in Chapter 9. This text is not to be intended to replace the many excellent textbooks dealing with the laboratory aspects of clinical immunology but to provide a simple outline of the main principles of this complex and difficult subject.

Investigation of hypersensitivity states

Antibodies in anaphylactic states

Hay fever and asthma sufferers characteristically have IgE antibodies in their blood. In 1921 Prausnitz and Kustner described a method for the detection of such 'reaginic' antibody performed by injecting a small quantity of serum from the hay fever patient into the skin of a normal subject. The IgE antibody fixes to the cells of the recipient close to the site of injection and, when the antigen (or allergen) to which the patient is sensitive (e.g. a pollen extract) is injected at the site, an inflammatory response takes place due to the release of histamine from mast cells (see p. 274). The same type of reaction can be elicited in the patient by introducing a small quantity of dilute antigen into the skin (prick test).

IgE antibodies can be quantitated by the radial immunodiffusion technique described on page 321. IgE directed at particular antigens can be assayed by coupling antigen to an insoluble material and mixing the complex with the patient's serum containing IgE antibody against the antigen. After allowing the binding of the IgE antibodies with antigen to take place, unbound serum proteins are washed away and the bound IgE antibody is detected with radiolabelled (^{125}I) anti-IgE antiserum.

Another laboratory procedure used in clinical practice is the determination of the histocompatibility antigen type (p. 243) of the peripheral blood leucocytes. In studies in the United States an association has been found between the occurrence of allergy to ragweed antigen (antigen E) and HLA haplotypes. These studies have been confined so far to a small number of families. The association has been found to occur within particular families, making it possible to identify within a particular family the members at risk and likely to develop the particular ragweed allergy. If these studies are confirmed, leucocyte typing may become a useful laboratory aid to the clinician.

Antibodies to inhaled organic material

A condition called 'extrinsic alveolitis' has been recognized in persons who inhale organic material such as fungal spores, dust from various birds or dust from mouldy hay or barley. The lung changes appear to be associated with IgG antibodies formed against the inhaled material and these antibodies are detected by gel diffusion precipitin tests, as described on page 318.

Pulmonary aspergillosis due to inhalation of spores of *Aspergillus fumigatus* sometimes develops in patients with asthma or with an old healed tuberculous cavity, and precipitating antibodies can be detected in their serum. *Candida albicans* respiratory infections can also result in similar antibodies.

Inhalation of *Micromonospora faeni* from mouldy hay can result in a form of alveolitis known as farmer's lung disease and mouldy barley containing *Aspergillus clavatus* can result in maltworker's lung disease. Gel diffusion tests for precipitating antibodies against antigenic extracts of the microorganisms have proved useful in the diagnosis of the conditions (see also p. 281).

Inhalation of antigens from birds is responsible for bird fancier's lung disease and here again precipitating IgG antibodies can be detected against avian antigens. The antigens are present in bird serum, feathers and droppings, and for the most reliable results material should be used from the particular species of bird to which the patient has been exposed — chickens, pigeons, budgerigars, parrots, and so on.

Antibodies against self-constituents (autoantibodies)

Organ (or tissue) specific autoantibodies

Autoantibodies against organ-specific antigens or non-organ-specific antigens are found in a wide range of disease states, as described in Chapter 9. Whilst their role, if any, in the disease process itself is not clear, their presence can be a useful guide as an aid in clinical diagnosis.

Amongst the more common organ-specific autoantibodies are those found in autoimmune haemolytic anaemia. Two main types of antibody have been found: (1) so-called 'warm antibodies' that combine at body temperature with red cells. These are usually of IgG class in contrast to IgM anti-red-cell autoantibodies responsible for 'cold antibody' haemolytic anaemia that can be shown to agglutinate red cells at 4°C . The detection of these antibodies usually depends on the use of the Coombs' antiglobulin test described in Fig. 10.9. (2) Leucocyte and platelet autoantibodies have also been described in some rare disease states and are occasionally induced by drugs that combine with these blood components (p. 278).

Organ-specific autoantibodies have been described in the serum of patients with thyroiditis, adrenal disease, pernicious anaemia and disease of the salivary glands (Sjogren's syndrome). The main test here is the fluorescent antibody method (p. 327) with tissue sections of the appropriate tissue but passive haemagglutination (p. 323) or gel diffusion tests are sometimes used in which red cells are coated with the tissue antigen or the antigen is placed in the wells for the immunodiffusion test (p. 319) with the patient's serum in opposite wells.

Non-organ-specific antibodies

In certain disease states, such as rheumatoid arthritis and systemic lupus erythematosus (discussed in Ch. 9), autoantibodies are found to widely distributed antigens not restricted to any one organ or tissue. Autoantibodies in this category are also found in various forms of chronic liver disease.

An agglutination test is widely used for the diagnosis of rheumatoid arthritis; the sera of 70 to 80% of patients with this disease contain an IgM antibody which is able to combine with the IgG globulin from various species. Detection of the antibody depends on the agglutination of sheep red cells or inert particles (polystyrene latex) coated with IgG globulin. Sheep red cells, for example, may be coated with specific rabbit antibody and will then be agglutinated by the IgM antibody in the rheumatoid patient's serum. The antibody is known as **rheumatoid factor**. Occasional low titres (less than 16) are found in normal sera (2 to 5%) and the test is not entirely specific for rheumatoid arthritis.

The fluorescent antibody test is the most commonly used method for the detection of the **antinuclear factor** (ANF) found in the majority of cases of systemic lupus erythematosus. Sections of tissue, e.g. rat liver, are used as the substrate and are layered with patient's serum. Binding of ANF to the liver cell nuclei is detected with fluorescein-labelled antihuman immunoglobulin (see p. 327).

In a liver disease known as primary biliary cirrhosis most patients have antibodies against mitochondrial antigens. These are detected by the fluorescent antibody test with unfixed tissue sections or sometimes by complement fixation tests with rat liver mitochondria. In chronic active hepatitis, and transiently in just over half of patients with infective hepatitis, antibodies are found against smooth muscle actinomyosin. The fluorescent antibody test is the method of choice using unfixed sections of rat stomach.

Immune deficiency states

The clinical and immunological aspects of these states are discussed in Chapter 9 and can be seen to involve one or more of the different components of the immune system: (1) the cells responsible for making circulating immunoglobulins, (2) the cells concerned with the cell-mediated immune response and (3) the bone marrow stem cells. A wide range of laboratory tests are available to investigate the various forms of deficiency.

Immunoglobulin production. Assay of circulating immunoglobulins can be assessed qualitatively by electrophoresis and quantitatively by immunodiffusion tests. These latter tests are capable of identifying deficiencies of particular classes of immunoglobulin, as described on page 319.

The ability of the patient to make specific immunoglobulin can be tested by **active immunization** with, for example, a bacterial antigen such as tetanus toxoid and the antibody response measured by a tube precipitation test (p. 317).

The presence of the cells involved in the humoral immune response can be assayed by making use of the fact that the particular cells concerned — the B-lymphocytes — have receptors on their surface for the Fc component of the Ig molecule and for the C3 complement component. In the test, sheep red blood cells coated with anti-sheep red cell antibody and complement (in non-lytic quantities) are mixed with peripheral blood leucocytes. The sheep red cells become attached to B-lymphocytes by means of the Fc and C3 receptors (that combine with the antibody and complement on the red cell) forming 'rosettes'. The proportion of leucocytes forming such rosettes gives an estimate of the number of B-lymphocytes and is normally about 25% of the lymphocytes in human peripheral blood.

Tests of the function of the cell-mediated immune system

Skin tests. The classical method for testing the responsiveness of the cells involved in cell-mediated immunity is the **delayed hypersensitivity skin test** described on page 124. The tuberculin response is the best-known example. It is induced by the intradermal injection of 0.1 ml of a 1:1000 dilution (or a greater dilution in a highly sensitive individual) of a protein extract of tubercle bacilli (purified protein derivative, PPD). The reaction is described on page 284; it is only one of a number of similar tests of delayed hypersensitivity such as that using lepromin (in leprosy) and brucellin (in brucellosis). One of the main uses of tests of this type is to detect sensitization to the relevant microorganism as, for example, prior to the use of the BCG vaccine (p. 223) in the prevention of tuberculosis. Clearly in the presence of a positive tuberculin test immunization with the vaccine will not be called for. A negative reaction in an adult, particularly in one known to have previously shown a positive test, raises the possibility of a defect of the cell-mediated immune system, which in the adult would be likely to be secondary to some disease state affecting the lymphoid tissues such as Hodgkin's disease, multiple myeloma, leukaemia and lymphosarcoma.

Lymphocyte function tests. The T-lymphocyte has been pointed to as the main effector cell in cell-mediated immune reactions (Ch. 4). The presence of the T-lymphocyte in the peripheral blood can be detected in very much the same way as B-lymphocytes can be detected. Instead of using antibody and complement-coated sheep red blood cells as is required for B-cells, sheep cells alone are all that is required. T-lymphocytes have receptors for sheep erythrocytes and can thus form rosettes when the two types of cell are mixed together. Between 40% and 60% of the human peripheral blood lymphocytes can form rosettes of this type. Monoclonal antibodies against T- and B-cell differentiation antigens are now widely used and can be used to estimate subclasses of T-cells and T- and B-cell ratios as in AIDS patients (see Fig. 1.2).

Lymphocyte transformation. A particularly useful and widely used assay of lymphocyte function is the lymphocyte transformation test. This is usually carried out using plant phytohaemagglutinin (PHA) as the stimulating agent; the process is described in some detail on p. 102. In other situations a transformation test may be performed with specific antigens to which the individual is believed to be sensitized (e.g. tuberculin). In contrast to the use of PHA, which stimulates a high proportion of T-lymphocytes, specific antigen will only stimulate those lymphocytes that are specifically 'committed' to the antigen in question and this is usually only a small portion of the total T-lymphocytes. A low level of lymphocyte transformation (when compared with control subjects), either with PHA or specific antigen, indicates impaired cell-mediated immunity (or perhaps absence of previous exposure to the antigen used), whilst increased transformation in the presence of a specific antigen may occur in certain hypersensitivity states, e.g. drug allergies (p. 278).

Migration inhibition. A modification of the macrophage migration inhibition test using human peripheral blood leucocytes (instead of guinea-pig peritoneal macrophages) can be used in the assessment of cell-mediated immunity. Peripheral blood leucocytes are collected in a small capillary tube in the same way as for the macrophage inhibition test and, when put in a culture chamber, grow out of the end of the tube in a fan shape. If, however, antigen, to which the cell donor has previously been sensitized, is put into the chamber the leucocytes fail to grow out of the tube. This inhibitory effect is due to a 'lymphokine' produced by the sensitized lymphocytes on exposure to antigen. This form of assessment of lymphocyte function has very much the same value as the transformation tests referred to above.

Cytokine production

Commercial kits are now widely available for the assay of a wide range of cytokines produced by lymphoid cells and are preferentially used to assess cell function and responses of cells to various stimuli. The most extensively used tests are those based on ELISA.

Tests of phagocytic cell activity. Defective phagocytic mechanisms are discussed in Chapter 9 and can be assayed in a variety of ways in the laboratory:

1. The ability of phagocytes to respond to a chemotactic agent (e.g. antigen/antibody (Ag/Ab) complexes in fresh serum) can be measured by inducing the phagocytes to migrate from a chamber through a millipore membrane towards an outer chamber containing the Ag/Ab complexes and serum. The number of phagocytes that respond can be estimated by removing the membrane, staining it with a suitable stain and, under the microscope, counting the number of cells either in the process of passing through the membrane or on the outer side of the membrane.

2. The ability of phagocytes to ingest and kill microorganisms (e.g. staphylococci) or ingest inert particles such as latex or oil droplets can be determined by microscopic examination of cell preparations mixed with the microorganism or inert particle. Killing of microorganisms within phagocytes can be estimated by disrupting the cells, e.g. by distilled water, and counting the colonies of microorganisms that can be grown on a suitable nutrient agar plate.

3. The normal functioning of phagocyte lysosomal enzyme activity can be assessed by a dye reduction test using tetrazolium nitroblue. A defect on the part of the patient's cells can be detected by a failure of the leucocytes to reoxidize the reduced colourless dye to its blue colour. A deficiency of this function is characteristic of chronic granulomatous disease (p. 286).

The complement system. Changes in the levels of this complex group of serum protein constituents (see Ch. 2) are often a reflection of an underlying disease process. **Raised** levels of the components are frequently found in acute inflammatory and infective disease states in conjunction with raised levels of 'acute phase proteins' such as C reactive protein.

Reduction in complement levels is a more useful guide to the understanding of disease pathogenesis and falls into two categories: (1) primary deficiencies — genetically determined deficiencies of complement components and (2) secondary deficiencies — as a consequence of complement consuming antibody–antigen interactions or associated with renal or liver disease.

The genetically determined deficiencies are rare conditions, the best known of which is the deficiency of C1 esterase inhibitor (see p. 286). Very rare deficiencies of other components (C3, C1, C5) have been described.

The secondary deficiencies are much more frequently found and most often occur in renal disease such as poststreptococcal nephritis, in the nephritis of systemic lupus erythematosus and in chronic membranoproliferative glomerulonephritis. Low levels also occur in serum sickness (immune complex disease), bacterial septicaemia, malaria and in various forms of liver disease.

In the laboratory two main types of assay are available: (1) functional tests of the haemolytic activity of the complement system and (2) immunochemical estimation of the levels of individual complement components.

Haemolytic activity of the complement system is usually assayed by the method described by Mayer, which measures the number of 'units' of complement per ml of serum. A unit of complement is defined as the quantity required to lyse 50% of a standard sheep cell suspension, optimally sensitized with anti-sheep cell antibody. The volume, buffer components and incubation condition are likewise defined. The test is sometimes referred to as a CH50 assay.

Estimation of individual components, whilst possible by assays of their functional activity, is usually performed by immunochemical methods utilizing specific antisera against individual components. The method of choice is the quantitative radial immunodiffusion test (p. 321) in which the antisera are incorporated in the agar and the serum specimens are placed in the wells. Commercially prepared plates are available for a wide range of complement components.

Immune complex detection. In the circulation the potentially pathogenic complexes are those found in antigen excess. There is now convincing evidence that they play a role in the pathogenesis of rheumatoid arthritis, glomerulonephritis, polyarteritis, rheumatic fever and a number of infective states discussed in Chapter 5. Detection of complexes is valuable in the diagnosis of bacterial endocarditis. In most instances, complement activation seems likely to be responsible for the inflammatory changes that occur, with chemotaxis of neutrophils and release of lysosomal enzymes as the prime factors involved (see Ch. 2, p. 30).

The following detection methods in general require specialized laboratory facilities:

1. Electron-microscopic demonstration of complexes in tissues, such as those found in the liver of patients with hepatitis B virus infections.

2. Precipitation of complexes in the cold, cryoprecipitation and subsequent identification of microbial antigens, e.g. hepatitis B antigens.

3. Detection of bound complement component (e.g. C1q) in the complexes, often after precipitation by polyethylene glycol. The principle of the assay is that the naturally bound C1q is removed with Na_2EDTA, a radiolabelled C1q is then added, followed by polyethylene glycol to precipitate the complexes. The C1q remaining in the supernatant is then measured, allowing the estimation of the bound C1q. A similar test commercially available involves the binding of bovine conglutinin to the bound complement.

4. Immunobiological tests such as aggregation of platelets and inhibition of antibody-mediated cytotoxicity. The latter test is quite widely used and involves inhibition of the killing by non-sensitized lymphocytes of target cells (e.g. Chang cells, a line of human liver cells) coated with antibody. If immune complexes are added to the lymphocytes, their Fc receptors are blocked by the antibody in the complexes so that the receptors cannot bind the antibody on the target cell.

5. Immunoblotting technique, or Western blotting, is a powerful method by which macromolecules, usually proteins, are separated by polyacrylamide gel electrophoresis and then transferred electrophoretically to a nitrocellulose membrane. It has largely superseded the traditional immunoelectrophoresis techniques and is used in all areas of immunological research and diagnostic serology. Immunoblot analysis is a valuable confirmatory test for HIV antibodies and its use is being extended to the detection of many hospital pathogens.

6. Laser-based flow cytometry which measures forward angle light scatter that is related to the size of cells being measured is increasingly used in immunology for the identification of cell populations (phenotyping) and for separation (sorting) on the basis of staining patterns with fluorescent ligands.

7. The polymerase chain reaction (PCR) is used for the direct detection of nucleic acids. It is particularly useful for the detection of viruses that are difficult to identify by conventional methods. The major requirement is that at least part of the sequence of the nucleic acid of the agent to be detected is known. In essence the technique is an in vitro technique for nucleic acid amplification specifically applied to a particular segment of DNA. Two synthetic oligonucleotide primers are required that will hybridize to the ends of opposite strands of the target sequence. The process is cyclical, involving three stages: (1) denaturation of target DNA by heating at 90–95°C, (2) cooling to 37–50°C at which point the primers anneal to the target DNA strands and (3) copying of the DNA and extension of the primers by means of a polymerase (Taq polymerase from *Thermus aquaticus* — a thermophilic bacterium). From 25 to 35 cycles can lead to a millionfold increase of the target DNA.

Table 10.1 Clinical immunology tests

Quantitation of immunoglobulins	Radial immunodiffusion Nephelometry for IgG, IgM and IgA quantitation
Evaluation of IgM function	Isohaemagglutination assay
Type 1 hypersensitivity	IgE quantitation by enzyme-linked immunosorbent assay (ELISA)
Complement activity	Haemolytic assays Radial immunodiffusion
Phagocytic function	Nitroblue tetrazolium (NBT) test Chemiluminescence Chemotaxis assays Quantitative intracellular killing
Cell-mediated immune function	Total T-cell and subclass estimation Mitogen responses Delayed hypersensitivity skin tests
Cytokine production	Cytokine assays, IL-1, IL-2, TNF

Table 10.1 lists some of the widely used tests in clinical immunology.

Other tests

A number of miscellaneous clinical immunological investigations are sometimes called for and include examination of biopsy material for deposits of antibody or complement by immunofluorescence, estimation of cryoglobulins, radioimmunoassay for the presence of hepatitis B antigen and characterization of monoclonal antibodies by immunoelectrophoresis or examination of bone marrow by immunofluorescence. In diagnosis of virus infection speed is important, enabling public health control measures to be started and more immediate care for the patient. Assays for cytokine production by lymphoid cells are now widely used in assessment of the activity of different lymphoid cell populations. The assays commonly use ELISA procedures and kits for the purpose are available commercially.

The ELISA assay has been discussed and is likely to have wide applications. Assay of specific IgM may be helpful in atypical measles or mumps and in certain arbovirus infections. Electron-microscopic examination is widely used for biopsy material as well as the fluorescent antibody technique. Laser nephelometry — the measurement of light scattered from a transmitted light source — is used for the determination of antigens by adding constant amounts of highly purified optically clear specific antibody to varying amounts of antigen.

Table 10.2 **Monoclonal antibodies — applications**

Lymphocyte subset and leucocyte determination
Detection of HLA antigens
Detection of viruses including typing
Microbial and parasite antigen detection
RIA for polypeptide hormones
Immunohistochemistry
Typing of leukaemias and lymphomas
Detection of tumour antigens

Monoclonal antibodies (p. 117) are widely available for the detection of cellular and soluble antigens with radioimmunoassays, enzyme linked assays and immunofluorescence (Table 10.2). Biotin–avidin techniques are being increasingly used in immunohistochemistry. Avidin, a glycoprotein from egg albumin, has a very high affinity for the vitamin biotin. Biotin is coupled to antibody covalently and interaction of the antibody with its antigen is demonstrated using fluorochrome-labelled avidin. The procedure can be used in the same way as in indirect fluorescent antibody tests (p. 327).

Most of these procedures required specialized laboratory facilities not generally available in the routine clinical pathology laboratory.

Summary of clinical applications

Quantitation of serum immunoglobulin levels

1. Patients with severe or repeated infection, e.g. actinomycosis, subacute bacterial endocarditis, infectious mononucleosis.
2. Liver disease.
3. To monitor immunotherapy of patients with immuno-proliferative disorders, e.g. monoclonal gammopathies of IgG, IgA or IgM (Ch. 9).
4. To distinguish transient changes, such as those following burns and in primary immunodeficiencies.
5. Estimation of immune responses following natural infection or immunization — IgA levels in patients with infections of mucosal surfaces or IgE levels in patients with allergies.
6. Levels of antibodies in cerebrospinal fluid of patients with infections or in demyelinating diseases.
7. To detect free heavy or light chains of immunoglobulins in the urine of patients with multiple myeloma.

Detection of levels of C reactive proteins

Used to follow the progress of treatment for an infection.

Detection of autoantibodies (Ch. 9)

Using immunofluorescence in tissue sections — thyroid sections for antithyroid antibodies, commercial assay kits for rheumatoid factor in rheumatoid arthritis and an antinuclear factor in systemic lupus erythematosus.

Detection of immune complexes in type III hypersensitivity states (Ch. 9)

Many methods are available — cryoprecipitation, precipitation by polyethylene glycol and detection of complement, if it is bound to the complexes.

Unfortunately the results tend to be variable and difficult to interpret. Valuable in bacterial endocarditis.

Skin tests for type I and type IV hypersensitivity states (Ch. 9)

There are various forms of the skin test:

1. **Intradermal injection** of dilute antigen (allergen).
2. **Prick tests**, in which test material is placed on the skin and needle pricks are made through the material.
3. **Patch tests**, in which the material is placed in absorbent materials and placed on the skin — particularly used for type IV hypersensitivity contact dermatitis.

Estimation of complement components

The most common procedure in the past was to measure total complement levels but individual components can be measured more conveniently with commercially available immunodiffusion plates.

Tests of lymphocyte function

1. **Lymphocyte transformation test** (see above) used for in vitro test of cell-mediated immunity in suspected immunodeficiency.
2. **Macrophage (leucocyte) migration inhibition test.** This is less commonly used than the transformation test above.

Tests of phagocyte function

For suspected chronic granulomatous disease in patients with unresolving infections:

1. **Intracellular enzyme activity** — ability to reduce the dye nitroblue tetrazolium (NBT) as an indicator of the activity of oxygen-dependent bactericidal activities.

2. **Phagocytosis** — ability to ingest inert particles (yeast or latex), opsonized red cells or bacteria to test for Fc receptor function.

3. **Chemotaxis** — ability to be attracted by a chemoattractant through a membrane filter.

4. **Chemiluminescence** — emission of light by phagocytes as a test for their ability to be activated.

5. **Cytokine production** by lymphocytes and monocytes using ELISA.

Diagnosis of infection

Many of the assays described above can be used to help in the diagnosis of infection. The availability of monoclonal antibodies has brought rapid progress to this area and they can be used, for example, to identify specific microorganisms in culture or in tissues and fluids from infected patients. Complement fixation tests, virus neuralization tests, ELISA assays, coagglutination tests, radioimmunoassay and immunofluorescence are widely used in the diagnostic laboratory. Immune complex detection can be valuable in the diagnosis of bacterial endocarditis. The development of simple and highly sensitive methods for the detection of nucleic acids is now being applied to the diagnosis of infection using nucleic acid hybridization and is likely to provide a valuable additional aid to immunoassays in the diagnostic laboratory.

FURTHER READING

Herzenberg L A, Weir D M, Blackwell C C (eds) 1997 Weir's Handbook of experimental immunology, 5th edn. Blackwell Science, Oxford, Boston

Hudson L, Hay F C 1989 Practical immunology, 3rd edn. Blackwell, Oxford

Rose N R (ed) 1997 Manual of clinical laboratory immunology, 5th edn. American Association of Microbiology, Washington

Shortman K (ed) 1991 Immunological techniques. Current Opinion in Immunology 3: 217

Weir D M (ed) 1990 Immunological techniques. Current Opinion in Immunology 2: 877

Index